Neuropsychological Neurology

The Neurocognitive Impairments of
Neurological Disorders

Neuropsychological Neurology

The Neurocognitive Impairments of Neurological Disorders

A. J. Larner

Consultant Neurologist, Cognitive Function Clinic,
Walton Centre for Neurology and Neurosurgery, Liverpool, UK

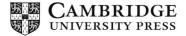

CAMBRIDGE
UNIVERSITY PRESS

CAMBRIDGE UNIVERSITY PRESS

Cambridge, New York, Melbourne, Madrid, Cape Town, Singapore, São Paulo, Delhi

Cambridge University Press
The Edinburgh Building, Cambridge CB2 8RU, UK

Published in the United States of America by Cambridge University Press, New York

www.cambridge.org
Information on this title: www.cambridge.org/9780521717922

First published 2008

Printed in the United Kingdom at the University Press, Cambridge

A catalogue record for this publication is available from the British Library

Library of Congress Cataloguing in Publication data

Larner, A. J.
 Neuropsychological neurology : the neurocognitive impairments of neurological disorders / A.J. Larner.
  p. ; cm.
 Includes bibliographical references and index.
 ISBN 978-0-521-71792-2 (pbk.)
 1. Cognition disorders. 2. Clinical neuropsychology. 3. Neurobehavioral disorders. I. Title.
 [DNLM: 1. Nervous System Diseases – complications. 2. Cognition Disorders – physiopathology. 3. Neuropsychology –
 methods. WL 140 L325n 2008]
 RC553.C64L37 2008
 616.8–dc22   2007049017

ISBN 978-0-521-71792-2 paperback

**To Jo – because no one has dedicated a book
to you before**

Disorders of intellect ... **happen much more
often than superficial observers will easily
believe.**

Samuel Johnson, *The History of Rasselas, Prince
of Abyssinia* (1759)

Contents

Acknowledgements

First and foremost I thank my wife Philippa, and children Thomas and Elizabeth, for their forbearance and moral support (perhaps involuntary) in allowing me to write another book.

I thank the many colleagues with whom I have worked and from whom I have learned much: Mark Doran, Eric Ghadiali, Daniel du Plessis, and Pavla Hancock in Liverpool; Alex Leff, Jonathan Schott, Nick Fox, Angus Kennedy, John Janssen, Lisa Cipolotti, Gail Robinson, Richard Wise, and Martin Rossor in London; and John Hodges in Cambridge.

I thank also the colleagues and friends who have offered advice on particular topics in this book: Rustam Al-Shahi, Alasdair Coles, Kalvinder Gahir, Desmond Kidd, Michael and Sally Mansfield, and Sivakumar Sathasivam.

All errors or misconceptions which remain are entirely my own work. I shall be pleased to hear from readers who detect errors or omissions.

Introduction

The aim of this book is to review what is known about the neuropsychological or neurocognitive impairments which occur in neurological disorders, and in some general medical conditions which may be seen by neurologists. Such neuropsychological deficits are of course relatively well defined in those disorders which present with, or whose clinical features are largely restricted to, cognitive impairment, specifically the dementia syndromes, of both neurodegenerative and vascular aetiology, and these account for a fair proportion of this book. However, cognitive dysfunction may also occur in other neurological disorders, an observation which may have implications for both clinical diagnosis and case management. Few texts have, to my knowledge, specifically addressed this area (e.g. Grant & Adams, 1996; Green, 2000; Harrison & Owen, 2002), and some only in passing. To be sure, there are a number of excellent texts which tackle the classical neuropsychological syndromes such as amnesia, aphasia, alexia, agraphia, apraxia, agnosia, and executive dysfunction (e.g. Baddeley *et al.*, 1995; Benson & Ardila, 1996; Kirshner, 2002; Heilman & Valenstein, 2003). The case-study approach to the neuropsychological features of neurological disorders (e.g. Kapur, 1996; Ogden, 2005) has even spilled over into populist texts, but though such in-depth case studies are informative, they may not immediately correspond to the case mix seen by clinical neurologists. Textbooks of neurology may mention dementia as a feature of certain neurological diseases, often in a rather diffuse way.

There is a perception in some quarters that neuropsychology is something rather separate from clinical neurology. The case may perhaps be persuasively made for academic cognitive neuropsychology, which aims to infer mental structure from neuropsychological test performance, often in single case studies of highly unusual but instructive patients (Shallice, 1988; Ellis & Young, 1996), and even 'clinical' neuropsychology texts (e.g. McCarthy & Warrington, 1990; Groth-Marnat, 2001; Halligan *et al.*, 2003; Devinsky & D'Esposito, 2004) may contain more than a practising clinician would require, or possibly desire. Nonetheless, clinical neurologists neglect cognitive function at their peril. It should not be forgotten that cognitive neuroscience has neurological foundations (D'Esposito 2003; Panegyres, 2004).

It is well recognized that the standard neurological examination is focused predominantly on functions mediated by the parietal and occipital lobes, with frontal and temporal lobe functions being relatively untested. Since, in the context of the clinical history, neurological signs help to focus on the likely locale of pathology (Larner, 2006), it would seem desirable to be able to tap the functions of these areas of the brain as well.

A neuropsychological examination provides the opportunity to do this; such assessment permits a more fine-grained analysis of cognitive function, a refinement which may have localizing and diagnostic value. Just as one would not contemplate omitting the visual field examination or the plantar responses when examining a patient suspected of harbouring neurological disease, so some form of higher cognitive testing should also be undertaken whenever the clinical history suggests possible cognitive impairment. The requirement is for a manual of 'neuropsychology in clinical practice'. Professor John Hodges' book on cognitive testing has pointed the way for clinical neurologists to do this without the need for highly specialized equipment or training (Hodges, 1994).

Not only are neuropsychological tests essential in the diagnosis of dementia disorders, but they may also be helpful in differential diagnosis, for example of movement disorders (Pillon et al., 1996). Neuropsychological features may contribute to disease morbidity even where outcome is judged good or excellent on neurological grounds, e.g. in multiple sclerosis (Feinstein, 1999) or subarachnoid haemorrhage (Hütter, 2000). Neuropsychological parameters may therefore be as appropriate as motor, sensory, or functional scales as outcome measures in the conduct of clinical trials. Early identification and treatment of cognitive impairments would seem the most likely time point at which interventions might show therapeutic efficacy. Part of the desire here, of course, is to identify conditions with neuropsychological deficits that may reverse with appropriate treatment of the underlying condition. Much has been written on the subject of 'reversible dementias', no less than 65 such conditions being alluded to in one review (Cummings et al., 1980), although it seems that the overall frequency of such reversible conditions is low, and falling (Barry & Moskovitz, 1988; Waldemar, 2002; Clarfield, 2003).

Part of the problem, of course, is the sophistication of neuropsychological testing, the plethora of possible tests available to bewilder the uninitiated (Lezak et al., 2004; Mitrushina et al., 2005; Strauss et al., 2006), and the lack of time devoted in clinical training to this subject. For this reason, a brief overview of cognitive function and neuropsychological evaluation prefaces the chapters devoted to the neuropsychological profiles of specific disease entities. This modest excursion into applied neuropsychology will in all probability horrify those trained in the art and science of neuropsychology,

but the aim has been entirely pragmatic, for the benefit of clinical practitioners. In the chapters which follow, the neuropsychological impairments of neurological and general medical disorders are considered. Detailed discussions of neurological features of the disorders covered are not included, although brief notes are given and, where possible, references to diagnostic criteria are cited. For more information on the clinical features of neurological disease, the reader is referred to other textbooks of neurology (for one of which the current author has a particular, and perhaps forgivable, predilection: Barker et al., 2005). A few comments on the treatment of cognitive impairments are given as a gentle rebuff to those who imagine neuropsychological neurology to be a purely descriptive undertaking.

This overview is no small undertaking (I have amongst my papers a draft plan of the book, not too dissimilar from the current contents, dated 27 August 1998), for which reason certain omissions have proved necessary. Perhaps the most important of these is the lack of coverage of neuropsychiatric features of neurological disease (mood disorders, delusions, hallucinations, depression, euphoria, etc.) which often coexist with, and may confound the examination of, neuropsychological deficits. (Pain is also a potential confounder of neuropsychological testing, as in mild traumatic brain injury or headache: Nicholson et al., 2001.) It seems to me that the domain of neuropsychiatry, or behavioural neurology, the overlap between neurological disorders and psychiatric features, has been relatively well addressed, both in general texts (e.g. Lishman, 1987; Trimble, 1996; Moore, 2001; Pincus & Tucker, 2002; Cummings & Mega, 2003; Feinberg & Farah, 2003) and in texts devoted to specific diseases (e.g. stroke: Robinson, 2006; multiple sclerosis: Feinstein, 1999; Parkinson's disease: Starkstein & Merello, 2002; Alzheimer's disease: Ballard et al., 2001). As a corollary to this, the grey area of depression-related dementia or depressive pseudodementia (Roose & Devanand, 1999; Kanner, 2005) has been referred to only briefly.

Given my personal clinical training and experience, the perspective is entirely that of adult neurological practice. For childhood disorders causing cognitive decline, standard texts are available (e.g. Lyon *et al.*, 1996; Brett, 1997; Clarke, 2002; Panteliadis & Korinthenberg, 2005). Learning disability (mental retardation), of which over 2000 different syndromes are described, is entirely eschewed. However, those 'childhood' neurodegenerative disorders that may on occasion present as dementia in adults (e.g. Coker, 1991; Doran, 1997; Panegyres, 2001; Sampson *et al.*, 2004) have been included. Some specific topics have not been tackled, again for lack of personal training and experience, most notably head injury and drug-induced cognitive problems (for the latter see Farlow & Hake, 1998; Moore & O'Keefe, 1999), with the exception of antiepileptic drugs, radiotherapy and chemotherapy treatment of brain tumours, and a passing mention of solvent exposure (Berent & Albers, 2005). Neither the management of dementia (e.g. Qizilbash *et al.*, 2002; Baldwin & Murray, 2003; Brown & Hillam, 2004; Curran & Wattis, 2004; Rabins *et al.*, 2006) nor neuropsychological rehabilitation (e.g. Wilson, 1999; Greenwood *et al.*, 2003; Halligan & Wade, 2005; Selzer *et al.*, 2006) is discussed. Since dementia syndromes have been relatively well covered, collectively (e.g. Parks *et al.*, 1993; Hodges, 2001; Mendez & Cummings, 2003; Burns *et al.*, 2005) and individually, the text is slightly weighted towards other neurological disorders. The arrangement of the chapters is somewhat arbitrary, with certain conditions potentially relevant to more than one, but hopefully those scanning rather than reading systematically will find what they are seeking without too much difficulty. Unavoidably, the author's own interests may appear overemphasized.

This book is envisaged as a reference text relevant to all neurologists, not only those with a declared interest in cognitive disorders; to old age psychiatrists and geriatricians who have to assess patients with cognitive decline; and also as a resource for general physicians and specialists who deal with any endocrine, metabolic, vascular, or infective disorders that may compromise cognitive function. Practitioners of professions allied to medicine which involve contact with cognitively impaired patients (mental health nursing, physiotherapy, occupational therapy, speech and language therapy) may also find material of interest and use.

REFERENCES

Baddeley A, Wilson BA, Watts FN (eds.). *Handbook of Memory Disorders*. Chichester: Wiley, 1995.

Baldwin R, Murray M (eds.). *Younger People with Dementia: a Multidisciplinary Approach*. London: Martin Dunitz, 2003.

Ballard CG, O'Brien J, James I, Swann A. *Dementia: Management of Behavioural and Psychological Symptoms*. Oxford: Oxford University Press, 2001.

Barker R, Rowe D, Scolding N, Larner AJ. *The A–Z of Neurological Practice: a Guide to Clinical Neurology*. Cambridge: Cambridge University Press, 2005.

Barry P, Moskovitz MA. The diagnosis of reversible dementia in the elderly: a critical review. *Arch Intern Med* 1988; **148**: 1914–18.

Benson DF, Ardila A. *Aphasia: a Clinical Perspective*. New York: Oxford University Press, 1996.

Berent S, Albers JW. *Neurobehavioral Toxicology: Neurological and Neuropsychological Perspectives. Volume I: Foundations and Methods*. London: Taylor & Francis, 2005: 101–33.

Brett EM. *Paediatric Neurology* (3rd edition). Edinburgh: Churchill Livingstone, 1997.

Brown J, Hillam J. *Dementia: Your Questions Answered*. Edinburgh: Churchill Livingstone, 2004.

Burns A, O'Brien J, Ames D (eds.). *Dementia* (3rd edition). London: Hodder Arnold, 2005.

Clarfield AM. The decreasing prevalence of reversible dementias: an updated meta-analysis. *Arch Intern Med* 2003; **163**: 2219–29.

Clarke JTR. *A Clinical Guide to Inherited Metabolic Disease* (2nd edition). Cambridge: Cambridge University Press, 2002.

Coker SB. The diagnosis of childhood neurodegenerative disorders presenting as dementia in adults. *Neurology* 1991; **41**: 794–8.

Cummings JL, Benson DF, LoVerme S Jr. Reversible dementia: illustrative cases, definition, and review. *JAMA* 1980; **243**: 2434–9.

Cummings JL, Mega MS. *Neuropsychiatry and Behavioral Neuroscience*. Oxford: Oxford University Press, 2003.

Curran S, Wattis JP (eds.). *Practical Management of Dementia: a Multi-Professional Approach*. Oxford: Radcliffe, 2004.

D'Esposito M (ed.). *Neurological Foundations of Cognitive Neuroscience*. Cambridge, MA: MIT Press, 2003.

Devinsky O, D'Esposito M. *Neurology of Cognitive and Behavioral Disorders*. Oxford: Oxford University Press, 2004.

Doran M. Diagnosis of presenile dementia. *Br J Hosp Med* 1997; **58**: 105–10.

Ellis AW, Young AW. *Human Cognitive Neuropsychology: a Textbook with Readings*. Hove: Psychology Press, 1996.

Farlow MR, Hake AM. Drug-induced cognitive impairment. In: Biller J (ed.), *Iatrogenic Neurology*. Boston: Butterworth-Heinemann, 1998: 203–14.

Feinberg TE, Farah MJ (eds.). *Behavioral Neurology and Neuropsychology* (2nd edition). New York: McGraw-Hill, 2003.

Feinstein A. *The Clinical Neuropsychiatry of Multiple Sclerosis*. Cambridge: Cambridge University Press, 1999.

Grant I, Adams KM (eds.). *Neuropsychological Assessment of Neuropsychiatric Disorders* (2nd edition). Oxford: Oxford University Press, 1996.

Green J. *Neuropsychological Evaluation of the Older Adult: a Clinician's Guidebook*. San Diego: Academic Press, 2000.

Greenwood RJ, Barnes MP, McMillan TM, Ward CD (eds.). *Handbook of Neurological Rehabilitation* (2nd edition). Hove: Psychology Press, 2003: 363–415.

Groth-Marnat G (ed.). *Neuropsychological Assessment in Clinical Practice: a Guide to Test Interpretation and Integration*. New York: Wiley, 2001.

Halligan PW, Kischka U, Marshall JC (eds.). *Handbook of Clinical Neuropsychology*. Oxford: Oxford University Press, 2003.

Halligan PW, Wade DT (eds.). *Effectiveness of Rehabilitation for Cognitive Deficits*. Oxford: Oxford University Press, 2005.

Harrison JE, Owen AM (eds.). *Cognitive Deficits in Brain Disorders*. London: Martin Dunitz, 2002.

Heilman KM, Valenstein E (eds.). *Clinical Neuropsychology* (4th edition). Oxford: Oxford University Press, 2003.

Hodges JR. *Cognitive Assessment for Clinicians*. Oxford: Oxford University Press, 1994.

Hodges JR (ed.). *Early-Onset Dementia: a Multidisciplinary Approach*. Oxford: Oxford University Press, 2001.

Hütter BO. *Neuropsychological Sequelae of Subarachnoid Hemorrhage and its Treatment*. Berlin: Springer, 2000.

Kanner AM. *Depression in Neurological Disorders*. Cambridge: Lundbeck Institute, 2005.

Kapur N. *Injured Brains of Medical Minds: Views from Within*. Oxford: Oxford University Press, 1996.

Kirshner HS. *Behavioral Neurology: Practical Science of Mind and Brain* (2nd edition). Boston: Butterworth-Heinemann, 2002.

Larner AJ. *A Dictionary of Neurological Signs* (2nd edition). New York: Springer, 2006.

Lezak MD, Howieson DB, Loring DW. *Neuropsychological Assessment* (4th edition). New York: Oxford University Press, 2004.

Lishman WA. *Organic Psychiatry* (2nd edition). Oxford: Blackwell Science, 1987.

Lyon G, Adams RD, Kolodny EH. *Neurology of Hereditary Metabolic Diseases of Children* (2nd edition). New York: McGraw-Hill, 1996.

McCarthy RA, Warrington EK. *Cognitive Neuropsychology: a Clinical Introduction*. San Diego: Academic Press, 1990.

Mendez MF, Cummings JL. *Dementia: a Clinical Approach* (3rd edition). Philadelphia: Butterworth-Heinemann, 2003.

Mitrushina M, Boone KB, Razani J, D'Elia LF. *Handbook of Normative Data for Neuropsychological Assessment* (2nd edition). Oxford: Oxford University Press, 2005.

Moore AR, O'Keefe ST. Drug-induced cognitive impairment in the elderly. *Drugs Aging* 1999; **15**: 15–28.

Moore DP. *Textbook of Clinical Neuropsychiatry*. London: Arnold, 2001.

Nicholson K, Martelli MF, Zasler ND. Does pain confound interpretation of neuropsychological test results? *Neuro Rehabilitation* 2001; **16**: 225–30.

Ogden JA. *Fractured Minds: a Case-Study Approach to Clinical Neuropsychology* (2nd edition). Oxford: Oxford University Press, 2005.

Panegyres PK. Dementia in young adults. In: Hodges JR (ed.), *Early-Onset Dementia: a Multidisciplinary Approach*. Oxford: Oxford University Press, 2001: 404–21.

Panegyres PK. The contribution of the study of neurodegenerative disorders to the understanding of human memory. *Q J Med* 2004; **97**: 555–67.

Panteliadis CP, Korinthenberg R (eds.). *Paediatric Neurology: Theory and Practice*. Stuttgart: Thieme, 2005.

Parks RW, Zec RF, Wilson RS (eds.). *Neuropsychology of Alzheimer's Disease and Other Dementias*. New York: Oxford University Press, 1993.

Pillon B, Dubois B, Agid Y. Testing cognition may contribute to the diagnosis of movement disorders. *Neurology* 1996; **46**: 329–34.

Pincus JH, Tucker GJ. *Behavioral Neurology* (4th edition), Oxford: Oxford University Press, 2002.

Qizilbash N, Schneider LS, Chui H, *et al.* (eds.). *Evidence-Based Dementia Practice*. Oxford: Blackwell, 2002.

Rabins PV, Lyketsos CG, Steele CD. *Practical Dementia Care* (2nd edition). Oxford: Oxford University Press, 2006.

Robinson RG. *The Clinical Neuropsychiatry of Stroke: Cognitive, Behavioral and Emotional Disorders Following Vascular Brain Injury* (2nd edition). Cambridge: Cambridge University Press, 2006.

Roose SP, Devanand DP. *The Interface Between Dementia and Depression*. London: Martin Dunitz, 1999.

Sampson EL, Warren JD, Rossor MN. Young onset dementia. *Postgrad Med J* 2004; **80**: 125–39.

Selzer ME, Clarke S, Cohen LG, Duncan PW, Gage FH (eds.). *Textbook of Neural Repair and Rehabilitation. Volume II: Medical Neurorehabilitation*. Cambridge: Cambridge University Press, 2006: 411–511.

Shallice T. *From Neuropsychology to Mental Structure*. Cambridge: Cambridge University Press, 1988.

Starkstein SE, Merello M. *Psychiatric and Cognitive Disorders in Parkinson's Disease*. Cambridge: Cambridge University Press, 2002.

Strauss E, Sherman EMS, Spreen O. *A Compendium of Neuropsychological Tests: Administration, Norms, Commentary* (3rd edition). Oxford: Oxford University Press, 2006.

Trimble MR. *Biological Psychiatry* (2nd edition). Chichester: Wiley, 1996.

Waldemar G. Reversible dementias: do they exist? *Pract Neurol* 2002; **2**: 138–43.

Wilson B. *Case Studies in Neuropsychological Rehabilitation*. Oxford: Oxford University Press, 1999.

Cognitive function, neuropsychological evaluation, and syndromes of cognitive impairment

This chapter seeks to elucidate briefly the various domains of cognitive function, their neuropsychological evaluation, and syndromes of cognitive impairment. It is aimed at the practising neurologist rather than the academic neuropsychologist.

Without necessarily subscribing to an explicitly modular concept of cerebral function, it is nonetheless convenient to think in terms of cognitive domains or functional systems ('a congeries of mental faculties') in the brain, specifically attention, memory, language, perception, praxis, and executive function. These subdivisions, all (hopefully) working in concert, not in isolation, to produce in sum what we understand by consciousness, may direct a structured approach to the clinical assessment of cognitive function. Nowadays, a model of distributed neural networks with nodal points more specialized for certain functions has supplanted the idea of particular brain centres (Mesulam, 1990).

The neurocognitive domains may be described as either localized, implying lateralization to one hemisphere of part thereof, focal damage to which may impair that specific function; or distributed, implying a non-localized function often involving both hemispheres and/or subhemispheric structures (basal ganglia, brainstem), widespread damage being required to impair these functions (Hodges, 1994). Moreover, particular domains may be subdivided, or fractionated, into subsystems or specific functions which may be selectively impaired, suggesting the existence of functionally distinct neuropsychological substrates.

There are many tests available to the neuropsychologist for the evaluation of cognitive function, either global function or individual domains (Lezak *et al.*, 2004; Mitrushina *et al.*, 2005, Strauss *et al.*, 2006). The variety of tests available may bewilder the non-specialist. Moreover, the choice of different test instruments in different studies may make direct comparisons difficult. Of course, it must be remembered that any neuropsychological test may have multiple sensory, motor, perceptual, and cognitive demands, and hence 'pure' tests of any single cognitive domain are the exception, rather than the rule.

Neuropsychologists insist, rightly, that special training is required in the administration and interpretation of neuropsychological tests. Clinical neurologists will therefore rely on their neuropsychologist colleagues for the performance and interpretation of these 'formal' tests, since they fall outwith neurologists' expertise, and may take substantial time to administer, incompatible with clinical schedules. Nonetheless, some form of neuropsychological testing, often labelled as 'bedside' to distinguish it from 'formal' testing, is within the scope of neurologists and may be of diagnostic use (Griffiths & Welch, 2003). Numerous test batteries which may be applied within 10–30 minutes are available, encompassing not only cognitive function but also functional, behavioural, and global assessment (Burns *et al.*, 1999, 2004). Because of the brevity which makes them clinically applicable, these instruments often have certain

shortcomings that neurologists need to bear in mind: a raw score derived from a series of tests is not necessarily 'diagnostic', although it may increase the likelihood of a particular diagnosis. The potential for incongruous or anomalous performance of tests in a medicolegal setting has been noted (Trimble, 2004).

It is also important to note that when evaluating cognitive disorders, particularly those involving memory impairment, obtaining some collateral history from a relative, friend, or carer familiar with the subject is a vital part of the evaluation (Tierney *et al.*, 1996; Jorm, 1997; Carr *et al.*, 2000; Shulman & Feinstein, 2003), even for early stages of disease (Isella *et al.*, 2006). Even the simple observation that a patient attends the clinic alone despite having been instructed to bring a relative or friend is of diagnostic relevance, arguing strongly against the presence of a cognitive disorder (Larner, 2005).

REFERENCES

Burns A, Lawlor B, Craig S. *Assessment Scales in Old Age Psychiatry*. London: Martin Dunitz, 1999.

Burns A, Lawlor B, Craig S. *Assessment Scales in Old Age Psychiatry* (2nd edition). London: Martin Dunitz, 2004.

Carr DB, Gray S, Baty J, Morris JC. The value of informant versus individual's complaints of memory impairment in early dementia. *Neurology* 2000; **55**: 1724–6.

Griffiths TD, Welch JL. How to do it: use a diagnostic neuropsychology service properly. *Pract Neurol* 2003; **3**: 170–5.

Hodges JR. *Cognitive Assessment for Clinicians*. Oxford: Oxford University Press, 1994.

Isella V, Villa L, Russo A, *et al.* Discriminative and predictive power of an informant report in mild cognitive impairment. *J Neurol Neurosurg Psychiatry* 2006; **77**: 166–71.

Jorm AF. Methods of screening for dementia: a meta-analysis of studies comparing an informant questionnaire with a brief cognitive test. *Alzheimer Dis Assoc Disord* 1997; **11**: 158–62.

Larner AJ. 'Who came with you?' A diagnostic observation in patients with memory problems? *J Neurol Neurosurg Psychiatry* 2005; **76**: 1739.

Lezak MD, Howieson DB, Loring DW. *Neuropsychological Assessment* (4th edition). New York: Oxford University Press, 2004.

Mesulam MM. Large-scale neurocognitive networks and distributed processing for attention, language, and memory. *Ann Neurol* 1990; **28**: 597–613.

Mitrushina M, Boone KB, Razani J, D'Elia LF. *Handbook of Normative Data for Neuropsychological Assessment* (2nd edition). Oxford: Oxford University Press, 2005.

Shulman K, Feinstein A. *Quick Cognitive Screening for Clinicians: Mini Mental, Clock Drawing and Other Brief Tests*. London: Martin Dunitz, 2003: 125–39.

Strauss E, Sherman EMS, Spreen O. *A Compendium of Neuropsychological Tests: Administration, Norms, and Commentary* (3rd edition). New York: Oxford University Press, 2006.

Tierney MC, Szalai JP, Snow WG, Fisher RH. The prediction of Alzheimer disease: the role of patient and informant perceptions of cognitive deficits. *Arch Neurol* 1996; **53**: 423–7.

Trimble M. *Somatoform Disorders: a Medicolegal Guide*. Cambridge: Cambridge University Press, 2004: 109–39.

1.1 Attention

It is perhaps redundant to point out that before any meaningful assessment of 'higher cognitive function' can be made, it should be ascertained that 'lower cognitive function' is intact, assuming that the workings of the nervous system are hierarchical in their operation. To indulge in *reductio ad absurdum*, it would not be reasonable to expect a comatose patient, or a sleeping subject, to perform well on tests of memory, although that memory function may be intact or impaired on recovery from coma or awakening from sleep. The nature of consciousness is an area of great interest to both neuroscientists and philosophers (e.g. Dennett, 1993; Penrose, 1995; Zeman, 2001, 2002; Libet, 2004), but other than to assume that it is an emergent property of brain function, nothing further about its possible neuro-anatomical and neurophysiological basis will be considered here. Dissociation between apparent preservation of consciousness and absence of cognitive function may occur, for example in vegetative states (Jennett, 2002).

Disturbance of consciousness may encompass both a quantitative and a qualitative dimension. Hence one may speak of a 'level' of consciousness, perhaps in terms of arousal, alertness, or vigilance, forming a continuum from coma to the awake state; and an 'intensity' or quality of consciousness, in terms of clarity of awareness of the environment, and ability to focus, sustain, or shift attention. Coma obviously implies a state of unresponsiveness from which a patient cannot be roused by verbal or mechanical stimuli. Lesser degrees of impaired consciousness, sometimes labelled clinically as stupor, torpor, or obtundation (although these terms lack precision, their meaning often varying between different observers) may also interfere with cognitive assessment. There are many causes of coma (Plum & Posner, 1980; Young *et al.*, 1998). These states may be obvious clinically, such as drowsiness, or difficulty rousing the patient, but may also be occult, perhaps manifesting as increased distractibility. Impairments in level of consciousness are a *sine qua non* for the diagnosis of delirium (see Section 1.10), as enshrined in the diagnostic criteria of DSM-IV and ICD10, although these deficits may be subtle and not immediately obvious at the bedside though yet sufficient to impair attentional mechanisms. These attentional deficits may be responsible for the impaired cognitive function that is also a diagnostic feature of delirium (Burns *et al.*, 2004; Larner 2004; Inouye, 2006).

Attention, or concentration, is a non-uniform, distributed cognitive function. It may be defined as that component of consciousness which distributes awareness to particular sensory stimuli. Bombarded as the nervous system is with stimuli in multiple sensory domains, only some reach awareness or salience, whilst many percepts are not consciously taken notice of. Attentional resources, which are finite, are devoted to some channels but not others. Attention is thus effortful, selective, and closely linked to intention. Distinction may be made between different types of attentional mechanism: sustained attention implies devotion of most attentional resources to one particular stimulus;

selective attention is the directing of attentional resources to one stimulus amongst many ('cocktail party phenomenon'); divided attention implies a division of attentional resources between competing stimuli. Neuroanatomical structures thought to be important in mediating attention include the reticular activating system in the brainstem, the thalamus, and prefrontal cerebral cortex of multimodal association type, particularly in the right hemisphere, since damage to any of these areas may result in impairments of attention. Dopaminergic and cholinergic pathways are thought to be the important neurotransmitters mediating attention (Perry *et al.*, 2002).

The term 'working memory' is used by neuropsychologists to describe a limited-capacity store for retaining information over a short term, 1–2 minutes, and for 'online' manipulation of that information. This system has a limited capacity wherein information rapidly degrades unless continuously rehearsed (hence 'unstable', compared to longer-term memory). Working memory may be fractionated into verbal (phonological or articulatory loop) and visual (visuospatial sketch pad) components, governed by a supervisory central executive (Baddeley, 1986). Working memory function is dissociable from 'long-term memory' function (see Section 1.3): for example, in patients with amnesia as a consequence of Wernicke–Korsakoff syndrome working memory is preserved (Section 8.3.1). Working memory is perhaps better envisaged as a component of the selective attention system (the 'specious present' of William James), and is certainly not congruent with the term 'short-term memory' often used by patients, which refers to recent long-term memory. Grammatical complexity, for example in sentence construction, is associated with working memory capacity, which mediates the need to keep many elements in play and not lose the train of thought before completing the sentence.

Neglect, sometimes known as inattention, is a failure to orient to, respond to, or report novel or meaningful stimuli in the absence of sensory or motor deficits such as hemiparesis or hemianopia that could explain such behaviour. Extinction, the failure to respond to a novel or meaningful sensory stimulus on one side when a homologous stimulus is given simultaneously to the contralateral side (i.e. double simultaneous stimulation), sometimes called 'suppression', may be a lesser degree of neglect. In the visual domain, neglect may be categorized as a disorder of spatial attention, which is more common after right rather than left brain damage, usually of vascular origin, an observation accounted for by the ability of the right hemisphere to attend to both sides of space whereas the left hemisphere attends to the right side of space only (i.e. there is some lateralization of function). The angular gyrus and parahippocampal gyrus may be the critical neuroanatomical substrates underpinning the development of visual neglect (Husain, 2002; Chatterjee, 2003; Heilman *et al.*, 2003).

The Glasgow Coma Scale (GCS) is the instrument most commonly used for monitoring level of consciousness (Teasdale & Jennett, 1974). Introduced to assess the severity of traumatic head injuries, it has subsequently been applied in other clinical situations (e.g. delirium, stroke) although its validity in some of these circumstances remains to be confirmed. In the individual patient, use of the individual components of the GCS (eye, verbal, motor response = EVM) is more useful than the summed score (out of 15), although for demographic research use of the summed score is preferable. A GCS score of 15/15 does not guarantee intact attention, since deficits may be subtle, and it may therefore be necessary to undertake tests of attentional function before any other neuropsychological instruments are administered.

Many tests of attention are available (Strauss *et al.*, 2006), such as the Trail Making Test, the Continuous Performance Test, the Paced Auditory Serial Addition Test (PASAT: Gronwall, 1977), and the Symbol Digit Modalities Test. Simple bedside tests which tap attentional mechanisms include orientation in time and place, digit span forwards and/or backwards (also WAIS-R Digit Span subtest), reciting the months of the year or the days of the week backwards, or counting back from 30 down to

1. Distractibility may be evident if the patient loses his or her way, or starts the more automatic forward recital. In the Mini-Mental State Examination (see Section 1.8), performing serial sevens (subtracting 7 from 100 repeatedly = 93, 86, 79, 72, 65, etc.) or spelling the word WORLD backwards are labelled as tests of attention or concentration, but it should be realized that failure in these tests may be for reasons other than impaired attention (e.g. poor mental arithmetic abilities in serial sevens).

Neglect may be clinically obvious, for example if a patient fails to dress one side of the body, but is sometimes more subtle, in which case its presence may be sought using cancellation tests (e.g. stars in an unstructured array, or letters in a structured array), figure copying (e.g. the Rey–Osterreith figure), line bisection tasks, numbering a clock face, or drawing from memory.

REFERENCES

Baddeley AD. *Working Memory.* Oxford: Oxford University Press, 1986.

Burns A, Gallagley A, Byrne J. Delirium. *J Neurol Neurosurg Psychiatry* 2004; **75**: 362–7.

Chatterjee A. Neglect: a disorder of spatial attention. In: D'Esposito M (ed.), *Neurological Foundations of Cognitive Neuroscience.* Cambridge, MA: MIT Press, 2003: 1–26.

Dennett DC. *Consciousness Explained.* London: Penguin, 1993.

Gronwall DMA. Paced Auditory Serial-Addition Task: a measure of recovery from concussion. *Percept Motor Skills* 1977; **44**: 367–73.

Heilman KM, Watson RT, Valenstein E. Neglect and related disorders. In: Heilman KM, Valenstein E (eds.), *Clinical Neuropsychology* (4th edition). Oxford: Oxford University Press, 2003: 296–346.

Husain M. Cognitive neuroscience of hemispatial neglect. *Cognit Neuropsychiatry* 2002; **7**: 195–209.

Inouye SK. Current concepts: delirium in older persons. *N Engl J Med* 2006; **354**: 1157–65.

Jennett B. *The Vegetative State: Medical Facts, Ethical and Legal Dilemmas.* Cambridge: Cambridge University Press, 2002.

Larner AJ. Delirium: diagnosis, aetiopathogenesis and treatment. *Adv Clin Neurosci Rehabil* 2004; **4** (2): 28–9.

Libet B. *Mind Time: the Temporal Factor in Consciousness.* Cambridge, MA: Harvard University Press, 2004.

Penrose R. *Shadows of the Mind.* London: Vintage, 1995.

Perry E, Ashton H, Young A (eds.). *Neurochemistry of Consciousness: Neurotransmitters in Mind.* Amsterdam: John Benjamins, 2002.

Plum F, Posner JB. *The Diagnosis of Stupor and Coma* (3rd edition). Philadelphia: Davis, 1980.

Strauss E, Sherman EMS, Spreen O. *A Compendium of Neuropsychological Tests: Administration, Norms, Commentary* (3rd edition). Oxford: Oxford University Press, 2006: 546–677.

Teasdale G, Jennett B. Assessment of coma and impaired consciousness: a practical scale. *Lancet* 1974; **2**: 81–4.

Young GB, Ropper AH, Bolton CF (eds.). *Coma and Impaired Consciousness: a Clinical Perspective.* New York: McGraw-Hill, 1998.

Zeman A. Consciousness. *Brain* 2001: **124**: 1263–89.

Zeman A. *Consciousness: a User's Guide.* New Haven: Yale University Press, 2002.

1.2   General intelligence, IQ

Formal neuropsychological assessment often involves testing of general intelligence, before any specific assessment of the individual domains of cognitive function. This is legitimate since a general intelligence factor, *g*, seems to account for a significant proportion of the individual differences among test scores for groups of people (Deary, 2001). General intellectual function is most often measured by administration of one of the Wechsler Intelligence Scales, most often the Wechsler Adult Intelligence Scale–Revised (WAIS-R: Wechsler, 1981) or the Wechsler Adult Intelligence Scale–III (WAIS-III: Wechsler, 1997). (There is a separate scale for children, the Wechsler Intelligence Scale for Children, WISC.) Updating of these tests is required periodically because of changes in the abilities of the normative group from which standardized scores are derived (Deary, 2001).

Administration of these tests may take anything up to 2 hours or more, sometimes necessitating more than one testing session to avoid patient fatigue. Subtests in these batteries fall into two categories, verbal and performance, the former including tests of general knowledge, vocabulary, comprehension, and verbal abstract thinking (e.g. Digit Span, Arithmetic, Similarities), and the latter including tests of perceptual organization, complex visuospatial function, and psychomotor speed (e.g. Digit Symbol, Picture Completion and Arrangement, Block Design, Object Assembly). These subtests yield an index of verbal intelligence, verbal IQ (VIQ), and of performance intelligence, performance IQ (PIQ), as well as an overall full-scale IQ (FSIQ). Based on extensive normative data from healthy North Americans and Europeans, these measures have a mean score of 100 and a standard deviation of 15 such that 95% of the population will fall within the range 70–130. Generally VIQ and PIQ are correlated, but occasional discrepancies may be seen in normal individuals. The belief that VIQ–PIQ split can be reliably used to infer the lateralization of brain pathology (VIQ more impaired in left-sided lesions, PIQ with right-sided lesions) should be viewed with caution (Iverson *et al.*, 2004).

For the assessment of individuals complaining of cognitive disorders, especially memory disorders, an IQ score per se may not be particularly helpful. Change in IQ, possibly reflecting cognitive decline, is more helpful, but it is seldom the case that an individual patient will have undergone previous testing with which to make comparison. Previous educational and occupational history may give clues to premorbid intelligence, as may performance on verbal subtests of the WAIS batteries. This difficulty may also be partially circumvented by administering a test specifically designed to estimate premorbid intellectual abilities, such as the National Adult Reading Test (NART: Nelson & Willison, 1991), since the overlearned ability to read a series of words with irregular spelling-to-sound correspondences is relatively preserved in a number of neurodegenerative disorders (there are exceptions, e.g. frontotemporal lobar degenerations causing linguistic syndromes, Sections 2.2.2 and 2.2.3). The NART IQ may then be compared with the Wechsler FSIQ to give some indication of whether general intellectual function is stable or has declined. A difference of 20 points is probably significant, of 40 points certainly so.

Non-verbal tests of general intelligence are also available, such as the Progressive Matrices described by Raven (1938, 1958). Other tests examining general cognitive functioning by means of neuropsychological batteries and assessment of premorbid intelligence are available (Strauss *et al.*, 2006).

REFERENCES

Deary IJ. *Intelligence: a Very Short Introduction*. Oxford: Oxford University Press, 2001.

Iverson GL, Mendrek A, Adams RL. The persistent belief that VIQ–PIQ splits suggest lateralized brain damage. *Appl Neuropsychol* 2004; **11**: 85–90.

Nelson HE, Willison J. *National Adult Reading Test (NART)* (2nd edition). Windsor: NFER-Nelson, 1991.

Raven JC. *Progressive Matrices: a Perceptual Test of Intelligence*. London: HK Lewis, 1938.

Raven JC. *Advanced Progressive Matrices, Set 1*. London: HK Lewis, 1958.

Strauss E, Sherman EMS, Spreen O. *A Compendium of Neuropsychological Tests: Administration, Norms, Commentary* (3rd edition). Oxford: Oxford University Press, 2006: 98–362.

Wechsler D. *Weschler Adult Intelligence Scale-Revised (WAIS-R)*. San Antonio: Psychological Corporation, 1981.

Wechsler D. *Weschler Adult Intelligence Scale, 3rd edition (WAIS-III)*. San Antonio: Psychological Corporation, 1997.

1.3 Memory

Memory is a non-uniform, distributed cognitive function. In other words, subdivisions in memory function may be discriminated, which involve various neuroanatomical substrates.

Current taxonomies of memory propose a distinction between declarative (also known as explicit or conscious memory) and non-declarative memory (implicit, procedural, unconscious memory). Declarative or explicit memories are intentional or conscious recollections of previous experience. Declarative memory may be further subdivided into episodic memory and semantic memory. Episodic memories are particular personal events, sometimes known as autobiographical memories, specific to time and place (context-specific), whereas semantic memories are facts, a database of culturally approved knowledge independent of any specific context (Schacter & Tulving, 1994; Hodges & Greene, 1995). Many tests are available to probe the specific areas of episodic and semantic long-term memory. A distinction may also be drawn between anterograde memory, the laying down of new memories, and retrograde memory, the store of previously encoded material. An autobiographical–semantic dissociation of retrograde memory loss may be noted (Kapur, 1993, 1997).

In contrast to explicit memory, implicit memories refer to a heterogeneous collection of faculties, such as skill learning, priming, and conditioning, which are not available to conscious thought or report (Schacter *et al.*, 1993). Generally, clinical examination of implicit memory functions is not undertaken.

In clinical practice, lay observers and primary care physicians frequently distinguish between problems with 'short-term memory' and 'long-term memory', most usually referring to material learned recently or in the more distant past, respectively. Such a division persists in professional terminology, although the meanings are different. Professional 'short-term memory' is analogous to 'working memory', best conceptualized as an attentional function (see Section 1.1). Patient 'short-term memory' is in fact one component of professional 'long-term memory' (which encompasses all the subdivisions previously mentioned), specifically that for the learning of new information. Amnesia is the syndrome of impaired memory and new learning, which may be characterized as anterograde or retrograde, acute/transient or chronic/persistent. Anterograde amnesia may be clinically manifest as repeated questioning about day-to-day matters, inability to carry out simple chores, or repeating the same information. A better distinction may be between 'recent' and 'remote' memory.

The neuroanatomical substrates of explicit memory are partially understood, based on studies of experimental animals and of patients developing memory problems as a consequence of focal brain lesions which may be examined by means of

neuropsychology and, more recently, neuroimaging. The literature makes reference to hippocampal, diencephalic, frontal, and basal forebrain amnesia, largely based on lesion and neuropathological studies. Structures in the medial temporal lobe, centred on the hippocampus, and in the diencephalon surrounding the third ventricle, are thought to be crucial to episodic memory (O'Keefe & Nadel, 1978; Cohen & Eichenbaum, 1993; Zola-Morgan & Squire, 1993). Lesions anywhere along the circuit described by Papez (entorhinal area of the parahippocampal gyrus, perforant and alvear pathways, hippocampus, fimbria and fornix, mammillary bodies, mammillothalamic tract, anterior thalamic nuclei, internal capsule, cingulate gyrus, and cingulum) may lead to anterograde and retrograde amnesia. The experience of the patient known as HM was a key indicator of the importance of these structures. Because of his medically refractory epilepsy, HM underwent bilateral medial temporal lobectomy, encompassing the amygdala, entorhinal cortex, anterior dentate gyrus, hippocampus, and subiculum, which operation was followed by a dense anterograde amnesia, and retrograde amnesia covering about a decade prior to the surgery (Scoville & Milner, 1957). HM has been followed up for many years with essentially no improvement in his neuropsychological deficits, such that he is 'marooned in the moment' (Ogden, 2005). Similar outcomes have been seen on occasion with unilateral surgery (Kapur & Prevett, 2003). Lesions confined to the hippocampus may be particularly associated with retrograde amnesia (Cipolotti *et al.*, 2001). Amnesia has been described in association with basal forebrain (Damasio *et al.*, 1985) and frontal lesions, the latter with a defect in memory encoding (Parkin, 1997a).

There are many causes of memory disorder (Kapur, 1994; Baddeley *et al.*, 1995; Hodges & Greene, 1995; Parkin, 1997b; Kopelman, 2002; Mega, 2003; Papanicolaou, 2006). Impairment of episodic memory is the most common presenting feature of Alzheimer's disease (AD: see Section 2.1), sometimes occurring in isolation, although other deficits may be apparent on clinical or neuropsychological assessment. For this reason, and because AD is the most common cause of dementia, neuropsychological test batteries, particularly 'bedside' tests, are often weighted toward memory testing to the relative exclusion of other cognitive domains such as executive function, leading to difficulty identifying other neurocognitive disorders in which memory is not the principal domain affected. Anterograde amnesia may also occur as a consequence of open or closed head injury (post-traumatic amnesia), Wernicke–Korsakoff syndrome (see Section 8.3.1), herpes simplex encephalitis (Section 9.1.1), limbic encephalitis of paraneoplastic or non-paraneoplastic origin (Sections 6.12.1 and 6.12.2, respectively), strategic brain infarcts (Section 3.4), and surgery to remove temporal lobe or third ventricle lesions (Section 7.2.3). Transient amnesias may be of epileptic origin (transient epileptic amnesia: Section 4.3.1) or, in transient global amnesia, of probable vascular aetiology (Section 3.7.3). Psychogenic amnesia may also enter the differential diagnosis of transient amnesias (Pujol & Kopelman, 2003; Butler & Zeman, 2006). A temporal gradient of retrograde amnesia may also be present in some of these conditions, but rare cases of focal retrograde amnesia with relative sparing of anterograde memory have been described, sometimes following head injury or an encephalitic illness (e.g. Stuss & Guzman, 1988; Kapur, 1993; Hunkin, 1997; Mackenzie-Ross, 2000; Larner *et al.*, 2004).

Many tests of memory are available (Strauss *et al.*, 2006). The Wechsler Memory Scale, now in its third edition (WMS-III), is a battery testing auditory and visual declarative (and working) memory. Other specific tests of episodic memory sometimes deployed include the Buschke Selective Reminding Test (Buschke & Fuld, 1974), the California Verbal Learning Test (Delis *et al.*, 2000), the Hopkins Verbal Learning Test (Brandt, 1991; Shapiro *et al.*, 1999), the Camden Recognition Memory Test and the Topographical Recognition Memory Test (Warrington, 1984, 1996), and the Rey Auditory Verbal Learning Test. Recall of the Rey–Osterrieth Complex Figure may be used as a test of visual memory. Retrograde memory may be investigated using the Autobiographical Memory Interview (Kopelman *et al.*, 1989),

which covers both personal semantic information and autobiographical incidents, although this may underestimate the true extent of retrograde amnesia, missing 'islands' of memory loss unique to the individual. The Famous Faces Test may be used to study remote memory (Hodges *et al.*, 1993). Integrity of the semantic network, including semantic memory, may be tested using category (or semantic) fluency tests (see Section 1.7). Reading words with irregular sound-to-spelling correspondence may produce surface dyslexia (regularization errors) in patients with impaired access to or breakdown of semantic networks. Other tests accessing associative semantic networks include the Pyramids and Palm Trees Test (Howard & Patterson, 1992). A semantic memory test battery involving subtests of category fluency, naming, naming to description, and picture–word matching in response to spoken word has also been described (Hodges *et al.*, 1992a,b).

Of the frequently used 'bedside' neuropsychological test instruments (see Section 1.8), the Mini-Mental State Examination has only perfunctory examination of memory function (registration and recall after distractor items of the names of three objects, e.g. ball, flag, tree). Longer (supraspan) word lists are used in the DemTect and the Hopkins Verbal Learning Test, and the latter includes both recall and recognition paradigms to try to ascertain whether failures result from encoding or retrieval defects. The Addenbrooke's Cognitive Examination (ACE) and its revision (ACE-R) add recall of a seven-item name and address, with a recognition paradigm in the ACE-R, and also a test of category fluency. The Queen Square Screening Test for Cognitive Deficits has a qualitative story recall test, and also picture recall to test visual memory.

REFERENCES

Baddeley AD, Wilson BA, Watts FN (eds.). *Handbook of Memory Disorders*. Chichester: Wiley, 1995.

Brandt J. The Hopkins Verbal Learning Test: development of a new memory test with six equivalent forms. *Clin Neuropsychol* 1991; **5**: 125–42.

Buschke H, Fuld PA. Evaluating storage, retention, and retrieval in disordered memory and learning. *Neurology* 1974; **24**: 1019–25.

Butler C, Zeman A. Syndromes of transient amnesia. *Adv Clin Neurosci Rehabil* 2006; **6** (4): 13–14.

Cipolotti L, Shallice T, Chan D, *et al.* Long-term retrograde amnesia: the crucial role of the hippocampus. *Neuropsychologia* 2001; **39**: 151–72.

Cohen NJ, Eichenbaum H. *Memory, Amnesia, and the Hippocampal System*. Cambridge, MA: MIT Press, 1993.

Damasio AR, Graff-Radford NR, Eslinger PJ, Damasio H, Kassell N. Amnesia following basal forebrain lesions. *Arch Neurol* 1985; **42**: 263–71.

Delis DC, Kramer JH, Kaplan E, Ober BA. *California Verbal Learning Test* (2nd edition, adult version). San Antonio: Psychological Corporation, 2000.

Hodges JR, Greene JDW. Disorders of memory. In: Kennard C (ed.). *Recent advances in clinical neurology 8*. Edinburgh: Churchill Livingstone, 1995: 151–69.

Hodges JR, Patterson K, Oxbury S, Funnell E. Semantic dementia: progressive fluent aphasia with temporal lobe atrophy. *Brain* 1992a; **115**: 1783–806.

Hodges JR, Salmon DP, Butters N. Semantic memory impairment in Alzheimer's disease: failure of access or degraded knowledge? *Neuropsychologia* 1992b; **30**: 301–14.

Hodges JR, Salmon DP, Butters NA. Recognition and naming of famous faces in Alzheimer's disease: a cognitive analysis. *Neuropsychologia* 1993; **31**: 775–88.

Howard D, Patterson K. *Pyramids and Palm Trees: a Test of Semantic Access From Pictures and Words*. Bury St Edmunds: Thames Valley Test Company, 1992.

Hunkin N. Focal retrograde amnesia: implications for the organisation of memory. In: Parkin AJ (ed.), *Case Studies in the Neuropsychology of Memory*. Hove: Psychology Press, 1997: 63–82.

Kapur N. Focal retrograde amnesia in neurological disease: a critical review. *Cortex* 1993; **29**: 219–34.

Kapur N. *Memory Disorders in Clinical Practice*. Hove: Lawrence Erlbaum, 1994.

Kapur N. Autobiographical amnesia and temporal lobe pathology. In: Parkin AJ (ed.), *Case Studies in the Neuropsychology of Memory*. Hove: Psychology Press, 1997: 37–62.

Kapur N, Prevett M. Unexpected amnesia: are there lessons to be learned from cases of amnesia following unilateral temporal lobe surgery? *Brain* 2003; **126**: 2573–85.

Kopelman MD. Disorders of memory. *Brain* 2002; **125**: 2152–90.

Kopelman MD, Wilson BA, Baddeley AD. The Autobiographical Memory Interview: a new assessment of autobiographical and personal semantic memory in amnesic patients. *J Clin Exp Neuropsychol* 1989; **11**: 724–44.

Larner AJ, Ghadiali EJ, Doran M. Focal retrograde amnesia: clinical, neuropsychological and neuroimaging study. *Neurobiol Aging* 2004; **25**: S128 (abstract P1–116).

Mackenzie-Ross S. Profound retrograde amnesia following mild head injury: organic or functional? *Cortex* 2000; **36**: 521–37.

Mega MS. Amnesia: a disorder of episodic memory. In: D'Esposito M (ed.), *Neurological Foundations of Cognitive Neuroscience*. Cambridge, MA: MIT Press, 2003: 41–66.

Ogden JA. *Fractured Minds: a Case-Study Approach to Clinical Neuropsychology* (2nd edition). Oxford: Oxford University Press, 2005: 46–63.

O'Keefe J, Nadel L. *The Hippocampus as a Cognitive Map*. Oxford: Clarendon Press, 1978.

Papanicolaou AC. *The Amnesias: a Clinical Textbook of Memory Disorders*. Oxford: Oxford University Press, 2006.

Parkin AJ. The long and winding road: twelve years of frontal amnesia. In: Parkin AJ (ed.), *Case Studies in the Neuropsychology of Memory*. Hove: Psychology Press, 1997a: 127–40.

Parkin AJ (ed.). *Case Studies in the Neuropsychology of Memory*. Hove: Psychology Press, 1997b.

Pujol M, Kopelman MD. Psychogenic amnesia. *Pract Neurol* 2003; **3**: 292–9.

Schacter DL, Chiu CYP, Ochsner KN. Implicit memory: a selective review. *Annu Rev Neurosci* 1993; **16**: 159–82.

Schacter DL, Tulving E. *Memory Systems*. Cambridge, MA: MIT Press, 1994.

Scoville W, Milner B. Loss of recent memory after bilateral hippocampal lesions. *J Neurol Neurosurg Psychiatry* 1957; **20**: 11–21.

Shapiro AM, Benedict RH, Schretlen D, Brandt J. Construct and concurrent validity of the Hopkins Verbal Learning Test-revised. *Clin Neuropsychol* 1999; **13**: 348–58.

Strauss E, Sherman EMS, Spreen O. *A Compendium of Neuropsychological Tests: Administration, Norms, Commentary* (3rd edition). Oxford: Oxford University Press, 2006: 678–890.

Stuss DT, Guzman DA. Severe remote memory loss with minimal anterograde amnesia: a clinical note. *Brain Cogn* 1988; **8**: 21–30.

Warrington EK. *Recognition Memory Test*. Windsor: NFER-Nelson, 1984.

Warrington EK. *The Camden Memory Tests Manual*. Hove: Psychology Press, 1996.

Zola-Morgan S, Squire LR. Neuroanatomy of memory. *Annu Rev Neurosci* 1993; **16**: 547–63.

1.4   Language

Historically, language disorder provided the first unequivocal evidence that loss of a higher brain function could be ascribed to damage to a specific brain region, based on the work of Broca and, possibly, Marc Dax in the mid nineteenth century (Schiller, 1993). The work of Wernicke was also seminal in establishing the neural substrates of language function, indicating that language is a localized function. Every medical student now knows that most individuals, whether left- or right-handed, have language in the dominant hemisphere, although around 30% of left-handers and < 1% of right-handers have language in the non-dominant hemisphere.

Aphasia, a primary disorder of language, is often mirrored by similar defects in reading (alexia) and writing (agraphia), all of which are amenable, within certain limitations (Willmes & Poeck, 1993), to clinical localization, often on the basis of simple bedside examination. In addition to the Broca (non-fluent, anterior, motor, expressive) and Wernicke (fluent, posterior, sensory, receptive) types of aphasia, clinical distinctions may also be drawn between conduction aphasia (impaired repetition) and transcortical aphasias (preserved repetition). A classification of aphasias as perisylvian (Broca, Wernicke, conduction) and extrasylvian has also been proposed. There are many texts and reviews devoted to the subject (e.g. Benson & Ardila, 1996; Brown & Hagoort, 2000; Basso, 2003; Caplan, 2003; Spreen & Risser, 2003).

It may be necessary to test auditory comprehension before undertaking any other neuropsychological testing of language, for example using the Token Test (De Renzi & Faglioni, 1978), in which commands of increasing length and complexity are given for manipulating a deck of coloured tokens of differing size and shape (some have objected to the word 'token', preferring 'item': Critchley, 1979). Sentence comprehension skills may be ascertained by performance of the Test for the Reception of Grammar (Bishop, 1983). Wernicke type aphasia typically has marked comprehension impairments, with fluent speech output but often with poverty of content, sometimes reduced to a meaningless jumble of words (jargon aphasia). Although Broca type aphasia is often characterized as having preserved comprehension, this may in fact be impaired for more complex syntax.

There are many tests of language available (Lezak *et al.*, 2004; Strauss *et al.*, 2006). Comprehensive batteries include the Boston Diagnostic Aphasia Examination (BDAE: Goodglass & Kaplan, 1983), the Western Aphasia Battery (WAB: Shewan & Kertesz, 1980), the Psycholinguistic Assessment of Language Processing in Aphasia (PALPA: Kay *et al.*, 1992), and the Comprehensive Aphasia Test (Swinburn *et al.*, 2004). Specific tests of naming often deployed include the Graded Naming Test (McKenna & Warrington, 1980, 1983) and the Boston Naming Test (Kaplan *et al.*, 2001).

At the bedside, listening to speech output will permit a simple classification of aphasia as fluent or non-fluent, and also detect paraphasias (phonemic or semantic) and neologisms. From questioning or instructing the patient during history taking and clinical examination, comprehension difficulties may be evident. Testing of repetition may differentiate aphasias in which this ability is relatively preserved (transcortical aphasias) or impaired (conduction aphasia). Naming skills have less localizing value, although marked anomia should raise the suspicion of semantic problems, either degradation of or access to semantic stores. Reading and writing function should also be examined, even if spoken language function seems intact, since various syndromes of alexia and agraphia are described (Benson & Ardila, 1996; Saver, 2002; Leff,

2004; Larner 2006). Idea density in written material reflects language processing ability.

Of the frequently used 'bedside' neuropsychological test instruments (see Section 1.8), most are heavily weighted for language function, such that patients with primarily linguistic disorders (e.g. semantic dementia, aphasic presentations of Alzheimer's disease) may find it difficult or impossible to complete them.

REFERENCES

Basso A. *Aphasia and its Therapy*. Oxford: Oxford University Press, 2003.

Benson DF, Ardila A. *Aphasia: a Clinical Perspective*. New York: Oxford University Press, 1996.

Bishop DVM. *Test for the Reception of Grammar*. Manchester: Chapel Press, 1983.

Brown CM, Hagoort P (eds.). *The Neurocognition of Language*. Oxford: Oxford University Press, 2000.

Caplan D. Aphasic syndromes. In: Heilman KM, Valenstein E (eds.), *Clinical Neuropsychology* (4th edition). Oxford: Oxford University Press, 2003: 14–34.

Critchley M. *The Divine Banquet of the Brain and Other Essays*. New York: Raven Press, 1979: 68.

De Renzi E, Faglioni P. Normative data and screening power of a shortened version of the Token Test. *Cortex* 1978; **14**: 41–9.

Goodglass H, Kaplan E. *Boston Diagnostic Aphasia Examination (BDAE)*. Philadelphia: Lea & Febiger, 1983.

Kaplan EF, Goodglass H, Weintraub S. *The Boston Naming Test* (2nd edition). Philadelphia: Lippincott Williams & Wilkins, 2001.

Kay J, Lesser R, Coltheart M. *Psycholinguistic Assessment of Language Processing in Aphasia*. Hove: Psychology Press, 1992.

Larner AJ. *A Dictionary of Neurological Signs* (2nd edition). New York: Springer, 2006: 10–1, 14–6, 32–3.

Leff A. Alexia. *Adv Clin Neurosci Rehabil* 2004; **4** (3): 18, 20, 22.

Lezak MD, Howieson DB, Loring DW. *Neuropsychological Assessment* (4th edition). New York: Oxford University Press, 2004: 501–30.

McKenna P, Warrington EK. Testing for nominal aphasia. *J Neurol Neurosurg Psychiatry* 1980; **43**: 781–8.

McKenna P, Warrington EK. *The Graded Naming Test*. Windsor: NFER-Nelson, 1983.

Saver JL. Approach to the patient with aphasia. In: Biller J (ed.), *Practical Neurology* (2nd edition). Philadelphia: Lippincott Williams & Wilkins, 2002: 27–39.

Schiller F. *Paul Broca: Founder of French Anthropology, Explorer of the Brain*. Oxford: Oxford University Press, 1993.

Shewan CM, Kertesz A. Reliability and validity characteristics of the Western Aphasia Battery (WAB). *J Speech Hear Disord* 1980; **45**: 308–24.

Spreen O, Risser AH. *Assessment of Aphasia*. Oxford: Oxford University Press, 2003.

Strauss E, Sherman EMS, Spreen O. *A Compendium of Neuropsychological Tests: Administration, Norms, Commentary* (3rd edition). Oxford: Oxford University Press, 2006: 891–962.

Swinburn K, Porter G, Howard D. *Comprehensive Aphasia Test*. Hove: Psychology Press, 2004.

Willmes K, Poeck K. To what extent can aphasic syndromes be localized? *Brain* 1993; **116**: 1527–40.

1.5   Perception

Higher-order deficits of sensory processing, not explicable in terms of a disorder of attention, intellectual decline, or a failure to name the stimulus (anomia), are known as agnosias, a term coined by Sigmund Freud (1891) and meaning literally 'not knowing' or 'without knowledge'. Lissauer (1890; abridged translation by Shallice & Jackson, 1988), speaking of *Seelenblindheit*, literally 'soul-blindness' or technically 'psychic blindness', drew a distinction between apperceptive deficits and associative deficits: in the former a defect of higher-order complex perceptual processing was deemed to be present, whereas in the latter perception was held to be intact but a defect in giving meaning to the percept was present. Earlier descriptions probably reporting agnosic defects had appeared (Meyer, 1974). The debate continues as to whether all agnosias, although clinically distinguishable as apperceptive or associative, are in fact attributable to faulty perception (Farah, 1995).

Although auditory and tactile agnosias are described, they seem to be relatively rare in comparison with visual agnosia, which has certainly been more extensively studied (Farah, 1995; Bauer & Demery, 2003; Ghadiali, 2004). The visual agnosias may be relatively selective, for example an inability to recognize previously known human faces or equivalent stimuli, known as prosopagnosia. This may be developmental (Nunn *et al.*, 2001; Larner *et al.*, 2003) or acquired in origin, the latter usually a consequence of cerebrovascular disease causing bilateral occipitotemporal lesions, but occasionally it occurs as a feature of neurodegenerative disease, sometimes in relative isolation associated with focal right temporal lobe atrophy (progressive prosopagnosia: Evans *et al.*, 1995). Pure alexia is an agnosia for words which results in a laborious letter-by-letter reading strategy to arrive at a word's identity, conceptualized as a consequence of damage to a brain region mediating whole-word recognition, which may be located in the medial left occipital lobe and posterior fusiform gyrus (Leff *et al.*, 2006). The rare syndrome of pure word deafness may be a form of auditory agnosia. Finger agnosia, the inability to identify which finger has been touched despite knowing that a finger has been touched, is a form of tactile agnosia, which may be seen as one feature of Gerstmann syndrome although it may occur in isolation (Della Sala & Spinnler, 1994). Likewise, Braille alexia may in some instances be a form of tactile agnosia (Larner, 2007).

The existence of two visual processing pathways within the brain was first proposed by Ungerlieder and Mishkin (1982): an occipitoparietal dorsolateral ('where') visual processing stream, and an occipitotemporal ventromedial ('what') stream. In rare cases, these pathways may be selectively affected: for instance the ventral stream, specifically the lateral occipital area, in a famous patient with 'visual form agnosia' following carbon monoxide poisoning. Her perceptual identification of shape and form was lost, although she could still perceive colour and the fine detail of surfaces (visual texture), and her visuomotor ('vision for action') skills were strikingly preserved (Milner & Goodale, 1995; Goodale & Milner, 2004). Optic ataxia, impaired voluntary reaching for a visually presented target with misdirection and dysmetria, is the sign typically evident in dorsal stream lesions. The workings of the visuomotor control system are not available to consciousness ('unconscious vision'), unlike the visual identification of objects.

A specific inability to see objects in motion, akinetopsia or cerebral visual motion blindness, despite preserved perception of other visual attributes such as colour, form, and depth, has been described in association with selective lesions to area V5 of the visual cortex (Zihl *et al.*, 1983; Zeki, 1991). Although exceptionally rare, such cases suggest a distinct neuroanatomical substrate for movement vision, as do cases in which motion vision is selectively spared in a scotomatous area (Riddoch's syndrome: Zeki & ffytche, 1998). Perception within a 'blind' visual field without conscious awareness has been termed blindsight (Weiskrantz, 1986). Visual neglect is considered as a disorder of attention (see Section 1.1).

Cases of isolated progressive visual agnosia were presented by De Renzi (1986). Benson *et al.* (1988) drew attention to a disorder comprising alexia, agraphia, visual agnosia, with or without components of Balint and Gerstmann syndromes, transcortical sensory aphasia, but with relative preservation of memory until late in the course, a disorder they named posterior cortical atrophy (PCA) in the absence of neuropathological data. It is now believed that most such cases have Alzheimer's disease pathology, hence the 'visual variant of Alzheimer's disease' (Levine *et al.*, 1993), although this might also be characterized, at least in its early stages, as focal onset AD or a non-amnestic form of mild cognitive impairment (MCI: Larner, 2004). Other pathologies have sometimes been found in PCA cases (Pantel & Schröder, 1996). Diagnostic criteria for PCA have been developed (Mendez *et al.*, 2002). Visual agnosic problems are a common finding in Alzheimer's disease, though usually less apparent than the mnemonic difficulties. Various visual processing disorders may occur in AD (Cronin-Golomb & Hof, 2004).

Various means may be used specifically to test visual perceptual and visuoconstructive functions (Strauss *et al.*, 2006). These may be individual tests such as Judgment of Line Orientation (thought to tap right occipital lobe function); copy of the Rey–Osterrieth Complex Figure (Rey, 1941; Osterrieth, 1944; translation by Corwin & Bylsma, 1993) or the Taylor Figure (Taylor, 1969); decoding embedded (Poppelreuter) figures; parts of test batteries, such as the WAIS-R Block Design (visuospatial construction); or dedicated batteries such as the Visual Object and Space Perception Battery (VOSP: Warrington & James, 1991).

Of the frequently used 'bedside' neuropsychological test instruments (see Section 1.8), the Mini-Mental State Examination has only perfunctory examination of visuospatial function, requiring copying a drawing of intersecting pentagons. Clock Drawing is, at least in part, a visuospatial test, but requires other skills. The Queen Square Screening Test for Cognitive Deficits calls for the identification of fragmented letters and pictures. The Addenbrooke's Cognitive Examination (ACE) adds copying a wire cube and clock drawing, and ACE-R adds counting dots and identifying fragmented letters. DemTect eschews specific visuoperceptual testing, other than in a number transcoding task.

REFERENCES

Bauer RM, Demery JA. Agnosia. In: Heilman KM, Valenstein E (eds.), *Clinical Neuropsychology* (4th edition). Oxford: Oxford University Press, 2003: 236–95.

Benson DF, Davis RJ, Snyder BD. Posterior cortical atrophy. *Arch Neurol* 1988; **45**: 789–93.

Corwin J, Bylsma FW. 'Psychological examination of traumatic encephalopathy' by A. Rey and 'The complex figure copy test' by P.A. Osterrieth. *Clin Neuropsychol* 1993; **7**: 3–21.

Cronin-Golomb A, Hof PR (eds.). *Vision in Alzheimer's Disease.* Basel: Karger, 2004.

Della Sala S, Spinnler H. Finger agnosia: fiction or reality? *Arch Neurol* 1994; **51**: 448–50.

De Renzi E. Slowly progressive visual agnosia or apraxia without dementia. *Cortex* 1986; **22**: 171–80.

Evans JJ, Heggs AJ, Antoun N, Hodges JR. Progressive prosopagnosia associated with selective right temporal lobe atrophy: a new syndrome? *Brain* 1995; **118**: 1–13.

Farah MJ. *Visual Agnosia: Disorders of Object Recognition and What They Tell Us About Normal Vision.* Cambridge, MA: MIT Press, 1995.

Freud S. *Zur Auffassung der Aphasien, eine Kritische Studie.* Leipizig: Deuticke, 1891.

Ghadiali E. Agnosia. *Adv Clin Neurosci Rehabil* 2004; **4** (5): 18–20.

Goodale MA, Milner AD. *Sight Unseen: an Exploration of Conscious and Unconscious Vision.* Oxford: Oxford University Press, 2004.

Larner AJ. 'Posterior cortical atrophy' or 'focal-onset Alzheimer's disease'? A clinical, neuropsychological and neuroimaging study. *J Neurol* 2004; **251** (suppl 3): III102 (abstract P385).

Larner AJ. Braille alexia: an apperceptive tactile agnosia? *J Neurol Neurosurg Psychiatry* 2007; **78**: 907–8.

Larner AJ, Downes JJ, Hanley JR, Tsivilis D, Doran M. Developmental prosopagnosia: a clinical and neuropsychological study. *J Neurol* 2003; **250** (suppl 2): II156 (abstract P591).

Leff AP, Spitsyna G, Plant GT, Wise RJS. Structural anatomy of pure and hemianopic alexia. *J Neurol Neurosurg Psychiatry* 2006; **77**: 1004–7.

Levine DN, Lee JM, Fisher CM. The visual variant of Alzheimer's disease: a clinicopathologic case study. *Neurology* 1993; **43**: 305–13.

Lissauer H. Ein Fall von Seelenblindheit nebst einem Beitrag zur Theorie derselben. *Arch Psychiatr Nervenkr* 1890; **21**: 222–70.

Mendez MF, Ghajarania M, Perryman KM. Posterior cortical atrophy: clinical characteristics and differences compared to Alzheimer's disease. *Dement Geriatr Cogn Disord* 2002; **14**: 33–40.

Meyer A. The frontal lobe syndrome, the aphasias and related conditions. *Brain* 1974; **97**: 565–600.

Milner AD, Goodale MA. *The Visual Brain in Action.* Oxford: Oxford University Press, 1995.

Nunn JA, Postma P, Pearson R. Developmental prosopagnosia: should it be taken at face value? *Neurocase* 2001; **7**: 15–27.

Osterrieth PA. Le test de copie d'une figure complex: contribution à l'étude de la perception et de la mémoire. *Arch Psychol* 1944; **30**: 286–356.

Pantel J, Schröder J. Posterior cortical atrophy: a new dementia syndrome or a form of Alzheimer's disease [in German]. *Fortschr Neurol Psychiatr* 1996; **64**: 492–508.

Rey A. L'examen psychologique dans les cas d'encéphalopathie traumatique. *Arch Psychol* 1941; **28**: 286–340.

Shallice T, Jackson M. Lissauer on agnosia. *Cogn Neuropsychol* 1988; **5**: 153–92.

Strauss E, Sherman EMS, Spreen O. *A Compendium of Neuropsychological Tests: Administration, Norms, Commentary* (3rd edition). Oxford: Oxford University Press, 2006: 963–1011.

Taylor LB. Localization of cerebral lesions by psychological testing. *Clin Neurosurg* 1969; **16**: 269–87.

Ungerlieder LG, Mishkin M. Two cortical visual systems. In: Ingle DJ, Goodale MA, Mansfield RJW (eds.), *Analysis of Visual Behavior*. Cambridge, MA: MIT Press, 1982: 549–86.

Warrington EK, James M. *The Visual Object and Space Perception Battery*. Bury St Edmunds: Thames Valley Test Company, 1991.

Weiskrantz L. *Blindsight: a Case Study and Implications*. Oxford: Clarendon Press, 1986.

Zeki S. Cerebral akinetopsia (cerebral visual motion blindness). *Brain* 1991; **114**: 811–24.

Zeki S, ffytche DH. The Riddoch syndrome: insights into the neurobiology of conscious vision. *Brain* 1998; **121**: 25–45.

Zihl J, Von Cramon D, Mai N. Selective disturbance of movement vision after bilateral brain damage. *Brain* 1983; **106**: 313–40.

1.6   Praxis

Apraxia, impairment of praxis, is an acquired disorder of higher-level motor control causing impaired purposeful voluntary motor skill (Grafton, 2003; Heilman & Gonzalez Rothi, 2003; Leiguarda, 2005), first defined as such and associated with left-sided lesions by Liepmann (1900). The disorder should not be explicable in terms of lower-motor deficits, such as pyramidal, extrapyramidal, cerebellar, or sensory dysfunction, nor in terms of other cognitive deficits such as language or perception. For example, deficits labelled as 'constructional apraxia' or 'dressing apraxia' are better explained as visuoperceptual and/or visuospatial deficits, as is the misdirected reaching for visual targets typical of optic ataxia.

Traditionally a distinction has been drawn between ideational and ideomotor apraxias, although both are often present in left hemisphere damage (De Renzi *et al.*, 1968). Ideomotor apraxia in Broca's aphasia may be conceptualized as a disconnection syndrome (see Section 1.12).

Cases of isolated progressive apraxia were presented by De Renzi (1986). Apraxia may be a feature of neurodegenerative disease, classically corticobasal degeneration (see Section 2.4.3), although Alzheimer's disease can on occasion present with a similar phenotype (biparietal atrophy: Section 2.1), even with alien limb behaviour.

Praxic difficulties may be tested for in various ways (Crutch, 2005), including gesture naming, decision and recognition; gesture to verbal command, to visual or tactile tool; imitation of real or nonsense gestures; and tool selection. There are test batteries, including the Florida Apraxia Screening Test-Revised (FAST-R: Gonzalez Rothi *et al.*, 1997).

REFERENCES

Crutch S. Apraxia. *Adv Clin Neurosci Rehabil* 2005; **5** (1): 16, 18.

De Renzi E. Slowly progressive visual agnosia or apraxia without dementia. *Cortex* 1986; **22**: 171–80.

De Renzi E, Pieczuro A, Vignolo LA. Ideational apraxia: a quantitative study. *Neuropsychologia* 1968; **6**: 41–52.

Gonzalez Rothi LJ, Raymer AM, Heilman KM. Limb praxis assessment. In: Gonzalez Rothi LJ, Heilman KM (eds.), *Apraxia: the Neuropsychology of Action*. Hove: Psychology Press, 1997: 61–74.

Grafton S. Apraxia: a disorder of motor control. In: D'Esposito M (ed.), *Neurological Foundations of Cognitive Neuroscience*. Cambridge, MA: MIT Press, 2003: 239–58.

Heilman KM, Gonzalez Rothi LJ. Apraxia. In: Heilman KM, Valenstein E (eds.), *Clinical Neuropsychology* (4th edition). Oxford: Oxford University Press, 2003: 215–35.

Leiguarda R. Apraxias as traditionally defined. In: Freund HJ, Jeannerod M, Hallett M, Leiguarda R (eds.), *Higher-Order Motor Disorders: from Neuroanatomy and Neurobiology to Clinical Neurology*. Oxford: Oxford University Press, 2005: 303–38.

Liepmann H. *Das Krankheitsbild der Apraxie ('motorischen Asymbolie')*. Berlin: Karger, 1900.

1.7   Executive function, 'frontal function'

The term 'executive function' is used to encompass various abilities, including the formulation of goals; organization, planning, execution, and monitoring of a sequence of actions; problem solving; and abstract thinking. It also overlaps with sustained attention. The term 'dysexecutive syndrome' may be used to describe dysfunction in any or all of these areas, which is most often associated with pathological processes in the frontal lobes (Filley, 2000; Chayer & Freedman, 2001; Miller & Cummings, 2007). Because of the heterogeneity of these functions, some authors dislike the umbrella term of 'executive function', and prefer to describe the specific function impaired. Moreover, frontal lobe damage may result in various clinical phenotypes, in which behavioural change is often the most salient feature. Orbitofrontal injury may result in disinhibition, as described in Phineas Gage, one of the most famous patients in the annals of clinical neuropsychology, who exhibited behavioural change following frontal lobe injury (Damasio *et al.*, 1994; Macmillan, 2000; Larner & Leach, 2002), although other patterns of clinical and cognitive change may be observed with frontal lobe injury (Loring & Meador, 2006): for example, apathetic (frontal convexity) and akinetic (medial frontal) syndromes are also described (Trimble, 1996).

Because of the overarching nature of the construct 'executive function', no single test is adequate to assess its integrity (Goldberg & Bougakov, 2005). A wide variety of tests known to be sensitive to aspects of executive dysfunction is available. At the bedside or in the clinic, 'Go–No Go' tests may be applied to assess failure of inhibitory responses, or stimulus-boundedness, for example asking the patient to tap twice in response to a single tap given by the examiner, and once in response to two taps. Repeating alternating sequences, for example of hand gestures (fist–palm) or of writing (m n m n m n), may be used to similar purpose. The Trails A and B test also requires a sequence, of letters or numbers, to be followed. Interpretation of proverbs is a popular bedside test, 'concrete' interpretation suggesting frontal lobe problems.

Oral tests of verbal fluency, or controlled oral word association tests (COWAT), may be divided into those testing phonological, letter, or lexical fluency, such as the FAS test (in one minute name as many words as possible beginning with the letter F, then another minute to name words beginning with A, then another minute to name words beginning with S), and those testing semantic or category fluency (in one minute name as many animals, or fruits, or musical instruments, or whatever category is chosen, as possible). Letter fluency has been characterized as a test of mental flexibility probing executive function, which is particularly impaired ('defective exemplification': Critchley, 1979) with left frontal lesions (without aphasia), whereas category fluency examines the integrity of the semantic network. Design fluency, a visual analogue of verbal fluency, may be more impaired with right frontal lesions (Jones-Gotman & Milner, 1977). Verbal fluency tasks are attractive because they are brief (1 minute each) and require no special equipment, but account may need to be taken of patient age and education when considering test norms (Mathuranath *et al.*, 2003). Verbal fluency tests are incorporated into test batteries such as the Dementia Rating Scale and the CERAD Battery, as well as the Addenbrooke's Cognitive Examination (see Section 1.8), and may be of diagnostic utility in Alzheimer's disease and vascular dementia (Cerhan *et al.*, 2002; Duff Canning *et al.*, 2004).

Perhaps the most frequently used tests probing executive functions are the Stroop Test (Stroop, 1935) and the Wisconsin Card Sorting Test (WCST) and the Modified Wisconsin Card Sorting Test (MWCST: Nelson, 1976). In the Stroop Test, patients are required to read a list of colour names, printed in colours which differ from the name, followed by naming the colours in which each name is printed, thus having to inhibit the reading of each colour name (i.e. inhibition of inappropriate responses). MWCST uses a set of cards marked with symbols of different shape, colour, and number which may be sorted in various ways. Sorting rules are changed by the examiner without informing the subject, requiring problem-solving skills. Difficulty switching category is typical of frontal lobe damage, leading to perseveration with previous categories. Clearly MWCST, unlike the Stroop Test, calls for novel responses. MWCST may not be specific to frontal lobe dysfunction, since patients with hippocampal lesions may commit perseverative errors (Corcoran & Upton, 1993).

There are many other tests probing executive functions, sometimes along with other domains (Strauss *et al.*, 2006). These include Raven's Progressive Matrices, the Porteus Mazes, the Tower of London Test (Shallice, 1982), the Tower of Hanoi Test, the Trail Making Test (especially Part B), the Halstead–Reitan Category Test, the Weigl Colour Form Sorting Test (Weigl, 1941), the Cognitive Estimates Test (Shallice & Evans, 1978), and the Verbal Switching Test (Warrington, 2000). The Hayling and Brixton Tests for sentence completion and spatial anticipation are tests of rule following and verbal suppression of a familiar response (Burgess & Shallice, 1996, 1997). Certain WAIS-R subtests are sensitive to aspects of executive/frontal lobe function, such as the Similarities test of verbal abstraction and the Digit Symbol test of psychomotor speed. Tests of decision making and risk taking, faculties which may also be encompassed under the rubric of executive function (Lehto & Elorinne, 2003) and mediated by the prefrontal cortex and amygdala, include the Iowa Gambling Test (Bechara *et al.*, 1994) and the Cambridge Gamble Task (Rogers *et al.*, 1999).

There are also batteries of tests such as the Behavioural Assessment of the Dysexecutive Syndrome (BADS: Wilson *et al.*, 1996) and the Delis–Kaplan Executive Function System (D-KEFS: Delis *et al.*, 2001), but since these take some time to administer they are best reserved for specific investigation of known frontal problems. The Frontal Lobe Personality Change Questionnaire (FLOPS) may be used to assess behavioural change and includes a carer version, useful for gaining collateral information.

Since most tests of executive function probe planning and strategy, mediated by dorsolateral prefrontal cortex, some patients with exclusive orbitofrontal damage, for example with frontal variant frontotemporal dementia, may complete these tests without conspicuous errors.

Of the 'bedside' neuropsychological test instruments (see Section 1.8), the Mini-Mental State Examination has been criticized for its lack of assessment of executive function, one shortcoming which the Addenbrooke's Cognitive Examination seeks to address by using letter and category verbal fluency tests. Moreover, a test subscore, the VLOM ratio, has been reported to distinguish frontotemporal dementia from Alzheimer's disease (Mathuranath *et al.*, 2000), although evidence to the contrary has been presented for some of these parameters (Bier *et al.*, 2004; Larner, 2005; Castiglioni *et al.*, 2006). Other batteries which tap executive function include the Frontal Assessment Battery (Dubois *et al.*, 2000; Slachevsky *et al.*, 2004), the Frontal Behavioural Inventory (Kertesz *et al.*, 2000), and the Middelheim Frontality Score (De Deyn *et al.*, 2005). Clock drawing may also discriminate FTD from AD, more errors being made in the latter (Blair *et al.*, 2006).

REFERENCES

Bechara A, Damasio AR, Damasio H, Anderson SW. Insensitivity to future consequences following damage to human prefrontal cortex. *Cognition* 1994; **50**: 7–15.

Bier JC, Ventura M, Donckels V, *et al.* Is the Addenbrooke's Cognitive Examination effective to detect frontotemporal dementia? *J Neurol* 2004; **251**: 428–31.

Blair M, Kertesz A, McMonagle P, Davidson W, Bodi N. Quantitative and qualitative analyses of clock drawing in frontotemporal dementia and Alzheimer's disease. *J Int Neuropsychol Soc* 2006; **12**: 159–65.

Burgess PW, Shallice T. Bizarre responses, rule detection and frontal lobe lesions. *Cortex* 1996; **32**: 241–59.

Burgess PW, Shallice T. *The Hayling and Brixton Tests*. Thurston: Thames Valley Test Company, 1997.

Castiglioni S, Pelati O, Zuffi M, *et al.* The Frontal Assessment Battery does not differentiate frontotemporal dementia from Alzheimer's disease. *Dement Geriatr Cogn Disord* 2006; **22**: 125–31.

Cerhan JH, Ivnik RJ, Smith GE, *et al.* Diagnostic utility of letter fluency, category fluency, and fluency difference scores in Alzheimer's disease. *Clin Neuropsychol* 2002; **16**: 35–42.

Chayer C, Freedman M. Frontal lobe functions. *Curr Neurol Neurosci Rep* 2001; **1**: 547–52.

Corcoran R, Upton D. A role for the hippocampus in card sorting? *Cortex* 1993; **29**: 293–304.

Critchley M. *The Divine Banquet of the Brain and Other Essays*. New York: Raven Press, 1979: 54.

Damasio H, Grabowski T, Frank R, Galaburda AM, Damasio AR. The return of Phineas Gage: clues about the brain from the skull of a famous patient. *Science* 1994; **264**: 1102–5.

De Deyn PP, Engelborghs S, Saerens J, *et al*. The Middelheim Frontality Score: a behavioural assessment scale that discriminates frontotemporal dementia from Alzheimer's disease. *Int J Geriatr Psychiatry* 2005; **20**: 70–9.

Delis D, Kaplan E, Kramer J. *Delis–Kaplan Executive Function System*. New York: Psychological Corporation, 2001.

Dubois B, Slachevsky A, Litvan I, Pillon B. The FAB: a Frontal Assessment Battery at bedside. *Neurology* 2000; **55**: 1621–6.

Duff Canning SJ, Leach L, Stuss D, Ngo L, Black SE. Diagnostic utility of abbreviated fluency measures in Alzheimer disease and vascular dementia. *Neurology* 2004; **62**: 556–62.

Filley CM. Clinical neurology and executive function. *Semin Speech Lang* 2000; **21**: 95–108.

Goldberg E, Bougakov D. Neuropsychologic assessment of frontal lobe dysfunction. *Psychiatr Clin North Am* 2005; **28**: 567–80.

Jones-Gotman M, Milner B. Design fluency: the invention of nonsense drawings after focal cortical lesions. *Neuropsychologia* 1977; **15**: 653–74.

Kertesz A, Nadkarni N, Davidson W, Thomas AW. The Frontal Behavioural Inventory in the differential diagnosis of frontotemporal dementia. *J Int Neuropsychol Soc* 2000; **6**: 460–8.

Larner AJ. An audit of the Addenbrooke's Cognitive Examination (ACE) in clinical practice. *Int J Geriatr Psychiatry* 2005; **20**: 593–4.

Larner AJ, Leach JP. Phineas Gage and the beginnings of neuropsychology. *Adv Clin Neurosci Rehabil* 2002; **2** (3): 26.

Lehto JE, Elorinne E. Gambling as an executive function task. *Appl Neuropsychol* 2003; **10**: 234–8.

Loring DW, Meador KJ. Case studies of focal prefrontal lesions in man. In: Risberg J, Grafman J (eds.), *The Frontal Lobes: Development, Function and Pathology*. Cambridge: Cambridge University Press, 2006: 163–77.

Macmillan M. *An Odd Kind of Fame: Stories of Phineas Gage*. Cambridge, MA: MIT Press, 2000.

Mathuranath P, George A, Cherian P, *et al*. Effects of age, education and gender on verbal fluency. *J Clin Exp Neuropsychol* 2003; **25**: 1057–64.

Miller BL, Cummings JL (eds.). *The Human Frontal Lobes: Functions and Disorders* (2nd edition). London: Guilford Press, 2007.

Nelson HE. A modified card sorting test sensitive to frontal lobe defects. *Cortex* 1976; **12**: 313–24.

Rogers RD, Everitt BD, Baldacchino A, *et al*. Dissociable deficits in the decision-making cognition of chronic amphetamine abusers, opiate abusers, patients with focal damage to prefrontal cortex, and tryptophan-depleted normal volunteers: evidence for monoaminergic mechanisms. *Neuropsychopharmacology* 1999; **20**: 322–39.

Shallice T. Specific impairments of planning. *Phil Trans R Soc Lond B Biol Sci* 1982; **298**: 199–209.

Shallice T, Evans ME. The involvement of the frontal lobes in cognitive estimation. *Cortex* 1978; **14**: 294–303.

Slachevsky A, Villalpando JM, Sarazin M, Hahn BV, Pillon B, Dubois B. Frontal assessment battery and differential diagnosis of frontotemporal dementia and Alzheimer disease. *Neurology* 2004; **61**: 1104–7

Strauss E, Sherman EMS, Spreen O. *A Compendium of Neuropsychological Tests: Administration, Norms, Commentary* (3rd edition). Oxford: Oxford University Press, 2006: 401–545.

Stroop J. Studies of interference in serial verbal reaction. *J Exp Psychol* 1935; **18**: 643–62.

Trimble MR. *Biological Psychiatry* (2nd edition). Chichester: Wiley, 1996: 147–56.

Warrington EK. Homophone meaning generation: a new test of verbal switching for the detection of frontal lobe dysfunction. *J Int Neuropsychol Soc* 2000; **6**: 643–8.

Weigl E. On the psychology of so-called processes of abstraction. *J Norm Soc Psychol* 1941; **36**: 3–33.

Wilson BA, Alderman N, Burgess PW, Emslie H, Evans JJ. *Behavioural Assessment of the Dysexecutive Syndrome*. Bury St Edmunds: Thames Valley Test Company, 1996.

1.8 'Bedside' neuropsychological test instruments

How should the practising clinician, perhaps untrained in the nuances of neuropsychology, and pressed for time, assess cognitive function at the bedside when the complaint of the patient and/or relatives suggests the possibility of cognitive disorder? Primary care practitioners may use simple clinical observations to give pointers to, or raise suspicion of, a diagnosis of dementia: patient age and suggestive collateral history are probably the most important factors (Fisher & Larner, 2006). Practitioners in secondary care settings will, in addition, use brief 'bedside' tests in the initial assessment of patients with cognitive complaints. ('Bedside' is a misnomer, since the bedside may be a far from ideal location in which to administer such tests, surrounded by the noise of a ward, spectators, and the imminent possibility of interruption.) There are many such instruments (Burns et al., 1999, 2006), some of the most widely used of which are briefly discussed here. These may be broadly categorized as 'simple' or 'complex'; or as 'mini', implying a performance time of 10 minutes or under, or 'midi', taking perhaps 15–30 minutes to perform. Batteries requiring 45–60 minutes or more are not discussed, as their use will in all likelihood be reserved to specialist clinics wherein the time factor is less of an issue. These tests have focused largely on identifying Alzheimer's disease (AD), since this is the commonest cause of dementia, and hence are weighted towards detecting memory deficits. Hence these instruments may be suboptimal for detecting disorders with prominent non-memory cognitive and/or behavioural symptoms.

Methodological standards to evaluate screening and diagnostic tests for dementia have been outlined, specifically their reliability and validity (Gifford & Cummings, 1999), and the principles of evidence-based diagnosis are well established (Qizilbash, 2002). Test sensitivity and specificity not less than 0.8 and positive predictive value approaching 0.9, the recommended criteria for molecular biomarkers for AD (Ronald and Nancy Reagan Research Institute of the Alzheimer's Association and the National Institute on Aging, 1998), would seem to be desirable attributes of bedside tests for dementia. Likelihood ratios, the ratio of pre-test to post-test odds and hence a measure of 'diagnostic gain', should desirably have values > 10 or < 0.1, meaning the test has a large diagnostic gain

(Deeks & Altman, 2004). Construction of a receiver operating characteristic (ROC) curve (Hanley & McNeil, 1982, 1983) is also desirable, with area under the curve (AUC), a measure of diagnostic accuracy, > 0.80, where $AUC = 0.5$ indicates a test providing no added information and $AUC = 1$ indicates a test providing perfect discrimination. Diagnostic odds ratio, a summary measure of test diagnostic performance, should be high. Such data are not available for all bedside tests.

Many bedside tests are available, all of which have their adherents. In primary care, where time is of the essence, guidelines have been published which recommend the use of formal cognitive testing as well as clinical judgment (Eccles et al., 1998). Very brief screens such as the Abbreviated Mental Test Score (AMTS: Hodkinson, 1972), the 6 Item Cognitive Impairment Test (6CIT, also sometimes known as the Kingshill Test: Brooke & Bullock, 1999), GPCOG (Brodaty et al., 2002), Memory Alteration Test (Rami et al., 2007), or some form of clock drawing task might be used. However, a recent survey suggested that cognitive test instruments were seldom used by general practitioners (c. 20%) prior to referral of patients to a dedicated cognitive function clinic, and that the Mini-Mental State Examination (MMSE; see below) was the instrument most commonly used (Fisher & Larner, 2007). However, in the primary care setting, Wind et al. (1997) found the MMSE to be of limited value in diagnosing dementia (sensitivity 0.65, specificity 0.93).

Both AMTS and 6CIT are derived from the Blessed Information Memory Concentration Test (BIMC: Blessed et al., 1968), one of a large number of tests available for clinical use. These include:

- Cognitive Capacity Screening Examination (CCSE: Jacobs et al., 1977)
- Telephone Interview for Cognitive Status (TICS: Brandt et al., 1988)
- Short Test of Mental Status (Kokmen et al., 1991)
- Structured Interview for the diagnosis of Dementia of the Alzheimer type, Multi-infarct dementia and dementias of other aetiology (SIDAM: Zaudig et al., 1991)

- Cognitive Abilities Screening Instrument (CASI: Teng *et al.*, 1994)
- Hasegawa Dementia Scale–Revised (HDS-R: Imai & Hasegawa, 1994; Kim *et al.*, 2005)
- Cambridge Cognitive Examination (CAMCOG: Huppert *et al.*, 1995)
- 7-minute screen (Solomon *et al.*, 1998)
- Memory Impairment Screen (Buschke *et al.*, 1999)
- Mini-Cog (Borson *et al.*, 2000)
- Visual Association Test (Lindeboom *et al.*, 2002)
- Kingston Standardized Cognitive Assessment (Hopkins *et al.*, 2004)
- TE4D-Cog (Mahoney *et al.*, 2005).

For dementia that has already progressed to a severe stage, the following instruments are available:

- Severe Impairment Battery (SIB: Saxton & Swihart, 1989)
- Middlesex Elderly Assessment of Mental State (MEAMS: Golding, 1989)
- Severe MMSE (Harrell *et al.*, 2000)
- mini-SIB (Qazi *et al.*, 2005).

Computerized test batteries are also available, such as the Cambridge Neuropsychological Test Automated Battery, from which the Paired Associates Learning test (CANTAB-PAL) may be useful for the early detection and diagnosis of dementia (Swainson *et al.*, 2001).

Tests measuring global function, behaviour, and activities of daily living (ADL) may also be undertaken in the assessment of patients with cognitive disorders (Burns *et al.*, 1999, 2006; McKeith, 1999). Popular global measures, not further discussed here, include the Functional Assessment Staging (FAST: Reisberg, 1988) and the Clinicians Interview-Based Impression of Change (CIBIC, or CIBIC+ if caregiver input is included). The Neuropsychiatric Inventory (NPI) is perhaps the most widely used measure of behaviour in dementia (Cummings *et al.*, 1994). Popular ADL scales include the Alzheimer's Disease Cooperative Study Activities of Daily Living Scale (ADCS-ADL), the Instrumental Activities of Daily Living (IADL) Scale (Lawton & Brody, 1969), the Functional Activities Questionnaire (FAQ: Pfeffer *et al.*, 1982), the Bristol Activities of Daily Living Scale (Bucks *et al.*, 1996), and the

Activities of Daily Living Questionnaire (Johnson *et al.*, 2004). Inclusion of global, behavioural, and ADL scales is now mandatory in clinical drug trials in dementia, whilst pharmacoeconomic assessments and quality of life scales are also thought desirable.

Informant questionnaires may also be used to gather collateral information not available from patient history (lone patient attendance in the clinic despite a request to bring a relative, carer, or friend is a strong indicator of the absence of dementia: Larner, 2004, 2005), particularly examining change from a premorbid level of functioning (Jorm, 1997). The Informant Questionnaire on Cognitive Decline in the Elderly (IQCODE: Jorm & Jacomb, 1989) is one such instrument, which has also been reported useful in the diagnosis of MCI (Isella *et al.*, 2006).

REFERENCES

Blessed G, Tomlinson BE, Roth M. The association between quantitative measures of dementia and of senile change in the cerebral grey matter of elderly subjects. *Br J Psychiatry* 1968; **114**: 797–811.

Borson S, Scanlan JM, Chen P, Ganguli M. The Mini-Cog: a cognitive 'vital signs' measure for dementia screening in multi-lingual elderly. *Int J Geriatr Psychiatry* 2000; **15**: 1021–7.

Brandt J, Spencer M, Folstein M. The Telephone Interview for Cognitive Status. *Neuropsychiatry Neuropsychol Behav Neurol* 1988; **1**: 111–17.

Brodaty H, Pond D, Kemp NM, *et al*. The GPCOG: a new screening test for dementia designed for general practice. *J Am Geriatr Soc* 2002; **50**: 530–4.

Brooke P, Bullock R. Validation of a 6 item Cognitive Impairment Test with a view to primary care usage. *Int J Geriatr Psychiatry* 1999; **14**: 936–40.

Bucks RS, Ashworth DL, Wilcock GK, Siegfried K. Assessment of activities of daily living in dementia: development of the Bristol Activities of Daily Living Scale. *Age Ageing* 1996; **25**: 113–20.

Burns A, Lawlor B, Craig S. *Assessment Scales in Old Age Psychiatry*. London: Martin Dunitz, 1999.

Burns A, Lawlor B, Craig S. *Assessment Scales in Old Age Psychiatry* (2nd edition). London: Martin Dunitz, 2006.

Buschke H, Kuslansky G, Katz M, *et al.* Screening for dementia with the Memory Impairment Screen. *Neurology* 1999; **52**: 231–8.

Cummings JL, Mega MS, Gray K, *et al.* The Neuropsychiatric Inventory: comprehensive assessment of psychopathology in dementia. *Neurology* 1994; **44**: 2308–14.

Deeks JJ, Altman DG. Diagnostic tests 4: likelihood ratios. *BMJ* 2004; **329**: 168–9.

Eccles M, Clarke J, Livingston M, Freemantle N, Mason J. North of England evidence based guidelines development project: guideline for the primary care management of dementia. *BMJ* 1998; **317**: 802–8.

Fisher CAH, Larner AJ. FAQs: memory loss. *Practitioner* 2006; **250** (1683): 14–16, 19, 21.

Fisher CAH, Larner AJ. Frequency and diagnostic utility of cognitive test instrument use by GPs prior to memory clinic referral. *Fam Pract* 2007; **24**: 495–7.

Gifford DR, Cummings JL. Evaluating dementia screening tests: methodologic standards to rate their performance. *Neurology* 1999; **52**: 224–7.

Golding E. *The Middlesex Elderly Assessment of Mental State.* Bury St Edmunds, Thames Valley Test Company, 1989.

Hanley JA, McNeil BJ. The meaning and use of the area under a receiver operating characteristic (ROC) curve. *Radiology* 1982; **143**: 29–36.

Hanley JA, McNeil BJ. A method of comparing the areas under a receiver operating characteristic curves derived from the same cases. *Radiology* 1983; **148**: 839–43.

Harrell LE, Marson D, Chatterjee A, Parrish JA. The Severe Mini-Mental State Examination: a new neuropsychological instrument for the bedside assessment of severely impaired patients with Alzheimer's disease. *Alzheimer Dis Assoc Disord* 2000; **14**: 168–75.

Hodkinson HM. Evaluation of a mental test score for assessment of mental impairment in the elderly. *Age Ageing* 1972; **1**: 233–8.

Hopkins R, Kilik L, Day D, Rows C, Hamilton P. The Revised Kingston Standardized Cognitive Assessment. *Int J Geriatr Psychiatry* 2004; **19**: 320–6.

Huppert FA, Brayne CA, Gill C, *et al.* CAMCOG: a concise neuropsychological test to assist dementia diagnosis. Sociodemographic determinants in an elderly population sample. *Br J Clin Psychol* 1995; **34**: 529–41.

Imai Y, Hasegawa K. The revised Hasegawa Dementia Scale (HDS-R): evaluation of its usefulness as a screening test for dementia. *J Hong Kong Coll Psychiatr* 1994; **4** (2): 20–4.

Isella V, Villa L, Russo A, *et al.* Discriminative and predictive power of an informant report in mild cognitive impairment. *J Neurol Neurosurg Psychiatry* 2006; **77**: 166–71.

Jacobs JW, Bernhard MR, Delgado A, Strain JJ. Screening for organic mental symptoms in the medically ill. *Ann Intern Med* 1977; **86**: 40–6.

Johnson N, Barion A, Rademaker A, Rehkemper G, Weintraub S. The Activities of Daily Living Questionnaire: a validation study in patients with dementia. *Alzheimer Dis Assoc Disord* 2004; **18**: 223–30.

Jorm AF. Methods of screening for dementia: a meta-analysis of studies comparing an informant questionnaire with a brief cognitive test. *Alzheimer Dis Assoc Disord* 1997; **11**: 158–62.

Jorm AF, Jacomb PA. The Informant Questionnaire on Cognitive Decline in the Elderly (IQCODE): sociodemographic correlates, reliability, validity and some norms. *Psychol Med* 1989; **19**: 1015–22.

Kim KW, Lee DY, Jhoo JH, *et al.* Diagnostic accuracy of mini-mental status examination and revised Hasegawa dementia scale for Alzheimer's disease. *Dement Geriatr Cogn Disord* 2005; **19**: 324–30.

Kokmen E, Smith GE, Petersen RC, Tangalos E, Ivnik RC. The Short Test of Mental Status: correlations with standardized psychometric testing. *Arch Neurol* 1991; **48**: 725–8.

Larner AJ. Getting it wrong: the clinical misdiagnosis of Alzheimer's disease. *Int J Clin Pract* 2004; **58**: 1092–4.

Larner AJ. 'Who came with you?' A diagnostic observation in patients with memory problems? *J Neurol Neurosurg Psychiatry* 2005; **76**: 1739.

Lawton MP, Brody EM. Assessment of older people: self-maintaining and instrumental activities of daily living. *Gerontologist* 1969; **9**: 176–85.

Lindeboom J, Schmand B, Tulner L, Walstra G, Jonker C. Visual association test to detect early dementia of the Alzheimer type. *J Neurol Neurosurg Psychiatry* 2002; **73**: 126–33.

McKeith IG (ed.). *Outcome Measures in Alzheimer's Disease.* London: Martin Dunitz, 1999.

Mahoney R, Johnston K, Katona C, Maxmin K, Livingston G. The TE4D-Cog: a new test for detecting early dementia in English-speaking populations. *Int J Geriatr Psychiatry* 2005; **20**: 1172–9.

Pfeffer RI, Kurosaki TT, Harrah CH, Chance JM, Filos S. Measurement of functional activities in older adults in the community. *J Gerontol* 1982; **37**: 323–9.

Qazi A, Richardson B, Simmons P, *et al.* The Mini-SIB: a short scale for measuring cognitive function in severe dementia. *Int J Geriatr Psychiatry* 2005; **20**: 1001–2.

Qizilbash N. Evidence-based diagnosis. In: Qizilbash N, Schneider LS, Chui H, *et al.* (eds.), *Evidence-Based Dementia Practice*. Oxford: Blackwell, 2002: 18–25.

Rami L, Molinuevo JL, Sanchez-Valle R, Bosch B, Villar A. Screening for amnestic mild cognitive impairment and early Alzheimer's disease with M@T (Memory Alteration Test) in the primary care population. *Int J Geriatr Psychiatry* 2007; **22**: 294–304.

Reisberg B. Functional assessment staging (FAST). *Psychopharmacol Bull* 1988; **24**: 653–9.

Ronald and Nancy Reagan Research Institute of the Alzheimer's Association and the National Institute on Aging. Consensus report of the Working Group on molecular and biochemical markers of Alzheimer's disease. *Neurobiol Aging* 1998; **19**: 109–16.

Saxton J, Swihart AA. Neuropsychological assessment of the severely impaired elderly patient. *Clin Geriatr Med* 1989; **5**: 531–43.

Solomon PR, Hirschoff A, Kelly B, *et al.* A 7-minute neurocognitive screening battery highly sensitive to Alzheimer's disease. *Arch Neurol* 1998; **55**: 349–55.

Swainson R, Hodges JR, Galton CJ, *et al.* Early detection and differential diagnosis of Alzheimer's disease and depression with neuropsychological tests. *Dement Geriatr Cogn Disord* 2001; **12**: 265–80.

Teng EL, Hasegawa K, Homma, A, *et al.* The Cognitive Abilities Screening Instrument (CASI): a practical test for cross-cultural epidemiological studies of dementia. *Int Psychogeriatr* 1994; **6**: 45–58.

Wind AW, Schellevis FG, Van Staveren G, *et al.* Limitations of the Mini-Mental State Examination in diagnosing dementia in general practice. *Int J Geriatr Psychiatry* 1997; **12**: 101–8.

Zaudig M, Mittelhammer J, Hiller W, *et al.* SIDAM: a structured interview for the diagnosis of dementia of the Alzheimer type, multi-infarct dementia and dementias of other aetiology according to ICD-10 and DSM-III-R. *Psychol Med* 1991; **21**: 225–36.

1.8.1   Mini-Mental State Examination (MMSE)

The Mini-Mental State Examination (MMSE) was originally designed to differentiate organic from functional disorders in psychiatric practice, and as a quantitative measure of cognitive impairment useful in monitoring change, but not primarily as a diagnostic tool (Folstein *et al.*, 1975). However, it has proved acceptable and useful in the assessment of cognitive status in general medical and neurological patients (Dick *et al.*, 1984; Tangalos *et al.*, 1996) and has become the most widely used brief cognitive assessment. (Surely no other medical investigation can claim to have been memorialized, at least in part, in a sonnet – by Rafael Campo: see Levin, 2001). The MMSE has good intra- and inter-rater reliability and internal consistency, although there has been debate about appropriate cutoff scores (Tombaugh & McIntyre, 1992). There are two demonstrable normative influences on MMSE scores, namely patient age and years of education, norms for which may be factored into the cutoffs (Crum *et al.*, 1993). MMSE may be useful in tracking cognitive decline in AD (Han *et al.*, 2000), falling on average 3 points per year, although there is variability, some patients remaining stable and some even improving (Holmes & Lovestone, 2003), meaning that this may be a less than ideal instrument on which to base therapeutic decisions, for example on the efficacy of cholinesterase inhibitors (even aside from the patient anxiety which foreknowledge of those judgments may engender, the 'Godot syndrome', which itself may influence test performance: Larner & Doran, 2002). It has also sometimes been objected that the MMSE takes too long to administer (c. 10 minutes: Tangalos *et al.*, 1996). Both expanded (Standardized MMSE, SMMSE: Molloy *et al.*, 1991; Modified MMSE, 3MS: Teng & Chui, 1987) and shortened (Galasko *et al.*, 1990) versions have been developed, as well as a version for severe disease (Harrell *et al.*, 2000).

One of the difficulties with the MMSE is determining where the cutoff(s) should be. For a cutoff < 24, Kukull *et al.* (1994) found a sensitivity of 0.63 and a specificity of 0.96 for the diagnosis of AD in a cohort of 133 patients (80 dementia, 53 no dementia); sensitivity increased at higher cutoff scores, unsurprisingly, leading to a recommendation that MMSE score of 26 or 27 should be used in symptomatic populations if the aim is to miss few true cases. Tangalos *et al.* (1996) found a sensitivity and specificity of 0.69 and 0.99 for a cutoff of 23 or less; use of age- and education-specific cutoff scores improved the sensitivity to 0.82 with no loss of specificity. In the author's clinic, in 154 consecutive patients, of whom 51% had a dementia syndrome, sensitivity and specificity for MMSE cutoff scores of 27 and 24 for a diagnosis of dementia were 0.91 and 0.70, and 0.73 and 0.86, respectively, giving positive and negative likelihood ratios (with 95% confidence intervals, log method) of 3.04 (2.14–4.31) and 0.13 (0.09–0.18), and 5.09 (2.90–8.95) and 0.32 (0.18–0.56), respectively, hence moderate values for MMSE > 27 excluding dementia and MMSE < 24 diagnosing dementia (Larner, 2005). Diagnostic odds ratio, a summary measure of test diagnostic performance, for MMSE cutoff of 27 was 23.5.

A subscore from the MMSE has been suggested to be helpful in the differential diagnosis of dementia, specifically of AD from dementia with Lewy bodies (DLB), based on the greater impairment of attentional and visuospatial function and the relative preservation of memory in DLB as compared to AD, calculated using the equation [attention − $5/3 \cdot$ memory $+ 5 \cdot$ construction]. A subscore of < 5 was reported in a small retrospective series of pathologically confirmed cases of AD and DLB to have sensitivity of 0.82 and specificity of 0.81 for DLB (Ala *et al.*, 2002), hence positive likelihood ratio (LR+) = 4.45 (small) and negative likelihood ratio (LR−) = 0.22 (small). This subscore has not been found helpful for differential diagnosis in a prospective study of a large ($n = 285$) clinically diagnosed cohort (Larner, 2003, 2004).

REFERENCES

Ala T, Hughes LF, Kyrouac GA, Ghobrial MW, Elble RJ. The Mini-Mental State exam may help in the differentiation of dementia with Lewy bodies and Alzheimer's disease. *Int J Geriatr Psychiatry* 2002; **17**: 503–9.

Crum RM, Anthony JC, Bassett SS, Folstein MF. Population-based norms for the Mini-Mental State Examination by age and educational level. *JAMA* 1993; **269**: 2386–91.

Dick JPR, Guiloff RJ, Stewart A, *et al.* Mini-mental state examination in neurological patients. *J Neurol Neurosurg Psychiatry* 1984; **47**: 496–9.

Folstein MF, Folstein SE, McHugh PR. 'Mini-Mental State': a practical method for grading the cognitive state of patients for the clinician. *J Psychiatr Res* 1975; **12**: 189–98.

Galasko D, Klauber MR, Hofstetter CR, *et al.* The Mini-Mental State Examination in the early diagnosis of Alzheimer's disease. *Arch Neurol* 1990; **47**: 49–52.

Han L, Cole M, Bellevance F, McCusker J, Primeau F. Tracking cognitive decline in Alzheimer's disease using the Mini-Mental State Examination: a meta-analysis. *Int Psychogeriatr* 2000; **12**: 231–47.

Harrell LE, Marson D, Chatterjee A, Parrish JA. The Severe Mini-Mental State Examination: a new neuropsychological instrument for the bedside assessment of severely impaired patients with Alzheimer's disease. *Alzheimer Dis Assoc Disord* 2000; **14**: 168–75.

Holmes C, Lovestone S. Long-term cognitive and functional decline in late onset Alzheimer's disease: therapeutic implications. *Age Ageing* 2003; **32**: 200–4.

Kukull WA, Larson EB, Teri L, *et al.* The Mini-Mental State Examination score and the clinical diagnosis of dementia. *J Clin Epidemiol* 1994; **47**: 1061–7.

Larner AJ. MMSE subscores and the diagnosis of dementia with Lewy bodies. *Int J Geriatr Psychiatry* 2003; **18**: 855–6.

Larner AJ. Use of MMSE to differentiate Alzheimer's disease from dementia with Lewy bodies. *Int J Geriatr Psychiatry* 2004; **19**: 1209–10.

Larner AJ. An audit of the Addenbrooke's Cognitive Examination (ACE) in clinical practice. *Int J Geriatr Psychiatry* 2005; **20**: 593–4.

Larner AJ, Doran M. Broader assessment needed for treatment decisions in AD. *Prog Neurol Psych* 2002; **6** (3): 5–6.

Levin P (ed.). *The Penguin Book of the Sonnet: 500 years of a classic tradition in English.* London: Penguin, 2001: 334.

Molloy DW, Alemayehu E, Roberts R. Reliability of a Standardized Mini-Mental State Examination compared with the traditional Mini-Mental State Examination. *Am J Psych* 1991; **148**: 102–5.

Tangalos EG, Smith GE, Ivnik RJ, *et al.* The Mini-Mental State Examination in general medical practice: clinical utility and acceptance. *Mayo Clin Proc* 1996; **71**: 829–37.

Teng EL, Chui HC. The modified Mini-Mental State (3MS) Examination. *J Clin Psychiatry* 1987; **48**: 314–18.

Tombaugh TN, McIntyre NJ. The Mini-Mental State Examination: a comprehensive review. *J Am Geriatr Soc* 1992; **40**: 922–35.

1.8.2   Clock drawing

Clock drawing has a long history as a test for cognitive impairment and remains popular (Freedman *et al.*, 1994; Shulman & Feinstein, 2003). It has the advantage of being quick and simple, and tests a wide range of cognitive domains (a 'diffuse' screening test) including auditory comprehension, memory, executive control (planning), and visuospatial abilities, as well as motor skills. However, this very breadth poses problems when interpreting and scoring clock drawing, to encompass both quantitative and qualitative features. Nonetheless, most scoring systems are reported to achieve a sensitivity and specificity of around 0.85. Clock drawing has been incorporated in other screening and diagnostic tests such as the CERAD (Morris *et al.*, 1989), CAMCOG (Huppert *et al.*, 1995), Mini-Cog (Borson *et al.*, 2000), and the ACE (Mathuranath *et al.*, 2000) and ACE-R (Mioshi *et al.*, 2006). It may address a deficiency in many other brief cognitive tests through its probing of executive function (Royall *et al.*, 1998), but it may have limitations in detecting mild dementia or MCI.

A Backward Clock Test, using the mirror image of a normal analogue clock, in which patients are required to read strings of times shown either backward (= backward clock, or normal analogue clock viewed, Alice *Through the Looking Glass* style, in a mirror) or forward (= normal analogue clock, or backward clock viewed in a mirror), may likewise be useful as a 'diffuse' test, differentiating patients with focal cognitive deficits from those with global impairments (i.e. dementia: Larner, 2007).

REFERENCES

Borson S, Scanlan JM, Chen P, Ganguli M. The Mini-Cog: a cognitive 'vital signs' measure for dementia screening in multi-lingual elderly. *Int J Geriatr Psychiatry* 2000; **15**: 1021–7.

Freedman M, Leach L, Kaplan E, *et al. Clock Drawing: a Neuropsychological Analysis*. New York: Oxford University Press, 1994.

Huppert FA, Brayne CA, Gill C, *et al*. CAMCOG: a concise neuropsychological test to assist dementia diagnosis. Sociodemographic determinants in an elderly population sample. *Br J Clin Psychol* 1995; **34**: 529–41.

Larner AJ. Of clocks and mirrors: the Backward Clock Test. *Eur J Neurol* 2007; **14** (suppl 1): 100 (abstract P1265).

Mathuranath PS, Nestor PJ, Berrios GE, Rakowicz W, Hodges JR. A brief cognitive test battery to differentiate Alzheimer's disease and frontotemporal dementia. *Neurology* 2000; **55**: 1613–20.

Mioshi E, Dawson K, Mitchell J, Arnold R, Hodges JR. The Addenbrooke's Cognitive Examination Revised (ACE-R): a brief cognitive test battery for dementia screening. *Int J Geriatr Psychiatry* 2006; **21**: 1078–85.

Morris J, Heyman A, Mohs R, *et al*. The Consortium to Establish a Registry for Alzheimer's Disease (CERAD). Part I. Clinical and neuropsychological assessment of Alzheimer's disease. *Neurology* 1989; **39**: 1159–65.

Royall DR, Cordes JA, Polk M. CLOX: an executive clock drawing task. *J Neurol Neurosurg Psychiatry* 1998; **64**: 588–94.

Shulman K, Feinstein A. *Quick Cognitive Screening for Clinicians: Mini Mental, Clock Drawing and Other Brief Tests*. London: Martin Dunitz, 2003: 43–78.

1.8.3   Queen Square Screening Test for Cognitive Deficits

For generations of neurological trainees at the National Hospital for Neurology and Neurosurgery in London, the Queen Square Screening Test for Cognitive Deficits (QSSTCD), often known as the 'green book', has been the standard bedside neuropsychology test instrument (Warrington, 1989). Although entirely qualitative, it is useful in giving pointers to the localization of any cognitive deficits.

REFERENCES

Warrington EK. *The Queen Square Screening Test for Cognitive Deficits*. London: Institute of Neurology, 1989.

1.8.4   Addenbrooke's Cognitive Examination (ACE) and Addenbrooke's Cognitive Examination–Revised (ACE-R)

This theoretically motivated development of the MMSE incorporates more material to address the acknowledged shortcomings of the MMSE, particularly with respect to testing of memory, visuospatial function, and executive function (Mathuranath *et al.*, 2000; Nestor & Hodges, 2001). The ACE has been widely adopted and translated into various languages (Mathuranath *et al.*, 2004; Bier *et al.*, 2005; Larner, 2005, 2006, 2007a; Garcia-Caballero *et al.*, 2006). The ACE is also reported to be useful in detecting the cognitive features of atypical parkinsonian syndromes (Bak *et al.*, 2005a,b) and in differentiating dementia from affective disorder (Dudas *et al.*, 2005).

For an ACE cutoff score of 88 the index paper reported sensitivity of 0.93 and specificity of 0.71, while for a cutoff score of 83 sensitivity was 0.82 and specificity 0.96, in a cohort of 139 patients (Mathuranath *et al.*, 2000). The study by Bier *et al.* (2004) ($n = 79$) also found high sensitivities (1.0 and 0.9 for cutoffs of 88 and 83, respectively) but lower specificities (0.46 and 0.64). In the author's clinic, in 154 consecutive patients, of whom 51% had a dementia syndrome, sensitivity and specificity for an ACE cutoff score of 88 were 0.97 and 0.47, with 0.92 and 0.62 for a cutoff score of 83, giving positive and negative likelihood ratios (with 95% confidence intervals, log method) of 1.83 (1.48–2.26) and 0.06 (0.05–0.07), and 2.45 (1.82–3.29) and 0.13 (0.10–0.17), respectively, hence large values for ACE > 88 excluding dementia (Larner, 2005). Diagnostic odds ratio for ACE cutoff of 88 was 32.9.

As well as proving useful for the early diagnosis of dementia, a subscore derived from the ACE, the VLOM ratio, may be calculated from the scores of the subtests [verbal fluency + language] / [orientation + delayed recall], to differentiate AD (VLOM ratio > 3.2) from FTD (VLOM ratio < 2.2). In the index paper (Mathuranath *et al.*, 2000), VLOM ratio > 3.2 showed sensitivity of 0.75 and specificity of 0.84 for the diagnosis of AD. Figures for the diagnostic utility of VLOM ratio > 3.2 for the diagnosis of AD were confirmed in independent cohorts but these studies also found low sensitivity of VLOM < 2.2 for the diagnosis of FTD (Bier *et al.*, 2004; Larner, 2005, 2007a).

Recently, a revised version of the ACE, ACE-R, has been published (Mioshi *et al.*, 2006), with excellent sensitivity and specificity in a selected university hospital clinic population. These results were largely replicated in a pragmatic study in an unselected clinic population (AUC = 0.95; 95% CI 0.90–0.99), but with the suggestion that a lower cutoff may be required, since day-to-day clinical practice permits no exclusion criteria and has no population preselected as 'normal' (Larner, 2007b).

REFERENCES

Bak TH, Crawford LM, Hearn VC, Mathuranath PS, Hodges JR. Subcortical dementia revisited: similarities and differences in cognitive function between progressive supranuclear palsy (PSP), corticobasal degeneration (CBD) and multiple system atrophy (MSA). *Neurocase* 2005b; **11**: 268–73.

Bak TH, Rogers TT, Crawford LM, *et al.* Cognitive bedside assessment in atypical parkinsonian syndromes. *J Neurol Neurosurg Psychiatry* 2005a; **76**: 420–2.

Bier JC, Ventura M, Donckels V, *et al.* Is the Addenbrooke's Cognitive Examination effective to detect frontotemporal dementia? *J Neurol* 2004; **251**: 428–31.

Bier JC, Donckels V, Van Eyll E, *et al.* The French Addenbrooke's Cognitive Examination is effective in detecting dementia in a French-speaking population. *Dement Geriatr Cogn Disord* 2005; **19**: 15–17.

Dudas RB, Berrios GE, Hodges JR. The Addenbrooke's Cognitive Examination (ACE) in the differential diagnosis of early dementias versus affective disorder. *Am J Geriatr Psychiatry* 2005; **13**: 218–26.

Garcia-Caballero A, Garcia-Lado I, Gonzalez-Hermida J, *et al.* Validation of the Spanish version of the Addenbrooke's Cognitive Examination in a rural community in Spain. *Int J Geriatr Psychiatry* 2006; **21**: 239–45.

Larner AJ. An audit of the Addenbrooke's Cognitive Examination (ACE) in clinical practice. *Int J Geriatr Psychiatry* 2005; **20**: 593–4.

Larner AJ. An audit of the Addenbrooke's Cognitive Examination (ACE) in clinical practice. 2. Longitudinal change. *Int J Geriatr Psychiatry* 2006; **21**: 698–9.

Larner AJ. Addenbrooke's Cognitive Examination (ACE) for the diagnosis and differential diagnosis of dementia. *Clin Neurol Neurosurg* 2007a; **109**: 491–4.

Larner AJ. Addenbrooke's Cognitive Examination-Revised (ACE-R) in day-to-day clinical practice. *Age Ageing* 2007b; **36**: 685–6.

Mathuranath PS, Nestor PJ, Berrios GE, Rakowicz W, Hodges JR. A brief cognitive test battery to differentiate Alzheimer's disease and frontotemporal dementia. *Neurology* 2000; **55**: 1613–20.

Mathuranath PS, Hodges JR, Mathew R, *et al.* Adaptation of the ACE for a Malayalam speaking population in southern India. *Int J Geriatr Psychiatry* 2004; **19**: 1188–94.

Mioshi E, Dawson K, Mitchell J, Arnold R, Hodges JR. The Addenbrooke's Cognitive Examination Revised (ACE-R): a brief cognitive test battery for dementia screening. *Int J Geriatr Psychiatry* 2006; **21**: 1078–85.

Nestor P, Hodges JR. The clinical approach to assessing patients with early onset dementia. In: Hodges JR (ed.), *Early-Onset Dementia: a Multidisciplinary Approach.* Oxford: Oxford University Press, 2001: 23–46.

1.8.5   DemTect

DemTect is a brief screening test for dementia comprising five subtests: repetition of 10-word list, number transcoding, semantic word fluency task, backward digit span, and delayed recall of the initial 10-word list. Raw scores are transformed to give a final score, maximum 18, which is independent of age and educational level, with classification as 'suspected dementia' (score ≤ 8), 'mild cognitive impairment' (9–12), and 'appropriate for age' (13–18) (Kalbe *et al.*, 2004). In the index study the sensitivity and specificity for AD were reported to be 100% and 92% respectively, and in a validation study ($n = 38$) with ^{18}FDG-PET imaging area under the ROC curve (AUC) was 0.85 (95% CI 0.73–0.97: Scheurich *et al.*, 2005). In the author's clinic, a study of 111 consecutive referrals, of whom 52% had a dementia syndrome, found sensitivity and specificity for dementia of 85% and 72% respectively, with AUC of 0.87 (95% CI 0.80–0.93: Larner 2006, 2007). Use of DemTect has also been reported in CADASIL, a subcortical dementia (Hennerici *et al.*, 2006).

REFERENCES

Hennerici MG, Daffertshofer M, Caplan LR, Szabo K. *Case Studies in Stroke: Common and Uncommon Presentations.* Cambridge: Cambridge University Press, 2006: 137 [Case 31].

Kalbe E, Kessler J, Calabrese P, *et al.* DemTect: a new, sensitive cognitive screening test to support the diagnosis of mild cognitive impairment and early dementia. *Int J Geriatr Psychiatry* 2004; **19**: 136–43.

Larner AJ. DemTect in the diagnosis of dementia: first 100 patients. *Alzheimers Dement* 2006; **2** (suppl 1): S375 (abstract P3–012).

Larner AJ. DemTect: 1-year experience of a neuropsychological screening test for dementia. *Age Ageing* 2007; **36**: 326–7.

Scheurich A, Muller MJ, Slessmeier T, *et al.* Validating the DemTect with 18-fluoro-2-deoxy-glucose positron emission tomography as a sensitive neuropsychological scree-ning test for early Alzheimer disease in patients of a memory clinic. *Dement Geriatr Cogn Disord* 2005; **20**: 271–7.

1.8.6   Dementia Rating Scale (DRS)

The Mattis Dementia Rating Scale (DRS: Mattis, 1976, 1992), and its successor DRS-2, comprise a number of subtests (attention, initiation, construction, conceptualization, memory) to give a global measure of dementia (score 0–144) and take about 30 minutes to perform. Normative data are available (Lucas *et al.*, 1998). DRS is useful in detecting cognitive impairment and is sensitive to the early stages of dementia. The assessment of a range of cognitive abilities suggests that the DRS may be useful in longitudinal tracking of cognitive change. Moreover, DRS was designed to assist in the differential diagnosis of dementia syndromes (e.g. Rosser & Hodges, 1994; Donnelly & Grohman, 1999; Lukatela *et al.*, 2000). It is reported to be able to distinguish subcortical diseases from AD (Bak *et al.*, 2005).

REFERENCES

Bak TH, Crawford LM, Hearn VC, Mathuranath PS, Hodges JR. Subcortical dementia revisited: similarities and differences in cognitive function between progressive supranuclear palsy (PSP), corticobasal degeneration (CBD) and multiple system atrophy (MSA). *Neurocase* 2005; **11**: 268–73.

Donnelly K, Grohman K. Can the Mattis Dementia Rating Scale differentiate Alzheimer's disease, vascular dementia, and depression in the elderly? *Brain Cogn* 1999; **39**: 60–3.

Lucas JA, Ivnik RJ, Smith GE, *et al.* Normative data for the Mattis Dementia Rating Scale. *J Clin Exp Neuropsychol* 1998; **20**: 536–47.

Lukatela K, Cohen RA, Kessler H, *et al.* Dementia Rating Scale performance: a comparison of vascular and Alzheimer's dementia. *J Clin Exp Neuropsychol* 2000; **22**: 445–54.

Mattis S. Mental status examination for organic mental syndrome in the elderly. In: Bellack R, Karasu B (eds.), *Geriatric Psychiatry.* New York: Grune & Stratton, 1976: 77–121.

Mattis S. *Dementia Rating Scale.* Windsor: NFER-Nelson, 1992.

Rosser AE, Hodges JR. The Dementia Rating Scale in Alzheimer's disease, Huntington's disease and progressive supranuclear palsy. *J Neurol* 1994; **241**: 531–6.

1.8.7 ADAS-Cog

The Alzheimer's Disease Assessment Scale–Cognitive Section (ADAS-Cog: Rosen *et al.*, 1984) has become a widely used reference measure, for example as an outcome measure of drug efficacy in clinical trials practice. Memory, attention, learning, and orientation are among the domains examined, the final score (0–70) being higher for more severe impairment. Since the ADAS-Cog takes significantly longer to perform than the MMSE (30–45 minutes) it may not be practical for use in day-to-day clinical practice. A 'calculator' to convert MMSE scores to equivalent ADAS-Cog scores is available, reflecting the strong correlation between ADAS-Cog and MMSE scores (Doraiswamy *et al.*, 1997).

REFERENCES

Doraiswamy PM, Bieber F, Kaiser L, *et al.* The Alzheimer's Disease Assessment Scale: patterns and predictors of baseline cognitive performance in multicenter Alzheimer's disease trials. *Neurology* 1997; **48**: 1511–7.

Rosen WG, Mohs RC, Davis KL. A new rating scale for Alzheimer's disease. *Am J Psych* 1984; **141**: 1356–64.

1.8.8 CERAD battery

The Consortium to Establish a Registry for Alzheimer's Disease (CERAD) battery (Morris *et al.*, 1989) incorporates the MMSE and other subtests of memory, naming, and verbal fluency.

REFERENCES

Morris J, Heyman A, Mohs R, *et al.* The Consortium to Establish a Registry for Alzheimer's Disease (CERAD). Part I. Clinical and neuropsychological assessment of Alzheimer's disease. *Neurology* 1989; **39**: 1159–65.

1.8.9 Clinical Dementia Rating (CDR)

Although this is a global staging measure, rather than a purely neuropsychological test instrument (Hughes *et al.*, 1982; Morris, 1993), it is included here because of the prominence which it has gained in the definition of mild cognitive impairment (MCI: see Section 2.6). It is based on both patient assessment and caregiver interview, rating memory, orientation, judgment and problem solving, community affairs, home and hobbies, and personal care. About 40 minutes is needed to gather the required information. Ratings range from 0 to 3. A CDR score of 0.5 (questionable dementia) correlates, although is not necessarily synonymous, with MCI. A CDR score of 1 has a good sensitivity and specificity in screening for dementia (Juva *et al.*, 1995), and the test is reliably and consistently scored (Schafer *et al.*, 2004).

REFERENCES

Hughes CP, Berg L, Danziger WL, Coben LA, Martin RL. A new clinical scale for the staging of dementia. *Br J Psychiatry* 1982; **140**: 566–72.

Juva K, Sulkava R, Erkinjuntti T, *et al.* Usefulness of the Clinical Dementia Rating scale in screening for dementia. *Int Psychogeriatr* 1995; **7**: 17–24.

Morris J. The CDR: current version and scoring rules. *Neurology* 1993; **43**: 2412–14.

Schafer KA, Tractenberg RE, Sano M, *et al.* Reliability of monitoring the clinical dementia rating in multicenter clinical trials. *Alzheimer Dis Assoc Disord* 2004; **18**: 219–22.

1.8.10 Global Deterioration Scale (GDS)

Like CDR, the Global Deterioration Scale (GDS) is a staging instrument for cognitive and functional capacity over a seven-point scale (Reisberg *et al.*, 1982). A GDS score of 3 has been used in some centres to define MCI, but similar caveats apply as with CDR = 0.5.

REFERENCES

Reisberg B, Ferris SH, de Leon MJ, Crook T. The Global Deterioration Scale (GDS) for assessment of primary degenerative dementia. *Am J Psych* 1982; **139**: 1136–9.

1.8.11 Instrumental Activities of Daily Living (IADL) scale

Since the canonical definition of dementia (see Section 1.10) encompasses not only cognitive impairment but also impairments in social and occupational function as a consequence of the cognitive decline, it might be argued that ADL scales could serve as independent diagnostic tests for dementia equally as well as cognitive tests. Certainly in epidemiological studies, loss of certain instrumental activities of daily living (such as independent use of the telephone, ability to travel alone on personal or public transport, and responsibility for supervising medications and finances) have proven predictive of a diagnosis of dementia (Barberger-Gateau *et al.*, 1992; De Lepeleire *et al.*, 2004). In a clinic-based population, however, use of the physical self-maintenance and instrumental activities of daily living scale of Lawton and Brody (1969), or parts thereof, had a low diagnostic accuracy for the diagnosis of dementia (AUC = 0.75), principally because many people adjudged demented by DSM-IV criteria were at ceiling on this scale (Hancock & Larner, 2007).

REFERENCES

Barberger-Gateau P, Commenges D, Gagnon M, *et al.* Instrumental activities of daily living as a screening tool for cognitive impairment and dementia in elderly community dwellers. *J Am Geriatr Soc* 1992; **40**: 1129–34.

De Lepeleire J, Aertgeerts B, Umbach I, *et al.* The diagnostic value of IADL evaluation in the detection of dementia in general practice. *Aging Ment Health* 2004; **8**: 52–7.

Hancock P, Larner AJ. The diagnosis of dementia: diagnostic accuracy of an instrument measuring activities of daily living in a clinic-based population. *Dement Geriatr Cogn Disord* 2007; **23**: 133–9.

Lawton MP, Brody EM. Assessment of older people: self-maintaining and instrumental activities of daily living. *Gerontologist* 1969; **9**: 176–85.

1.9   Normal aging

Various changes in neurological function occur with increasing age, motor, sensory, and cognitive (Larner, 2006; Peters, 2006). To what extent these changes reflect 'normal aging', however that may be defined, or to what extent they reflect an increasing burden of age-related neurological disease, remains uncertain. In consequence, the inevitable physiological changes that occur in cognition with increasing age may be difficult to distinguish from the earliest stages of pathological brain disorders causing cognitive impairments.

A distinction may be drawn between 'crystallized intelligence', characterized by practical problem-solving skills, knowledge gained from experience, and vocabulary, and 'fluid intelligence', characterized by the ability to acquire and use new information, as measured by the solution of abstract problems and speeded performance (Horn & Cattell, 1967). Crystallized intelligence is assumed to be cumulative: longitudinal studies of vocabulary, for example, show no decline through old age. By contrast, fluid intelligence does change with age: performance on tests such as Raven's Progressive Matrices and Digit Symbol substitution declines marginally up to the age of 40 years and then more rapidly (Salthouse, 1982). There is general consensus that typical cognitive aging involves losses in processing speed, cognitive flexibility, and the efficiency of working memory (sustained attention). In other words, it may take more time and/or more trials to learn new information. Cognitive domains such as access to remotely learned information, including semantic networks, and retention of well-encoded new information are spared with typical aging; this may permit testing of these domains to be used as sensitive indicators of disease processes (Smith & Ivnik, 2003). It may be that memory decline in healthy aging is secondary to decline in processing speed and efficiency, since controlling for processing speed may attenuate or eliminate age-related differences in memory performance, unlike the situation with memory impairment in dementia (Sliwinski *et al.*, 2003).

Longitudinal studies of neuropsychological function in older Americans indicate that there is considerable variability in normal older adults across different skills, and consistency across different domains may not necessarily be observed (Smith & Ivnik, 2003). Clearly this needs to be taken into account when assessing whether perceived cognitive decline is pathological or normal, that is in defining neuropsychological norms for aging. Furthermore, norms for IQ are increasing over time (Deary, 2001). Likewise, norms may need to be age-weighted rather than age-corrected to detect cognitive impairment related to Alzheimer's disease (Sliwinski *et al.*, 2003), the prevalence of which increases exponentially with increasing age. Many other situational influences may also impact on testing of cognitive skills, such as fatigue, emotional status, medication use, pain (Nicholson *et al.*, 2001), and stress. These also need to be taken into account when considering the results of cognitive testing, as may factors such as educational and background experience. Many norms are also culturally weighted.

Notwithstanding these difficulties, the definition of a syndrome or syndromes of cognitive impairment greater than expected for age, which are the harbingers of progressive cognitive decline, the prodromal phases of neurodegenerative disorder, may now be identifiable, with all the consequent ramifications for potential therapeutic intervention (see Section 2.6).

REFERENCES

Deary IJ. *Intelligence: a Very Short Introduction*. Oxford: Oxford University Press, 2001: 102–13.

Horn JL, Cattell RB. Age difference in fluid and crystallized intelligence. *Acta Psychol* 1967; **26**: 107–29.

Larner AJ. Neurological signs of aging. In: Pathy MSJ, Sinclair AJ, Morley JE (eds.), *Principles and Practice of Geriatric Medicine* (4th edition). Chichester: Wiley, 2006: 743–50.

Nicholson K, Martelli MF, Zasler ND. Does pain confound interpretation of neuropsychological test results? *Neuro Rehabilitation* 2001; **16**: 225–30.

Peters R. Ageing and the brain. *Postgrad Med J* 2006; **82**: 84–8.

Salthouse TA. *Adult Cognition*. New York: Springer, 1982.

Sliwinski M, Lipton R, Buschke H, Wasylyshyn C. Optimizing cognitive test norms for detection. In: Petersen RC (ed.), *Mild Cognitive Impairment: Aging to Alzheimer's Disease*. Oxford: Oxford University Press, 2003: 89–104.

Smith GE, Ivnik RJ. Normative neuropsychology. In: Petersen RC (ed.), *Mild Cognitive Impairment: Aging to Alzheimer's Disease*. Oxford: Oxford University Press, 2003: 63–88.

1.10   Dementia, delirium, depression

The diagnosis of dementia is currently based on fulfilment of clinical diagnostic criteria, for example those in the generic *Diagnostic and Statistical Manual* (DSM), the *International Classification of Diseases* (ICD), or dedicated criteria for specific dementia subtypes. DSM-IV (American Psychiatric Association, 1994), for example, requires the development of multiple cognitive deficits that include memory impairment, of gradual onset and progressive course, sufficiently severe to cause impairment in occupational or social functioning, not better accounted for by another diagnosis. However, application of such criteria to large cohorts of patients may classify different numbers of patients as having dementia, with differences up to a factor of 10 found in one study (Erkinjuntti *et al.*, 1997). One reason for this variability is that many of these criteria are heavily weighted toward memory impairment. Because memory impairment is the most salient feature in Alzheimer's disease, the most common cause of dementia, many diagnostic criteria, for example those for vascular dementia, have been inadvertently 'Alzheimerized', with undue emphasis placed on memory loss at the expense of other clinical features (Bowler & Hachinski, 2003).

A 'type 2 dementia', which unlike 'type 1 dementia' is lacking cortical features such as amnesia, has been proposed, in which demonstrable executive control function impairments are sufficient to cause disability (Royall, 2006). Another potentially confusing outcome of the emphasis of diagnostic criteria on memory is that syndromes with a diagnostic label of dementia, such as frontotemporal dementia, may not fulfil diagnostic crtieria for dementia in their early stages because the initial features are executive (frontal) dysfunction and non-cognitive behavioural change (Mendez et al., 2006). Tautology may also occur simply as a reflection of the fact that unequivocal cognitive deficits may not be sufficient to meet criteria for dementia (e.g. in mild cognitive impairment: see Section 2.6).

Other diagnoses may also be confused with dementia, necessitating consideration in the differential diagnosis, most particularly delirium and depression. Cognitive deficits, particularly those of acute onset in an elderly person, should not immediately lead to a diagnosis of dementia unless delirium has been excluded, since a degree of reversibility of cognitive deficits may be possible with correction of the precipitating factors of delirium. Impairments of consciousness, a *sine qua non* for the diagnosis of delirium (see Section 1.1), may be subtle. Furthermore, delirium may be the presenting feature of an underlying dementia syndrome (Robertsson et al., 1998; Rockwood et al., 1999). In other words, dementia may be a predisposing factor for delirium, presumably because cerebral reserve is reduced and hence the brain is less able to cope with additional precipitating factors, of which infection or metabolic derangement are the most common (Lindesay et al., 2002; Larner, 2004). One study found that around one quarter of AD patients had an episode of delirium during the course of their illness (Baker et al., 1999). Guidelines for the prevention, diagnosis, and treatment of delirium have been published (e.g. Royal College of Physicians, 2006).

It may also be pointed out that since dementia may be defined as an acquired syndrome of cognitive impairment in a clear sensorium, it might be imagined that attentional mechanisms in dementia are normal, thereby permitting a clear-cut distinction between delirium and dementia. This is not the case: attentional mechanisms may not be normal in dementia syndromes (e.g. divided and selective attention in Alzheimer's disease); indeed in some (e.g. dementia with Lewy bodies), attentional dysfunction is central to the diagnosis.

Affective disorder, principally in the form of major depression, may be associated with impairment of cognitive functions. Terms used to describe this clinical entity have included pseudodementia, dementia syndrome of depression, and depression-related cognitive dysfunction (Kiloh, 1961; Wells, 1979; Roose & Devanand, 1999; Shanmugham & Alexopoulos, 2005). To ascertain with certainty whether manifest cognitive decline, particularly in elderly patients, results from depression or from an underlying neurodegenerative disorder is one of the greatest challenges facing the clinician in the memory clinic (Christensen et al., 1997). Moreover, depression may be an integral part of many neurological disorders, including dementia syndromes, not simply a reaction to diagnosis and neurological impairment (Kanner, 2005). Neuropsychological test results may not reliably discriminate, although some have been claimed to do so (e.g. ACE: Dudas et al., 2005; CANTAB-PAL: Swainson et al., 2001). An empirical trial of antidepressant medication may be given, but even clinical improvement may not absolutely establish the diagnosis; prolonged follow-up may be required. Progressive cognitive decline may also be a feature of the natural history of schizophrenia (Almeida & Howard, 2005; Al-Uzri et al., 2006; Morrison et al., 2006).

REFERENCES

Almeida OP, Howard R. Schizophrenia, cognitive impairment and dementia. In: Burns A, O'Brien J, Ames D (eds.), *Dementia* (3rd edition). London: Hodder Arnold, 2005: 750–3.

Al-Uzri MM, Reveley MA, Owen L, *et al.* Measuring memory impairment in community-based patients with schizophrenia. *Br J Psychiatry* 2006; **189**: 132–6.

American Psychiatric Association. *Diagnostic and Statistical Manual of Mental Disorders.* Washington, DC: American Psychiatric Association, 1994.

Baker FM, Wiley C, Kokmen E, Chandra V, Schoenberg BS. Delirium episodes during the course of clinically diagnosed Alzheimer's disease. *J Natl Med Assoc* 1999; **91**: 625–30.

Bowler JV, Hachinski V. Current criteria for vascular dementia: a critical appraisal. In: Bowler JV, Hachinski V (eds.), *Vascular Cognitive Impairment: Reversible Dementia.* Oxford: Oxford University Press, 2003: 1–11.

Christensen H, Griffiths K, MacKinnon A. A quantitative review of cognitive deficits in depression and Alzheimer-type dementia. *J Int Neuropsychol Soc* 1997; **3**: 631–51.

Dudas RB, Berrios GE, Hodges JR. The Addenbrooke's Cognitive Examination (ACE) in the differential diagnosis of early dementias versus affective disorder. *Am J Geriatr Psychiatry* 2005; **13**: 218–26.

Erkinjuntti T, Ostbye T, Steenhuis R, Hachinski V. The effect of different diagnostic criteria on the prevalence of dementia. *N Engl J Med* 1997; **337**: 1667–74.

Kanner AM. *Depression in Neurological Disorders.* Cambridge: Lundbeck, 2005.

Kiloh L. Pseudodementia. *Acta Psychiatr Scand* 1961; **37**: 336–51.

Larner AJ. Delirium: diagnosis, aetiopathogenesis and treatment. *Adv Clin Neurosci Rehabil* 2004; **4** (2): 28–9.

Lindesay J, Rockwood K, Macdonald A (eds.). *Delirium in Old Age.* Oxford: Oxford University Press, 2002.

Mendez MF, McMurtray A, Licht EA, Saul RE, Miller BL. Is early frontotemporal dementia a dementia? *Alzheimers Dement* 2006; **2** (suppl 1): S548 (abstract P4–112).

Morrison G, O'Carroll R, McCreadie R. Long-term course of cognitive impairment in schizophrenia. *Br J Psychiatry* 2006; **189**: 556–7.

Robertsson B, Blennow K, Gottfries CG, Wallin A. Delirium in dementia. *Int J Geriatr Psychiatry* 1998; **13**: 49–56.

Rockwood K, Cosway S, Carver D, *et al.* The risk of dementia and death following delirium. *Age Ageing* 1999; **28**: 551–6.

Roose SP, Devanand DP. *The Interface Between Dementia and Depression.* London: Martin Dunitz, 1999.

Royal College of Physicians. *The Prevention, Diagnosis and Management of Delirium in Older People.* London: Royal College of Physicians, 2006.

Royall DR. Executive control function in 'mild' cognitive impairment and Alzheimer's disease. In: Gauthier S, Scheltens P, Cummings JL (eds.), *Alzheimer's Disease and Related Disorders Annual 5.* London: Taylor & Francis, 2006: 35–62.

Shanmugham B, Alexopoulos G. Depression with cognitive impairment. In: Burns A, O'Brien J, Ames D (eds.), *Dementia* (3rd edition). London: Hodder Arnold, 2005: 731–7.

Swainson R, Hodges JR., Galton CJ, *et al.* Early detection and differential diagnosis of Alzheimer's disease and depression with neuropsychological tests. *Dement Geriatr Cogn Disord* 2001; **12**: 265–80.

Wells CE. Pseudodementia. *Am J Psych* 1979; **136**: 895–900.

1.11 Cortical versus subcortical dementias, thalamic dementia

Albert *et al.* (1974) first used the term 'subcortical dementia' to describe the cognitive impairments seen in progressive supranuclear palsy: forgetfulness, slowness of thought processes (bradyphrenia), alteration of personality with marked apathy and depression, and an impaired ability to manipulate acquired knowledge. These deficits were felt to be qualitatively distinct from those seen in cortical dementias, typically Alzheimer's disease, which include impairments in language (aphasia), memory (amnesia), perception (agnosia), and skilled learned movements (apraxia). The term 'limbic dementia' has sometimes been used for syndromes with marked amnesia and evidence for limbic system pathology such as Alzheimer's disease.

Whereas cueing or recognition paradigms could improve performance in delayed recall memory tests in subcortical dementias, suggesting ineffective retrieval but with relatively preserved encoding of material, in cortical dementias such strategies were ineffective, suggesting impaired encoding as well as retrieval. The term 'subcortical' was selected because of the resemblance of the deficits to those seen with bifrontal lobe disease, also reflected in the concurrent emotional and movement deficits in the two types: subcortical dementias tended to be associated with apathy and depression and prominent disorders of muscle tone, posture, and gait, whereas cortical dementias were attended with cognitive anosognosia and disinhibition and an absence of movement disorder (Cummings, 1990).

Prototypical subcortical dementias were said to occur in Huntington's disease (McHugh & Folstein, 1975) and Parkinson's disease (Starkstein & Merello, 2002). It has been hypothesized that the basal ganglia, in addition to their role in movement, support a basic attentional mechanism, facilitating the synchronization of cortical activity underlying the selection and promulgation of an appropriate sequence of thoughts; this 'focused attention' differs from arousal, vigilance, or alertness. Basal ganglia damage thus results in a failure of synchronization, manifest as abulia and bradyphrenia (Brown & Marsden, 1998). The 'white matter' dementia occurring in, for example, some patients with multiple sclerosis may have similar neuropsychological features (Rao, 1996). White matter cognitive impairments have been extensively documented by Filley (2001).

An entity called thalamic dementia is also mentioned in the literature (Stern, 1939), referring to cognitive impairments in conditions with relatively selective thalamic damage. Most commonly this is due to vascular lesions (see Section 3.3.3) or neoplasia, but in addition relatively selective degeneration of the thalamus may occur. This may mostly be due to prion disease (Petersen et al., 1992) such as fatal familial insomnia (Gallassi et al., 1996), although cases of selective thalamic degeneration with the pathology of multiple system atrophy (Petersen et al., 1992) or motor neurone disease (Deymeer et al., 1989), or without evidence of prion disease (Janssen et al., 2000), have been reported. The neuropsychological features may include forgetfulness, apathy, and hypersomnia. Cognitive impairment may also occur in patients with isolated brainstem lesions of vascular, inflammatory, infective, or metabolic origin (Garrard et al., 2002; for examples, see Sections 3.3.8, 8.2.1, 9.4.2).

Evidence for and against the cortical/subcortical dichotomy has been debated (Brown & Marsden, 1988), and objections have been raised to the concept of subcortical dementia. Cortical and subcortical areas are not functionally independent, but overlapping. Since white matter has an essentially integrative function, reciprocally linking cortical and subcortical structures, white matter pathology might be expected to result in functional disconnection of brain areas, and disordered brain function at a site distant from a lesion (diaschisis) is a well-recognized phenomenon (see Section 1.12). This may be seen with frontal lobe dysfunction in multiple sclerosis (Foong et al., 1997) and has also been suggested in X-linked adrenoleukodystrophy (Larner, 2003a). Identical or similar clinical phenotypes may result from pathologies affecting either grey matter or subjacent white matter (e.g. subcortical aphasias: Benson & Ardila, 1996). Against this argument, however, false localization of neurological signs usually deemed indicative of higher, cortical cognitive function (e.g. agnosia, neglect) is rarely reported (Larner, 2003b, 2005).

Whatever the precise physiological relationship, nonetheless, the cortical/subcortical terminology may still have some clinical utility in the differential diagnosis of dementia syndromes (e.g. Neary & Snowden, 2002; Bak et al., 2005).

REFERENCES

Albert ML, Feldman RG, Willis AL. The 'subcortical dementia' of progressive supranuclear palsy. *J Neurol Neurosurg Psychiatry* 1974; **37**: 121–30.

Bak TH, Crawford LM, Hearn VC, Mathuranath PS, Hodges JR. Subcortical dementia revisited: similarities and differences in cognitive function between progressive supranuclear palsy (PSP), corticobasal degeneration (CBD) and multiple system atrophy (MSA). *Neurocase* 2005; **11**: 268–73.

Benson DF, Ardila A. *Aphasia: a Clinical Perspective.* New York: Oxford University Press, 1996: 166–79.

Brown P, Marsden CD. What do the basal ganglia do? *Lancet* 1998; **351**: 1801–4.

Brown RG, Marsden CD. 'Subcortical dementia': the neuropsychological evidence. *Neuroscience* 1988; **25**: 363–87.

Cummings JL. *Subcortical Dementias.* London: Oxford University Press, 1990.

Deymeer F, Smith TW, De Girolami U, Drachman DA. Thalamic dementia and motor neuron disease. *Neurology* 1989; **39**: 58–61.

Filley CM. *The Behavioral Neurology of White Matter*. New York: Oxford University Press, 2001.

Foong J, Rozewicz L, Quaghebeur G, *et al*. Executive function in multiple sclerosis: the role of frontal lobe pathology. *Brain* 1997; **120**: 15–26.

Gallassi R, Morreale A, Montagna P, *et al*. Fatal familial insomnia: behavioral and cognitive features. *Neurology* 1996; **46**: 935–9.

Garrard P, Bradshaw D, Jäger HR, *et al*. Cognitive dysfunction after isolated brainstem insult: an under-diagnosed cause of long-term morbidity. *J Neurol Neurosurg Psychiatry* 2002; **73**: 191–4.

Janssen JC, Lantos PL, Al Sarraj S, Rossor MN. Thalamic degeneration with negative prion protein immunostaining. *J Neurol* 2000; **247**: 48–51.

Larner AJ. Adult-onset dementia with prominent frontal lobe dysfunction in X-linked adrenoleukodystrophy with R152C mutation in ABCD1 gene. *J Neurol* 2003a; **250**: 1253–4.

Larner AJ. False localising signs. *J Neurol Neurosurg Psychiatry* 2003b; **74**: 415–8.

Larner AJ. A topographical anatomy of false-localising signs. *Adv Clin Neurosci Rehabil* 2005; **5** (1): 20–1.

McHugh PR, Folstein MF. Psychiatric symptoms of Huntington's chorea: a clinical and phenomenological study. In: Benson DF, Blumer D (eds.), *Psychiatric Aspects of Neurological Disease*. New York: Raven Press, 1975: 267–85.

Neary D, Snowden JS. Sorting out the dementias. *Pract Neurol* 2002; **2**: 328–39.

Petersen RB, Tabaton M, Berg L, *et al*. Analysis of the prion protein gene in thalamic dementia. *Neurology* 1992; **42**: 1859–63.

Rao SM. White matter disease and dementia. *Brain Cogn* 1996; **31**: 250–68.

Starkstein SE, Merello M. *Psychiatric and Cognitive Disorders in Parkinson's Disease*. Cambridge: Cambridge University Press, 2002: 59–66.

Stern K. Severe dementia associated with bilateral symmetrical degeneration of the thalamus. *Brain* 1939; **62**: 157–71.

1.12 Disconnection syndromes

Disconnection syndromes may be defined as conditions in which there is an interruption of inter- and/or intra-hemispheric fibre tracts. The concept was originally advanced in the 1890s, but was revived and developed by Norman Geschwind in the 1960s (Geschwind, 1965; Absher & Benson, 1993; Catani & ffytche, 2005). Disconnection syndromes essentially result either from interruption of fibres within the corpus callosum or commissures (inter-hemispheric disconnection syndromes), or of fibres within a hemisphere (intrahemispheric disconnection syndromes). The former is most graphically seen in patients who have undergone surgical commissurotomy for intractable seizure disorders ('split-brain' patients: Sperry, 1982; Zaidel *et al.*, 2003), whilst the latter syndromes are best described in the domain of language. Although mass lesions and iatrogenesis (surgery) are obvious causes of disconnection, functional disconnection may also result from inflammatory disorders of white matter (see Section 1.11). A 'callosal dementia' has been postulated, characterized by callosal disconnection, Balint syndrome, gaze apraxia, and neurobehavioural features such as alternating apathy and agitation (Ghika Schmid *et al.*, 1999).

With complete interhemispheric disconnection, for example with a tumour or following surgical section of the corpus callosum, a blindfolded patient can correctly name objects placed in the right hand, but not those in the left, and objects in the left visual hemifield cannot be named or matched to a similar object in the right hemifield. With posterior callosal section at the splenium, for example following left posterior cerebral artery occlusion, patients cannot read or name colours, since information cannot pass to the left hemispheric language areas. Copying of words and writing, both spontaneously and to dictation, is intact, as information may pass to the left hemisphere anterior to the site of damage (aphasia without agraphia).

Various intrahemispheric disconnection syndromes have been described. In conduction aphasia, the patient has fluent but paraphasic speech and writing, with greatly impaired repetition despite relatively normal comprehension of the spoken and written word. This has traditionally been explained as due to a lesion in the arcuate fasciculus/supramarginal gyrus disconnecting the sensory (Wernicke) and motor (Broca) language areas. Ideomotor apraxia in Broca's aphasia, an apraxia of left hand movements to command, is ascribed to lesions disconnecting the cortical motor areas anterior to the primary motor cortex. In pure word deafness, patients are able to hear and identify non-verbal sounds but unable to understand spoken language, due to lesions in the white matter of the left temporal lobe which isolate Wernicke's area from the auditory cortex.

Alzheimer's disease may be viewed as a disconnection syndrome (Lakmache *et al.*, 1998; Delbeuck *et al.*, 2003). AD pathology isolates the hippocampus from association cortices, basal forebrain, thalamus, and hypothalamus (Hyman *et al.*, 1984). Disconnection of cortical regions caused by white matter lesions and cerebral atrophy due to internal carotid artery occlusive disease has been suggested (Yamauchi *et al.*, 1996). Speculations that unusual delusional syndromes (e.g. Capgras', Cotard's) might also represent disconnection syndromes have been advanced.

REFERENCES

Absher JR, Benson DF. Disconnection syndromes: an overview of Geschwind's contributions. *Neurology* 1993; **43**: 862–7.

Catani M, ffytche DH. The rises and falls of disconnection syndromes. *Brain* 2005; **128**: 2224–39.

Delbeuck X, van der Linden M, Collette F. Alzheimer's disease as a disconnection syndrome? *Neuropsychol Rev* 2003; **13**: 79–92.

Geschwind N. Disconnexion syndromes in animals and man. *Brain* 1965; **88**: 237–94, 585–644.

Ghika Schmid F, Ghika J, Assal G, Bogousslavsky J. Callosal dementia: behavioural disorders related to central and extrapontine myelinolysis [in French]. *Rev Neurol Paris* 1999; **155**: 367–73.

Hyman BT, van Hoesen GW, Damasio AR, Barnes CL. Alzheimer's disease: cell-specific pathology isolates the hippocampal formation. *Science* 1984; **225**: 1168–70.

Lakmache Y, Lassonde M, Gauthier S, Frigon JY, Lepore F. Interhemispheric disconnection syndrome in Alzheimer's disease. *Proc Natl Acad Sci USA* 1998; **95**: 9042–6.

Sperry RW. Some effects of disconnecting the cerebral hemispheres. *Science* 1982; **217**: 1223–6.

Yamauchi H, Fukuyama H, Nagahama Y, *et al.* Atrophy of the corpus callosum associated with cognitive impairment and widespread cortical hypometabolism in carotid artery occlusive disease. *Arch Neurol* 1996; **53**: 1103–9.

Zaidel E, Iacoboni M, Zaidel DW, Bogen JE. The callosal syndromes. In: Heilman KM, Valenstein E (eds.), *Clinical Neuropsychology* (4th edition). Oxford: Oxford University Press, 2003: 347–403.

Postscript

In the chapters which follow, the deficits in the various cognitive domains discussed in this chapter which have been observed in neurological disorders are discussed. These may be localized or discrete deficits, or part of more widespread impairments which add up to a diagnosis of dementia. It should, however, be added that many attending memory clinics with a complaint of impaired memory prove, after careful clinical, neuropsychological, and imaging evaluation, to have no evidence for underlying neurological disorder. Such individuals, who may account for up to 50% of patients seen in the clinic (Larner, 2005), sometimes labelled as 'memory complainers' or 'worried well', but perhaps better described as those with 'purely subjective memory impairment', pose a significant diagnostic challenge. Some, to be sure, may represent missed diagnoses of incipient neurodegenerative disease ('mild cognitive impairment': see Section 2.6); others may have primary affective disorders, sleep-related disorders, problems with drug misuse (prescription or recreational), or any combination thereof to account for their complaints. Others may perhaps have intuited their physiological age-related decline in cognitive function (see Section 1.9). If doubt persists, such patients should ideally be followed up for longitudinal assessment.

REFERENCES

Larner AJ. An audit of the Addenbrooke's Cognitive Examination (ACE) in clinical practice. *Int J Geriatr Psychiatry* 2005; **20**: 593–4.

Neurodegenerative disorders

2.1 Alzheimer's disease (AD)

Alzheimer's disease (AD) is the archetypal neuro-degenerative cognitive disorder (Larner, 2008). Alois Alzheimer's critical contribution, which later prompted Emil Kraepelin to bestow the eponym upon the condition, was to link the clinical phenotype of cognitive decline with specific neuropathological findings, namely neurofibrillary tangles (Hodges, 2006; Larner 2006a).

Initially conceived of as a rare disease of the presenium, it was not until the 1960s that neuropsychological (Blessed *et al.*, 1968) and neuropathological (Tomlinson *et al.*, 1968, 1970) studies showed that most cases of 'senile dementia' were identical to AD. Clinical diagnostic criteria for AD have been developed by the National Institute of Neurologic and Communicative Disorders and Stroke, and the Alzheimer's Disease and Related Disorders Association (NINCDS-ADRDA) workgroup, with definite, probable, and possible categories (McKhann *et al.*, 1984). Clinical criteria are also available from the American Psychiatric Association's (1994) *Diagnostic and Statistical Manual* (DSM-IV). Generally these criteria perform well, with >80% accuracy of clinical diagnosis, hence highly sensitive for an antemortem diagnosis of AD, although specificity is poorer such that other dementias may erroneously be identified as AD. Neuropathological criteria are also available for AD, based on the quantitation and distribution of the hallmark features, senile plaques and neurofibrillary tangles (Mirra *et al.*, 1991; Braak & Braak, 1991; National Institute on Aging, 1997).

Epidemiological studies have shown that the prevalence of AD increases steeply with increasing age, with over 50% of over-85-year-olds being affected. Early-onset AD, that is presenting at or before 65 years of age, may be differentiated from late-onset disease (McKhann *et al.*, 1984), although this distinction is probably arbitrary since the underlying pathobiology is identical. More useful, in terms of elucidating aetiology, has been the distinction of sporadic AD, where there is no family history of the condition, from familial AD, where at least one first-degree family relative is affected, and autosomal dominant AD, where at least three family members are affected in at least two generations. Autosomal dominant AD is most usually of early-onset type, sometimes manifesting as early as the third or fourth decade of life. To date, mutations deterministic for AD have been discovered in three genes, encoding the amyloid precursor protein (APP), presenilin-1 (PS1), and presenilin-2 (PS2). Multiple mutations have been identified in each gene (Alzheimer Disease and Frontotemporal Dementia Mutation Database, www.molgen.ua.ac.be/Admutations), around 150 in PS1 (Larner & Doran, 2006), which is the commonest site for genetic mutations causing AD (Cruts *et al.*, 1998). Virtually all of these mutations appear to alter the metabolism of APP such that production of the amyloid β-peptide, the major protein component of amyloid plaques, is increased. These findings have raised hopes for the development of disease-modifying therapy for AD, particularly if cases can be identified early in the disease course. To date, however, only symptomatic treatments for AD are available, namely cholinesterase inhibitors and memantine.

Diagnosis hinges on appropriate clinical features aided by ancillary investigations (Waldemar *et al.*, 2000, 2006; Knopman *et al.*, 2001). Structural brain imaging may show generalized brain atrophy, but this finding is non-specific, and over-reliance on it may lead to incorrect diagnosis of AD (Larner, 2004). Volumetric magnetic resonance imaging showing hippocampal atrophy, progressing with longitudinal follow-up, may be a more secure sign (Fox *et al.*, 1996). Imaging of amyloid deposits themselves has been demonstrated and may soon be applicable clinically (Klunk *et al.*, 2004). EEG changes of background slowing and loss of signal synchronization between different brain regions may be seen (Hegerl & Möller, 1997; Stam, 2006).

The neuropsychological features of AD have been extensively studied (Parks *et al.*, 1993; Morris & Becker, 2004). Disturbance of memory, particularly recent memory, is the commonest presenting symptom, often manifested as repeating the same information or questions within a short space of time, accompanied by difficulty learning new information, for example use of new household appliances. Although this may be an isolated amnesic syndrome, usually with a temporal gradient with more recent information more significantly affected, more often than not other cognitive domains are found to be affected when formally tested, particularly language and visuospatial function.

On occasion, AD may present with complaints other than memory decline, representing other variants – not subtypes (Jorm, 1985) – of AD. Presentation with primarily visuoperceptual dysfunction is well recognized, described as posterior cortical atrophy (PCA) or the visual variant of AD (Benson et al., 1988; Levine et al., 1993), although other pathologies can on occasion be the substrate of PCA (Pantel & Schröder, 1996). Diagnostic criteria for PCA have been suggested (Mendez et al., 2002). Slowly progressive apraxia has been described as a presentation of AD, either bilateral with biparietal atrophy (Mackenzie Ross et al., 1996; Galton et al., 2000) or, rarely, unilateral (Crystal et al., 1982). AD cases which overlap clinically with corticobasal degeneration are described (Doran et al., 2003), even with the alien limb phenomenon (Ball et al., 1993). Slowly progressive aphasia has been reported on occasion to be the presentation of AD, rather than one of the focal frontotemporal lobar degeneration syndromes (see Section 2.2), often with non-fluent aphasia (Section 2.2.3) but sometimes fluent aphasia with the characteristics approximating a transcortical sensory aphasia (Pogacar & Williams, 1984; Mendez & Zander, 1991; Galton et al., 2000; Godbolt et al., 2004a; Hodges et al., 2004). Acute, post-operative, presentation of isolated aphasia resembling a cerebrovascular event but subsequently evolving to AD has also been reported (Larner, 2005). A frontal variant of AD has been postulated (Johnson et al., 1999), based on the retrospective finding of early and disproportionately severe impairments on tests of frontal lobe functioning in a subset of definite AD cases with higher neurofibrillary tangle (NFT) load in frontal cortex. Behavioural variants of AD with a clinical phenotype overlapping frontal variant frontotemporal dementia (fvFTD) have also been recorded in association with certain PS1 mutations (Larner & Doran, 2006), cases which might be labelled as fvAD. Whether such a phenotype ever occurs in sporadic AD is uncertain, although possible cases have been presented (Brun & Gustafson, 2006; Larner, 2006b). The frequency of these clinical variants is uncertain, but may constitute up to 10% of AD presentations in a specialist cognitive disorders clinic with a particular interest in early-onset cases, the agnosic (PCA) and aphasic presentations being the most common (Larner, 2006c). However, even in this selected population, amnesic presentations greatly outnumber variant cases.

Although cognitive decline is the dominant phenotypic manifestation of AD, other neurological features may occur such as epileptic seizures (Mendez & Lim, 2003; Lozsadi & Larner, 2006) and movement disorders, particularly myoclonus (Kurlan et al., 2000), most often in the later stages of the disease. Extrapyramidal signs such as parkinsonism are reported (Tsolaki et al., 2001; Scarmeas et al., 2004), though confounding by concurrent Lewy body pathology (see Section 2.4) or use of neuroleptic medications is possible. Sleep-related disorders may likewise become more common with disease progression. Although behavioural and psychological symptoms are common in AD, presentation with prominent features of this kind has been reported only occasionally (Rippon et al., 2003; Doran & Larner, 2004).

Neuropsychological profile

The neuropsychological deficits of AD are summarized in Table 2.1 and are discussed in more detail below.

Attention

Attentional mechanisms are impaired in AD (Perry & Hodges, 1999; Parasuraman, 2004). Tests of selective attention such as the Stroop Test are

Table 2.1. Neuropsychological deficits in Alzheimer's disease (AD).

Attention	↓ Selective, divided; sustained attention relatively preserved
General intelligence, IQ	↓ FSIQ vs. premorbid IQ; PIQ typically more impaired than VIQ
Memory	↓ Episodic memory (encoding, storage) with temporal gradient; +/− semantic memory impairment (category verbal fluency)
Language	Semantic naming errors, circumlocutions; phonology, syntax relatively spared. Aphasic presentations rare
Perception	Agnosic presentations may occur (PCA): Balint syndrome, topographical agnosia, dressing apraxia; object agnosia, pure alexia, prosopagnosia
Praxis	Ideomotor, ideational apraxia: modest. Apraxic presentations rare
Executive function	May be early impairments of judgment, abstract reasoning, problem solving

impaired early in the disease course, possibly reflecting pathological involvement of the cingulate gyrus and/or the basal forebrain cholinergic system (Lawrence & Sahakian, 1995). Tests of divided attention such as dual-task performance tests also show impairment (Baddeley *et al.*, 2001). In contrast, sustained attention is relatively preserved in the early stages, as evidenced by preserved performance on tests of 'working memory' (Cherry *et al.*, 2002), although these may show progressive decline. The greater preservation of attentional functions may be one feature assisting in the differential diagnosis of AD from dementia with Lewy bodies (see Section 2.4).

General intelligence, IQ
Typically patients with AD show disparity between their current full-scale IQ scores and estimates of premorbid IQ based on the NART or educational/occupational achievement, especially for performance IQ, indicating a decline in intellectual functioning. Estimates of premorbid IQ using the NART may be difficult or impossible if there is marked aphasia.

Memory
Memory decline is the commonest complaint of patients and, more often, of their caregivers in AD. This is most commonly seen in the domain of anterograde episodic memory, that is the encoding, storage, retention, and recall of new information about day-to-day personal experiences, in other

words memories with an autobiographical referent (Overman & Becker, 2004). Tests requiring the learning and recall of supraspan word lists are very sensitive to the episodic memory impairment in early AD; examples include the Buschke Selective Reminding Test, the Rey Auditory Verbal Learning Test, the California Verbal Learning Test, and the Hopkins Verbal Learning Test. (It is of note that the MMSE word list contains only three items and is therefore a less stringent test; this has been addressed in other bedside instruments such as the CERAD, ACE, and DemTect.) The learning curve is virtually flat (i.e. many trials are required to learn the new information), intrusion errors are common (i.e. reporting words which were not on the list to be remembered, although these may be semantically related), and recognition paradigms are little better than recall. There may be an accelerated rate of forgetting (Christensen *et al.*, 1998). In other words, the findings are typical of a cortical, as opposed to subcortical, disorder: encoding and storage deficits are paramount, rather than a primary deficit of memory retrieval.

Although it is a common clinical observation that patients' distant, long-term, (remote) memory is spared, evaluation of retrograde memory is not entirely normal, with a temporal gradient such that more distant memories are most intact (Bright & Kopelman, 2004).

The deficits of episodic memory reflect pathological change in the mesial temporal regions, particularly the hippocampal formation, which is also evident on volumetric brain imaging (Fox *et al.*, 1996). That these are typically the earliest changes in AD is confirmed by their observation in individuals carrying deterministic genetic mutations for AD who are tracked from the pre-symptomatic stages (Fox *et al.*, 1998). This is also the area earliest affected by neurofibrillary pathological change (Braak & Braak, 1991; Delacourte *et al.*, 1999).

Semantic memory impairments may also be detected in AD (Hodges *et al.*, 1992; Garrard *et al.*, 2004). On tests of verbal fluency, category fluency is more impaired than letter fluency, indicating difficulty accessing the semantic lexicon of word meanings (Cerhan *et al.*, 2002; Henry *et al.*, 2004). Naming difficulties may also be semantic in their origin.

The pattern of implicit memory impairments in AD differs from that in Huntington's disease, with verbal priming severely impaired but motor (pursuit rotor) skill normally acquired (Salmon & Fennema-Notestine, 2004).

Language

Language deficits in AD have been extensively studied (Kertesz, 2004). The language disorder of AD varies with the stage of the disease, initially remaining fluent with lexicosemantic deficits predominating, but ultimately evolving to global aphasia (Cummings *et al.*, 1985; Faber-Langendoen *et al.*, 1988; Emery, 2000).

Word-finding difficulties are common in the early stages of AD. The tip-of-the-tongue phenomenon may be evident: for example, on picture naming the first letter or phoneme may be generated but not the rest of the word, sometimes with the use of circumlocutions (anomia). Naming errors are largely semantic, rarely phonological or visual (Huff *et al.*, 1986; Hodges *et al.*, 1991). Naming may be relatively preserved in some PS1 mutations (e.g. M139V: Fox *et al.*, 1997; Warrington *et al.*, 2001; Larner & du Plessis 2003), whereas other PS1 mutations may present with aphasia (Godbolt *et al.*, 2004a).

Progressive loss of the richness of language may be evident to the point that speech production may be described as 'empty', lacking in specific content and impoverished in both conveying and obtaining information. Some semantic information about items which cannot be named may be generated, for example 'a beautiful thing which jumps' for kangaroo (Garrard *et al.*, 2005). As previously mentioned, verbal fluency is typically more impaired in the category (semantic) than in the letter (phonological) paradigm (Henry *et al.*, 2004). In comparison with the semantic aspects of language, phonological and syntactic abilities are relatively preserved early in AD, although they may break down as the disease progresses (Croot *et al.*, 2001). Repetition and motor speech may be relatively intact whilst increasingly impaired comprehension of the spoken or written word is evident. Attempts have been made to fit the language disturbance of AD into established aphasia categories (e.g. anomic aphasia in the early stages, extrasylvian or transcortical sensory aphasia in the later stages) but the implication that AD-related language dysfunction is congruent with one of these 'typical' aphasia syndromes may not be justified.

Slowly progressive aphasia has occasionally been reported as the presenting symptom of AD. Such aphasia at onset may lead to confusion with the linguistic variants of frontotemporal lobar degeneration (see Section 2.2). Presence or absence of deficits in other cognitive domains may give clues to the correct diagnosis, as may structural and functional brain imaging. Sometimes, however, only with the passage of time and the evolution of symptoms does diagnostic clarity emerge, or even only at postmortem.

Perception

Visuoperceptual and visuospatial deficits are seldom clinically evident in the early stages of AD, with the notable exception of those patients who present with visual agnosia, the visual variant of AD (Levine *et al.*, 1993), or posterior cortical atrophy (PCA: Mendez *et al.*, 2002), with evidence from functional imaging of visual cortical hypoperfusion and hypometabolism (Nestor *et al.*, 2003). Impaired naming is not thought to result from perceptual deficits. Tests which tap aspects of visual cognition, such as drawing the Rey–Osterrieth Complex Figure, overlapping pentagons (from the MMSE), the Necker cube, and clock drawing, may be impaired early in AD, although performance may also be degraded by concurrent apraxia and/or planning difficulties.

Various visual processing disorders may occur in AD (Mendez *et al.*, 2002; Cronin-Golomb & Hof, 2004), their exact nature depending upon the relative involvement of right or left hemisphere, and the two streams of visual processing (Ungerlieder & Mishkin, 1982; see Section 1.5), namely dorsal (occipitoparietal, 'where') or ventral (occipitotemporal, 'what': Mackenzie Ross *et al.*, 1996). These may occur with relative preservation of memory and language in posterior cortical atrophy. Dorsal stream involvement, the most commonly observed pattern in one series of PCA patients (Nestor *et al.*, 2003), results in Balint syndrome and dressing apraxia, whereas ventral stream involvement may produce object agnosia, pure alexia, and prosopagnosia. However, segregation of cases into dorsal and ventral stream involvement may be clinically difficult (Mendez *et al.*, 2002). Predominant right hemisphere involvement may produce left visual hemineglect, whereas predominant left hemisphere involvement is associated with Gerstmann syndrome, pure alexia, and right hemiachromatopsia. Cortical blindness and Anton's syndrome (visual anosognosia) have also been recorded.

Praxis

Both ideomotor and ideational apraxia may occur in AD, prevalence increasing with disease severity (Edwards *et al.*, 1991; Derouesne *et al.*, 2000). However, this is usually inapparent or of modest severity, rarely producing symptoms (Rapcsak *et al.*, 1989), in comparison with cognitive impairments in other areas. Limb transitive actions (e.g. asking the patient to show how he/she would use a comb/toothbrush/pair of scissors) are most likely

to show impairment; imitation of meaningless gestures may be a sensitive early measure of apraxia. Apraxia as the earliest symptom of AD is rare (Green *et al.*, 1995; Galton *et al.*, 2000). However, apraxia sufficient to cause diagnostic confusion with corticobasal degeneration does rarely occur (Boeve *et al.*, 1999; Doran *et al.*, 2003). Conceptual apraxia, defined by Ochipa *et al.* (1992) as impaired knowledge of what tools and objects are needed to perform a skilled movement, is said to be common in AD.

Executive function

Executive abilities may be impaired in AD, producing impairments of judgment, abstract reasoning, and problem solving, as evidenced by difficulties with verbal fluency, the Wisconsin Card Sorting Test (WCST), and trail-making tests. These changes may occur early in the disease course in some patients, and are commonly observed when specifically sought (Lafleche & Albert, 1995; Binetti *et al.*, 1996; Collette *et al.*, 1999; Royall, 2000; Chen *et al.*, 2000, 2001; Swanberg *et al.*, 2004). Verbal fluency measures have sometimes been proposed as diagnostic tests for AD (Cerhan *et al.*, 2002; Duff Canning *et al.*, 2004). The possible impact of executive dysfunction on tests which also tap language and perceptual functions has already been noted. Very prominent executive dysfunction, sufficient to prompt a clinical diagnostic label of 'frontotemporal dementia', has been reported in some familial AD cases with certain PS1 gene mutations, but whether this phenotype ever occurs in sporadic AD is doubtful.

Presymptomatic Alzheimer's disease

Patients with mild cognitive impairment (MCI: see Section 2.6) may be in the prodromal phase of AD, but to examine presymptomatic AD patients one needs either to test large numbers of normal individuals, ideally in a community sample, follow them up over a period of years until some develop a diagnosis of AD, and then look back at their pre-diagnosis cognitive profile; or, perhaps easier, to study asymptomatic individuals known to be carrying highly penetrant genetic mutations deterministic for AD. In individuals harbouring genetic mutations, episodic memory deficit was the earliest change detected, along with decline in general intelligence, whilst perceptual, naming, and spelling skills were relatively preserved (Newman *et al.*, 1994; Fox *et al.*, 1998; Godbolt *et al.*, 2004b).

Community-based studies have suggested that tests of both memory and executive function, and possibly perceptual speed, show the greatest declines over time in individuals destined to manifest AD, and these may be apparent several years prior to diagnosis (Chen *et al.*, 2000, 2001; Bäckman *et al.*, 2001, 2004; Amieva *et al.*, 2005). These domains are similar to those which decline in 'normal' cognitive aging (see Section 1.9).

Treatment of neuropsychological deficits

Cholinesterase inhibitors (ChEIs) are licensed for the symptomatic treatment of mild to moderate AD in many jurisdictions, the rationale being that they help to restore the cholinergic deficits that are a neurochemical feature of AD brain. The evidence base for their modest efficacy is relatively strong, as evidenced by meta-analyses (Lanctôt *et al.*, 2003; Ritchie *et al.*, 2004; Whitehead *et al.*, 2004). These show stability or even improvement in cognitive scales such as the MMSE and ADAS-Cog as compared with placebo-treated patients over periods of 6–12 months. Whether this reflects genuine mnemonic improvement, or simply better attentional function, is debatable. Behavioural improvements are also noted with ChEIs, but cognitive domains other than attention and memory are little affected. A report of improved visuospatial function following ChEI treatment in a case of PCA (Kim *et al.*, 2005) would seem to be exceptional. Whether ChEIs have disease-modifying effects, or alter the natural history of AD, for example by reducing the rate of nursing home placement, remains debatable (Lopez *et al.*, 2002; Larner, 2007). Memantine, an antagonist at the NMDA type of glutamate receptors, has also been shown to benefit cognitive domains (Reisberg *et al.*, 2003, 2006) and is licensed for use in moderate to severe AD, although not reimbursed in some jurisdictions.

REFERENCES

American Psychiatric Association. *Diagnostic and Statistical Manual of Mental Disorders*. Washington, DC: American Psychiatric Association, 1994.

Amieva H, Jacqmin-Gadda H, Orgogozo JM, *et al*. The 9 year cognitive decline before dementia of the Alzheimer type: a prospective population-based study. *Brain* 2005; **128**: 1093–101.

Bäckman L, Jones S, Berger AK, Laukka EJ, Small BJ. Multiple cognitive deficits during the transition to Alzheimer's disease. *J Intern Med* 2004; **256**: 195–204.

Bäckman L, Small BJ, Fratiglioni L. Stability of the preclinical episodic memory deficit in Alzheimer's disease. *Brain* 2001; **124**: 96–102.

Baddeley AD, Baddeley HA, Bucks RS, Wilcock GK. Attentional control in Alzheimer's disease. *Brain* 2001; **124**: 1492–508.

Ball JA, Lantos PL, Jackson M, *et al*. Alien hand sign in association with Alzheimer's histopathology. *J Neurol Neurosurg Psychiatry* 1993; **56**: 1020–3.

Benson DF, Davis RJ, Snyder BD. Posterior cortical atrophy. *Arch Neurol* 1988; **45**: 789–93.

Binetti G, Magni E, Padovani A, *et al*. Executive dysfunction in early Alzheimer's disease. *J Neurol Neurosurg Psychiatry* 1996; **60**: 91–3.

Blessed G, Tomlinson BE, Roth M. The association between quantitative measures of dementia and of senile change in the cerebral grey matter of elderly subjects. *Br J Psychiatry* 1968; **114**: 797–811.

Boeve BF, Maraganore MD, Parisi JE, *et al*. Pathologic heterogeneity in clinically diagnosed corticobasal degeneration. *Neurology* 1999; **53**: 795–800.

Braak H, Braak E. Neuropathological stageing [*sic*] of Alzheimer-related changes. *Acta Neuropathol (Berl)* 1991; **82**: 239–59.

Bright P, Kopelman MD. Remote memory in Alzheimer's disease. In: Morris RG, Becker JT (eds.), *Cognitive Neuropsychology of Alzheimer's Disease* (2nd edition). Oxford: Oxford University Press, 2004: 141–51.

Brun A, Gustafson L. Clinical symptoms and neuropathology in organic dementing disorders affecting the frontal lobes. In: Risberg J, Grafman J (eds.), *The Frontal Lobes: Development, Function and Pathology*. Cambridge: Cambridge University Press, 2006: 199–221 [at 212–13].

Cerhan JH, Ivnik RJ, Smith GE, *et al*. Diagnostic utility of letter fluency, category fluency, and fluency difference scores in Alzheimer's disease. *Clin Neuropsychol* 2002; **16**: 35–42.

Chen P, Ratcliff G, Belle SH, *et al*. Cognitive tests that best discriminate between presymptomatic AD and those who remain nondemented. *Neurology* 2000; **55**: 1847–53.

Chen P, Ratcliff G, Belle SH, *et al*. Patterns of cognitive decline in presymptomatic Alzheimer disease: a prospective community study. *Arch Gen Psychiatry* 2001; **58**: 853–8.

Cherry BJ, Buckwalter JG, Henderson VW. Better preservation of memory span relative to supraspan immediate recall in Alzheimer's disease. *Neuropsychologia* 2002; **40**: 846–52.

Christensen H, Kopelman MD, Stanhope N, Lorentz I, Owen P. Rates of forgetting in Alzheimer dementia. *Neuropsychologia* 1998; **36**: 547–57.

Collette F, van der Linden M, Salmon E. Executive dysfunction in Alzheimer's disease. *Cortex* 1999; **35**: 57–72.

Cronin-Golomb A, Hof PR (eds.). *Vision in Alzheimer's Disease*. Basel: Karger, 2004.

Croot K, Hodges JR, Xuereb JH, Patterson K. Phonological and articulatory impairment in Alzheimer's disease: a single case series. *Brain Lang* 2001; **75**: 277–309.

Cruts M, van Duijn CM, Backhovens H, *et al*. Estimation of the genetic contribution of presenilin-1 and -2 mutations in a population-based study of presenile Alzheimer disease. *Hum Mol Genet* 1998; **7**: 43–51.

Crystal HA, Horoupian DS, Katzman R, Jotkowicz S. Biopsy-proved Alzheimer disease presenting as a right parietal lobe syndrome. *Ann Neurol* 1982; **12**: 186–8.

Cummings JL, Benson DF, Hill MA, Read S. Aphasia in dementia of the Alzheimer type. *Neurology* 1985; **35**: 394–7.

Delacourte A, David JP, Sergeant N, *et al*. The biochemical pathway of neurofibrillary degeneration in aging and Alzheimer's disease. *Neurology* 1999; **52**: 1158–65.

Derouesne C, Lagha-Pierucci S, Thibault S, Baudouin-Madec V, Lacomblez L. Apraxic disturbances in patients with mild to moderate Alzheimer's disease. *Neuropsychologia* 2000; **38**: 1760–9.

Doran M, du Plessis DG, Enevoldson TP, *et al*. Pathological heterogeneity of clinically diagnosed corticobasal degeneration. *J Neurol Sci* 2003; **216**: 127–34.

Doran M, Larner AJ. Prominent behavioural and psychiatric symptoms in early-onset Alzheimer's disease in a sib pair with the presenilin-1 gene R269G mutation. *Eur Arch Psychiatry Clin Neurosci* 2004; **254**: 187–9.

Duff Canning SJ, Leach L, Stuss D, Ngo L, Black SE. Diagnostic utility of abbreviated fluency measures in Alzheimer disease and vascular dementia. *Neurology* 2004; **62**: 556–62.

Edwards DF, Deuel RK, Baum CM, Morris JC. A quantitative analysis of apraxia in senile dementia of Alzheimer type: stage-related differences in prevalence and type. *Dementia* 1991; **2**: 142–9.

Emery VO. Language impairment in dementia of the Alzheimer type: a hierarchical decline? *Int J Psychiatry Med* 2000; **30**: 145–64.

Faber-Langendoen K, Morris JC, Knesevich JW, *et al*. Aphasia in senile dementia of the Alzheimer type. *Ann Neurol* 1988; **23**: 365–70.

Fox NC, Kennedy AM, Harvey RJ, *et al*. Clinicopathological features of familial Alzheimer's disease associated with the M139V mutation in the presenilin 1 gene. Pedigree but not mutation specific age at onset provides evidence for a further genetic factor. *Brain* 1997; **120**: 491–501.

Fox NC, Warrington EK, Freeborough PA, *et al*. Presymptomatic hippocampal atrophy in Alzheimer's disease: a longitudinal MRI study. *Brain* 1996; **119**: 2001–7.

Fox NC, Warrington EK, Seiffer AL, Agnew SK, Rossor MN. Presymptomatic cognitive deficits in individuals at risk of familial Alzheimer's disease: a longitudinal prospective study. *Brain* 1998; **121**: 1631–9.

Galton CJ, Patterson K, Xuereb JH, Hodges JR. Atypical and typical presentations of Alzheimer's disease: a clinical, neuropsychological, neuroimaging and pathological study of 13 cases. *Brain* 2000; **123**: 484–98.

Garrard P, Maloney LM, Hodges JR, Patterson K. The effects of very early Alzheimer's disease on the characteristics of writing by a renowned author. *Brain* 2005; **128**: 250–60.

Garrard P, Patterson K, Hodges JR. Semantic processing in Alzheimer's disease. In: Morris RG, Becker JT (eds.), *Cognitive Neuropsychology of Alzheimer's Disease* (2nd edition). Oxford: Oxford University Press, 2004: 179–96.

Godbolt AK, Beck JA, Collinge J, *et al*. A presenilin 1 R278I mutation presenting with language impairment. *Neurology* 2004a; **63**: 1702–4.

Godbolt AK, Cipolotti L, Watt H, *et al*. The natural history of Alzheimer disease: a longitudinal presymptomatic and symptomatic study of a familial cohort. *Arch Neurol* 2004b; **61**: 1743–8.

Green RC, Goldstein FC, Mirra SS, *et al.* Slowly progressive apraxia in Alzheimer's disease. *J Neurol Neurosurg Psychiatry* 1995; **59**: 312–15.

Hegerl U, Möller HJ. Electroencephalography as a diagnostic instrument in Alzheimer's disease: reviews and perspectives. *Int Psychogeriatr* 1997; **9** (suppl 1): 237–46.

Henry JD, Crawford JR, Phillips LH. Verbal fluency performance in dementia of the Alzheimer type: a meta-analysis. *Neuropsychologia* 2004; **42**: 1212–22.

Hodges JR. Alzheimer's centennial legacy: origins, landmarks and the current status of knowledge concerning cognitive aspects. *Brain* 2006; **129**: 2811–22.

Hodges JR, Davies RR, Xuereb JH, *et al.* Clinicopathological correlates in frontotemporal dementia. *Ann Neurol* 2004; **56**: 399–406.

Hodges JR, Salmon DP, Butters N. The nature of the naming deficit in Alzheimer's and Huntington's disease. *Brain* 1991; **114**: 1547–58.

Hodges JR, Salmon DP, Butters N. Semantic memory impairment in Alzheimer's disease: failure of access or degraded knowledge? *Neuropsychologia* 1992; **30**: 301–14.

Huff FJ, Corkin S, Growden JH. Semantic impairment and anomia in Alzheimer's disease. *Brain Lang* 1986; **28**: 235–49.

Johnson JK, Head E, Kim R, Starr A, Cotman CW. Clinical and pathological evidence for a frontal variant of Alzheimer disease. *Arch Neurol* 1999; **56**: 1233–9.

Jorm AF. Subtypes of Alzheimer's disease: a conceptual analysis. *Psychol Med* 1985; **15**: 543–53.

Kertesz A. Language in Alzheimer's disease. In: Morris RG, Becker JT (eds.), *Cognitive Neuropsychology of Alzheimer's Disease* (2nd edition). Oxford: Oxford University Press, 2004: 197–218.

Kim E, Lee Y, Lee J, Han SH. A case with cholinesterase inhibitor responsive asymmetric posterior cortical atrophy. *Clin Neurol Neurosurg* 2005; **108**: 97–101.

Klunk WE, Engler H, Nordberg A, *et al.* Imaging brain amyloid in Alzheimer's disease with Pittsburgh Compound-B. *Ann Neurol* 2004; **55**: 306–19.

Knopman DS, DeKosky ST, Cummings JL, *et al.* Practice parameter: diagnosis of dementia (an evidence-based review). Report of the Quality Standards Subcommittee of the American Academy of Neurology. *Neurology* 2001; **56**: 1143–53.

Kurlan R, Richard IH, Papka M, Marshall F. Movement disorders in Alzheimer's disease: more rigidity of definitions is needed. *Mov Disord* 2000; **15**: 24–9.

Lafleche G, Albert MS. Executive function deficits in mild Alzheimer's disease. *Neuropsychology* 1995; **9**: 313–20.

Lanctôt KL, Hermann N, Yau KK, *et al.* Efficacy and safety of cholinesterase inhibitors in Alzheimer's disease: a meta-analysis. *CMAJ* 2003; **169**: 557–64.

Larner AJ. Getting it wrong: the clinical misdiagnosis of Alzheimer's disease. *Int J Clin Pract* 2004; **58**: 1092–4.

Larner AJ. 'Dementia unmasked': atypical, acute aphasic, presentations of neurodegenerative dementing disease. *Clin Neurol Neurosurg* 2005; **108**: 8–10.

Larner AJ. Alzheimer 100. *Adv Clin Neurosci Rehabil* 2006a; **6** (5): 24.

Larner AJ. 'Frontal variant Alzheimer's disease': a reappraisal. *Clin Neurol Neurosurg* 2006b; **108**: 705–8.

Larner AJ. Frequency of agnosic, apraxic and aphasic presentations of Alzheimer's disease. *Eur J Neurol* 2006c; **13** (suppl 2): 193 (abstract P2098).

Larner AJ. Do cholinesterase inhibitors alter the course of dementia? *Prog Neurol Psych* 2007; **11** (5): 26–8.

Larner AJ. Alzheimer's disease. In: Cappa S, Abutalebi J, Demonet JF, Fletcher P, Garrard P (eds.), *Cognitive Neurology: a Clinical Textbook.* Oxford: Oxford University Press, 2008: in press.

Larner AJ, Doran M. Clinical phenotypic heterogeneity of Alzheimer's disease associated with mutations of the presenilin-1 gene. *J Neurol* 2006; **253**: 139–58.

Larner AJ, du Plessis DG. Early-onset Alzheimer's disease with presenilin-1 M139V mutation: clinical, neuropsychological and neuropathological study. *Eur J Neurol* 2003; **10**: 319–23.

Lawrence AD, Sahakian BJ. Alzheimer's disease, attention, and the cholinergic system. *Alzheimer Dis Assoc Disord* 1995; **9** (suppl 2): 43–9.

Levine DN, Lee JM, Fisher CM. The visual variant of Alzheimer's disease: a clinicopathologic case study. *Neurology* 1993; **43**: 305–13.

Lopez OL, Becker JT, Wisniewski S, *et al.* Cholinesterase inhibitor treatment alters the natural history of Alzheimer's disease. *J Neurol Neurosurg Psychiatry* 2002; **72**: 310–14.

Lozsadi DA, Larner AJ. Prevalence and causes of seizures at the time of diagnosis of probable Alzheimer's disease. *Dement Geriatr Cogn Disord* 2006; **22**: 121–4.

McKhann G, Drachman D, Folstein M, *et al.* Clinical diagnosis of Alzheimer's disease. Report of the NINCDS-ADRDA work group under the auspices of the Department of Health and Human Service Task forces on Alzheimer's disease. *Neurology* 1984; **34**: 939–44.

Mackenzie Ross SJ, Graham N, Stuart-Green L, *et al.* Progressive biparietal atrophy: an atypical presentation of Alzheimer's disease. *J Neurol Neurosurg Psychiatry* 1996; **61**: 388–95.

Mendez MF, Ghajarania M, Perryman KM. Posterior cortical atrophy: clinical characteristics and differences compared to Alzheimer's disease. *Dement Geriatr Cogn Disord* 2002; **14**: 33–40.

Mendez MF, Lim GTH. Seizures in elderly patients with dementia: epidemiology and management. *Drugs Aging* 2003; **20**: 791–803.

Mendez MF, Zander BA. Dementia presenting with aphasia: clinical characteristics. *J Neurol Neurosurg Psychiatry* 1991; **54**: 542–5.

Mirra SS, Heyman A, McKeel D, *et al.* The Consortium to Establish a Registry for Alzheimer's Disease (CERAD). Part II. Standardization of the neuropathologic assessment of Alzheimer's disease. *Neurology* 1991; **41**: 479–86.

Morris RG, Becker JT (eds.). *Cognitive Neuropsychology of Alzheimer's Disease* (2nd edition). Oxford: Oxford University Press, 2004.

National Institute on Aging and Reagan Institute Working Group on Diagnostic Criteria for the Neuropathological Assessment of Alzheimer Disease. Consensus recommendations for the post-mortem diagnosis of Alzheimer's disease. *Neurobiol Aging* 1997; **18** (suppl 4): S1–2.

Nestor PJ, Caine D, Fryer TD, Clarke J, Hodges JR. The topography of metabolic deficits in posterior cortical atrophy (the visual variant of Alzheimer's disease) with FDG-PET. *J Neurol Neurosurg Psychiatry* 2003; **74**: 1521–9.

Newman SK, Warrington EK, Kennedy AM, Rossor MN. The earliest cognitive change in a person with familial Alzheimer's disease: presymptomatic neuropsychological features in a pedigree with familial Alzheimer's disease confirmed at necropsy. *J Neurol Neurosurg Psychiatry* 1994; **57**: 967–72.

Ochipa C, Rothi LJG, Heilman KM. Conceptual apraxia in Alzheimer's disease. *Brain* 1992; **115**: 1061–71.

Overman AA, Becker JT. Information processing defects in episodic memory in Alzheimer's disease. In: Morris RG, Becker JT (eds.), *Cognitive Neuropsychology of Alzheimer's Disease* (2nd edition). Oxford: Oxford University Press, 2004: 121–40.

Pantel J, Schröder J. Posterior cortical atrophy: a new dementia syndrome or a form of Alzheimer's disease [in German]. *Fortschr Neurol Psychiatr* 1996; **64**: 492–508.

Parasuraman R. Attentional functioning in Alzheimer's disease. In: Morris RG, Becker JT (eds.), *Cognitive Neuropsychology of Alzheimer's Disease* (2nd edition). Oxford: Oxford University Press, 2004: 81–102.

Parks RW, Zec RF, Wilson RS (eds.). *Neuropsychology of Alzheimer's Disease and Other Dementias.* New York: Oxford University Press, 1993.

Perry RJ, Hodges JR. Attention and executive deficits in Alzheimer's disease: a critical review. *Brain* 1999; **122**: 383–404.

Pogacar S, Williams RS. Alzheimer's disease presenting as slowly progressive aphasia. *R I Med J* 1984; **67**: 181–5.

Rapcsak SZ, Croswell SC, Rubens A. Apraxia in Alzheimer's disease. *Neurology* 1989; **39**: 664–8.

Reisberg B, Doody R, Stöffler A, *et al.*, for the Memantine Study Group. Memantine in moderate-to-severe Alzheimer's disease. *N Engl J Med* 2003; **348**: 1333–41.

Reisberg B, Doody R, Stöffler A, *et al.* A 24-week open-label extension study of memantine in moderate to severe Alzheimer disease. *Arch Neurol* 2006; **63**: 49–54.

Rippon GA, Crook R, Baker M, *et al.* Presenilin 1 mutation in an African American family presenting with atypical Alzheimer dementia. *Arch Neurol* 2003; **60**: 884–8.

Ritchie CW, Ames D, Clayton T, Lai R. Metaanalysis of randomized trials of the efficacy and safety of donepezil, galantamine and rivastigmine for the treatment of Alzheimer disease. *Am J Geriatr Psychiatry* 2004; **12**: 358–69.

Royall DR. Executive cognitive impairment: a novel perspective on dementia. *Neuroepidemiol* 2000; **19**: 293–9.

Salmon DP, Fennema-Notestine C. Implicit memory in Alzheimer's disease: priming and skill learning. In: Morris RG, Becker JT (eds.), *Cognitive Neuropsychology of Alzheimer's Disease* (2nd edition). Oxford: Oxford University Press, 2004: 153–78.

Scarmeas N. Hadjigeorgiou GM, Papadimitriou A, *et al.* Motor signs during the course of Alzheimer disease. *Neurology* 2004; **63**: 975–82.

Stam CJ. Modern applications of electroencephalography in dementia diagnosis. In: Gauthier S, Scheltens P, Cummings JL (eds.), *Alzheimer's Disease and Related Disorders Annual 5.* London: Taylor & Francis, 2006: 191–206.

Swanberg MM, Tractenberg RE, Mohs R, Thal LJ, Cummings JL. Executive dysfunction in Alzheimer disease. *Arch Neurol* 2004; **61**: 556–60.

Tomlinson BE, Blessed G, Roth M. Observations on the brains of non-demented old people. *J Neurol Sci* 1968; **7**: 331–56.

Tomlinson BE, Blessed G, Roth M. Observations on the brains of demented old people. *J Neurol Sci* 1970; **11**: 205–42.

Tsolaki M, Kokarida K, Iakovidou V, *et al.* Extrapyramidal symptoms and signs in Alzheimer's disease: prevalence and correlation with the first symptom. *Am J Alzheimers Dis Other Demen* 2001; **16**: 268–78.

Ungerlieder LG, Mishkin M. Two cortical visual systems. In: Ingle DJ, Goodale MA, Mansfield RJW (eds.), *Analysis of Visual Behavior*. Cambridge, MA: MIT Press, 1982: 549–86.

Waldemar G, Dubois B, Emre M, *et al.* Diagnosis and management of Alzheimer's disease and other disorders associated with dementia: the role of neurologists in Europe. European Federation of Neurological Societies. *Eur J Neurol* 2000; **7**: 133–44.

Waldemar G, Dubois B, Emre M, *et al.* Alzheimer's disease and other disorders associated with dementia. In: Hughes R, Brainin M, Gilhus NE (eds.), *European Handbook of Neurological Management*. Oxford: Blackwell, 2006: 266–98 [also *Eur J Neurol* 2007; **14**: e1–26].

Warrington EK, Agnew SK, Kennedy AM, Rossor MN. Neuropsychological profiles of familial Alzheimer's disease associated with mutations in the presenilin 1 and amyloid precursor protein genes. *J Neurol* 2001; **248**: 45–50.

Whitehead A, Perdomo C, Pratt RD, *et al.* Donepezil for the symptomatic treatment of patients with mild to moderate Alzheimer's disease: a meta-analysis of individual patient data from randomised controlled trials. *Int J Geriatr Psychiatry* 2004; **19**: 624–33.

2.2 Frontotemporal lobar degenerations (FTLD)

Arnold Pick, in the 1890s, was the first clinician to describe syndromes related to focal lobar degeneration of the brain, both frontal degeneration associated with behavioural change and temporal degeneration associated with linguistic decline (Graham & Hodges, 2005). The term 'Pick's disease' came later, based on the neuropathological finding (by Alzheimer) of ballooned achromatic neurones (Pick cells) and neuronal inclusions (Pick bodies) in some, but not all, cases of lobar degeneration.

A potentially bewildering profusion of names has become attached to these focal degenerative disorders, based on clinical, pathological, and clinicopathological observations. Although some investigators have tried to label these, and related, conditions as 'Pick's complex' (Kertesz & Munoz, 1998), the term 'frontotemporal lobar degenerations' (FTLD) seems preferable (Snowden *et al.*, 1996), of which frontotemporal dementia (FTD) is one specific type. Clinical and neuropathological diagnostic criteria have been suggested (Gregory & Hodges, 1993; Brun *et al.*, 1994; Neary *et al.*, 1998; McKhann *et al.*, 2001), but not all have been evaluated for their validity and reliability (Miller *et al.*, 1997). Moreover, it has been suggested that most cases of FTD also meet diagnostic criteria for AD (Varma *et al.*, 1999): it is known that AD criteria have good sensitivity but poor specificity, hence misidentifying other dementias as AD. If so, FTLD cases may be misdiagnosed, and incidence and prevalence underestimated. Reported prevalence rates of FTLD are around 15/100 000 (Ratnavalli *et al.*, 2002; Rosso *et al.*, 2003).

Besides the clinical phenotype of primary behavioural (frontal) or linguistic (temporal) decline, neuropsychological findings may be helpful in differentiating FTD from AD (Hodges *et al.*, 1999; Bozeat *et al.*, 2000; Perry & Hodges, 2000). Subscores from the Addenbrooke's Cognitive Examination (ACE), a bedside test of neuropsychological function, are claimed to facilitate the distinction (Mathuranath *et al.*, 2000; see Section 1.8). Neuropsychiatric features may also help to differentiate FTD from AD, such as stereotypic behaviours, changes in eating preference, disinhibition, and poor social awareness (Bozeat *et al.*, 2000; Bathgate *et al.*, 2001).

Other investigations may help with the diagnosis: structural brain imaging (CT, MRI) may show focal frontal and/or temporal atrophy, often asymmetric, and functional neuroimaging (SPECT, PET) may show frontotemporal hypoperfusion or hypometabolism. The EEG has been said to be normal, despite clinically evident dementia (this is one of the investigational diagnostic criteria of Neary *et al.*,

1998), in contrast to the situation in AD, although a recent study suggested that EEG abnormalities were in fact present in more than 60% of FTLD patients, increasing with dementia severity (Chan *et al.*, 2004).

Although a universally acceptable nomenclature and taxonomy is not currently available, perhaps the most significant distinction (at time of writing) is between those FTLDs with neuropathological appearances characterized by inclusions immuno-positive for tau protein, and those without tau inclusions but with ubiquitin immunopositive inclusions (FTLD-U: Hodges *et al.*, 2004; Cairns, 2006). Amongst the former group may be included 'true' Pick's disease (European Concerted Action on Pick's (ECAPD) Consortium, 1998), and fronto-temporal dementia with parkinsonism linked to chromosome 17 (FTDP-17), associated with muta-tions in the tau gene. In the FTLD-U group may be included some sporadic FTLD cases, FTD associ-ated with or without clinical evidence of motor neurone disease (FTLD-MND and motor neurone disease inclusion dementia, MNDID, respectively: see Section 2.3), and rare entities such as pure hip-pocampal sclerosis (Section 2.3.3) and FTD with inclusion body myopathy and Paget's disease (Sec-tion 5.1.8). Some cases lack either tau or ubiquitin pathology and are labelled as 'dementia lacking distinctive histology' (Knopman *et al.*, 1990). Corti-cobasal degeneration and progressive supranuclear palsy may also be subsumed under the rubric of FTLDs with tau inclusions (Kertesz & Munoz, 1998; Hodges *et al.*, 2004; Cairns, 2006).

Neurogenetic studies also confirm the hetero-geneity of FTLDs. FTDP-17 may be associated with mutations of either the tau or progranulin genes (see Section 2.2.4). Besides FTDP-17, familial FTLDs have also been described linked to chromosomes 3 and 9. The former, in a Danish kindred (Brown *et al.*, 1995), was eventually found to have mutations in the charged multivesicular body protein 2B gene (*CHMP2B*: Skibinski *et al.*, 2005); the latter, in a family with FTLD and motor neurone disease (MND), in the dynactin gene (Munch *et al.*, 2005).

Since this text is oriented to clinical practice, FTLDs will be considered according to clinical presentation (behavioural, linguistic: Snowden *et al.*, 1996), followed by some additional notes about specific neuropathological entities. Cortico-basal degeneration and progressive supranuclear palsy are considered under atypical parkinsonian syndromes (Section 2.4.2 and 2.4.3, respectively).

REFERENCES

Bathgate D, Snowden JS, Varma A, Blackshaw A, Neary D. Behaviour in frontotemporal dementia, Alzheimer's disease and vascular dementia. *Acta Neurol Scand* 2001; **103**: 367–78.

Bozeat S, Gregory CA, Lambon Ralph MA, Hodges JR. Which neuropsychiatric and behavioural features dis-tinguish frontal and temporal variants of frontotem-poral dementia from Alzheimer's disease? *J Neurol Neurosurg Psychiatry* 2000; **69**: 178–86.

Brown J, Ashworth A, Gydesen S, *et al.* Familial non-specific dementia maps to chromosome 3. *Hum Mol Genet* 1995; **4**: 1625–8.

Brun A, Englund B, Gustafson L, *et al.* Clinical and neuropathological criteria for frontotemporal dementia. *J Neurol Neurosurg Psychiatry* 1994; **57**: 416–18.

Cairns NJ. Neuropathology of frontotemporal lobar degenerations. In: Strong MJ (ed.), *Dementia and Motor Neuron Disease*. Abingdon: Informa Healthcare, 2006: 147–66.

Chan D, Walters RJ, Sampson EL, *et al.* EEG abnormalities in frontotemporal lobar degeneration. *Neurology* 2004; **62**: 1628–30.

European Concerted Action on Pick's (ECAPD) Consor-tium. Provisional clinical and neuroradiological criteria for the diagnosis of Pick's disease. *Eur J Neurol* 1998; **5**: 519–20.

Graham A, Hodges J. Pick's disease: its relationship to progressive aphasia, semantic dementia and fronto-temporal dementia. In: Burns A, O'Brien J, Ames D (eds.), *Dementia* (3rd edition). London: Hodder Arnold, 2005: 678–88.

Gregory CA, Hodges JR. Dementia of frontal type and the focal lobar atrophies. *Int Rev Psychiatry* 1993; **5**: 397–406.

Hodges JR, Davies RR, Xuereb JH, *et al.* Clinicopatholo-gical correlates in frontotemporal dementia. *Ann Neurol* 2004; **56**: 399–406.

Hodges JR, Patterson K, Ward R, *et al.* The differentiation of semantic dementia and frontal lobe dementia (temporal and frontal variants of frontotemporal dementia) from early Alzheimer's disease: a comparative neuropsychological study. *Neuropsychology* 1999; **13**: 31–40.

Kertesz A, Munoz DG (eds.). *Pick's Disease and Pick Complex.* New York: Wiley-Liss, 1998.

Knopman DS, Mastri AR, Frey WH, Sung JH, Rustan T. Dementia lacking distinctive histologic features: a common non-Alzheimer degenerative dementia. *Neurology* 1990; **40**: 251–6.

McKhann GM, Albert MS, Grossman M, *et al.* Clinical and pathological diagnosis of frontotemporal dementia. Report of the Work Group on Frontotemporal Dementia and Pick's disease. *Arch Neurol* 2001; **58**: 1803–9.

Mathuranath PS, Nestor PJ, Berrios GE, Rakowicz W, Hodges JR. A brief cognitive test battery to differentiate Alzheimer's disease and frontotemporal dementia. *Neurology* 2000; **55**: 1613–20.

Miller BL, Ikonte C, Ponton M, *et al.* A study of the Lund–Manchester research criteria for frontotemporal dementia: clinical and single-photon emission CT correlations. *Neurology* 1997; **48**: 937–42.

Munch C, Rosenbohm A, Sperfeld AD, *et al.* Heterozygous R1101K mutation of the DCTN1 gene in a family with ALS and FTD. *Ann Neurol* 2005; **58**: 777–80.

Neary D, Snowden JS, Gustafson L, *et al.* Frontotemporal lobar degeneration: a consensus on clinical diagnostic criteria. *Neurology* 1998; **51**: 1546–54.

Perry RJ, Hodges JR. Differentiating frontal and temporal variant frontotemporal dementia from Alzheimer's disease. *Neurology* 2000; **54**: 2277–84.

Ratnavalli E, Brayne C, Dawson K, Hodges JR. The prevalence of frontotemporal dementia. *Neurology* 2002; **58**: 1615–21.

Rosso SM, Donker KL, Baks T, *et al.* Frontotemporal dementia in the Netherlands: patient characteristics and prevalence estimates from a population-based study. *Brain* 2003; **126**: 2016–22.

Skibinski G, Parkinson NJ, Brown J, *et al.* Mutations in the endosomal ESCRTIII complex subunit CHMP2B in frontotemporal dementia. *Nat Genet* 2005; **37**: 806–8.

Snowden JS, Neary D, Mann DMA. *Fronto-Temporal Lobar Degeneration: Fronto-Temporal Dementia, Progressive Aphasia, Semantic Dementia.* New York: Churchill Livingstone, 1996.

Varma AR, Snowden JS, Lloyd JJ, *et al.* Evaluation of the NINCDS-ADRDA criteria in the differentiation of Alzheimer's disease and frontotemporal dementia. *J Neurol Neurosurg Psychiatry* 1999; **66**: 184–8.

2.2.1 Frontotemporal dementia (FTD), dementia of frontal type (DFT), frontal variant of frontotemporal dementia (fvFTD), behavioural variant of frontotemporal dementia (bvFTD)

This syndrome, variously known as FTD, DFT, fvFTD, or bvFTD, is defined on the basis of a behavioural disorder, featuring declines in social interpersonal conduct and the regulation of personal conduct, emotional blunting, and loss of insight (Neary *et al.*, 1998). Characteristics may include neglect of personal hygiene, transgression of social mores, mental rigidity and inflexibility (increased adherence to routines, rituals, clockwatching), changes in dietary habits with a predilection for sweet foods, motor and verbal perseverations, disinhibition, or inertia. The syndrome is not homogeneous, and clinical subtypes may be defined on the basis of the most prominent behavioural and motor features: disinhibited type, with predominant orbitofrontal lobe involvement, apathetic type, with predominant dorsolateral convexity involvement, and stereotypic type, with predominant striatal involvement (Snowden *et al.*, 1996). Early diagnosis may be difficult, since neuropsychological tests and structural and functional neuroimaging may not be sensitive to the early changes in fvFTD (Gregory *et al.*, 1999), which may be associated with various pathologies (Hodges *et al.*, 2004).

Neuropsychological profile

The neuropsychological deficits of fvFTD are summarized in Table 2.2 and discussed in more detail below.

Attention

Poor sustained attention, manifest as distractibility or motor restlessness, may be an evident behavioural feature in fvFTD (cf. AD). 'Don't know' responses may be frequent, especially for effortful tasks, one feature of the lack of mental application, or economy of effort, evident on clinical testing. Responses may be rapid and impulsive, with lack

Table 2.2. Neuropsychological deficits in frontal variant frontotemporal dementia (fvFTD).

Attention	↓ Sustained attention; distractibility, apathy, economy of effort, poor self-monitoring, impulsive
General intelligence, IQ	FSIQ may be normal or ↓ due to lack of mental effort
Memory	Absence of amnesia may be a requirement for diagnosis; amnesia generally not prominent but reported in some cases; better performance with cueing, and specific as opposed to open-ended questions
Language	↓ Verbal fluency (letter and category)
Perception	Typically normal
Praxis	Generally preserved; imitation and utilization behaviour may be seen
Executive function	Lack of insight; impaired planning, judgment, abstraction, organization, and problem solving; perseveration, failure to inhibit inappropriate responses

of attention to accuracy, or slowed in apathetic patients.

General intelligence, IQ
Performance may be normal on test batteries such as the WAIS-R or MMSE, despite the change in behaviour. More usually, however, performance is impaired. This may sometimes affect all areas, reflecting lack of mental application to tests, or may sometimes favour performance over verbal subtests.

Memory
Some clinical diagnostic criteria require no amnesia (Neary *et al.*, 1998). However, severe rapidly progressive anterograde amnesia has been recorded on occasion in pathologically confirmed FTD with prominent involvement of the hippocampi (Caine *et al.*, 2001), and marked amnesia at presentation has been noted in other pathologically confirmed cases (Hodges *et al.*, 2004; Graham *et al.*, 2005). Semantic memory is stable in fvFTD (Perry & Hodges, 2000).

Performance on memory tests is, however, often impaired for both recall and recognition, despite patients, ability to provide autobiographical information and orientation in time (i.e. not evidently amnesic clinically; cf. AD). Memory performance may benefit from cues and from the use of specific as opposed to open-ended questions. Poor performance may be related to the generalized economy of effort in performing tests and poor sustained attention.

Language
In conversation, spontaneous speech output may be reduced, brief, and concrete in character. Stereotyped words or phrases ('catchphrases') and verbal perseverations may be evident; repetition is relatively preserved. Output is fluent although prosody may be lost. Comprehension is preserved at the individual word level but may be impaired on tests of more complex items, perhaps related to lack of mental effort or self-monitoring, and impulsive responding. Object naming is generally preserved, in contrast to difficulties with verbal fluency, both letter and category. Progression to eventual mutism may occur. Preservation of calculation skills despite dissolution of language has been reported (Rossor *et al.*, 1995). Acute aphasic presentation of clinically diagnosed frontal variant FTD, following cardiac surgery, has been reported (Larner, 2005).

Perception
Some clinical diagnostic criteria require no perceptual deficit (Neary *et al.*, 1998). Visual agnosia is not apparent, and spatial skills are intact. Patients may take long walks without becoming lost. Impaired performance on tests such as drawing the Rey–Osterrieth Complex Figure may reflect cursory

performance with lack of attention to detail. Dot counting and line orientation, undemanding tasks of visuospatial function, are typically normal. Enhancement of artistic ability has been noted in FTD (Miller *et al.*, 1998).

Praxis

Manual skills are generally well preserved. Tests of praxis may reveal perseveration of gestures, writing, and alternating hand movements or motor sequences, although copying of hand postures is generally performed better. Use of body part as object is typical when pantomiming actions. Contextually inappropriate use of objects, utilization behaviour, may occur. Dependent upon the topographical distribution of pathology, a phenotype resembling corticobasal degeneration may occur occasionally (Doran *et al.*, 2003).

Executive function

A dysexecutive syndrome is typical of fvFTD, manifest as lack of insight and impaired planning, judgment, abstraction, organization, and problem solving. Tests deemed sensitive to frontal lobe function are performed poorly. For example, in the WAIS-R, the Similarities subtest may be impaired due to difficulties in abstracting similarities between objects, and Picture Arrangement to tell a story may not be completed, although individual elements can be identified and described. Proverb interpretation is concrete and cognitive estimates may be wildly inaccurate. As previously mentioned, verbal fluency is impaired for both letter and category; design fluency, the visual analogue of verbal fluency, is also impaired, with multiple rule violations. Sorting rules are not identified and perseverative errors common in both the Weigl and the Wisconsin Card Sorting Test. Failure to inhibit inappropriate responses may be encountered on the Stroop Colour Word Test. In mild fvFTD, however, risk-taking behaviour with increased deliberation time may be the only finding, with other tests sensitive to frontal lobe function remaining normal (Rahman *et al.*, 1999). FvFTD presenting with pathological gambling has been reported (Lo Coco & Nacci, 2004).

Treatment of neuropsychological deficits

Currently there are no licensed treatments for the neuropsychological deficits of fvFTD, although empirical treatments for behavioural features (e.g. mood stabilizers for disinhibition) might temporarily improve some aspects of cognitive function. A trial of the serotonin reuptake inhibitor paroxetine impaired cognition in fvFTD (Deakin *et al.*, 2004).

REFERENCES

Caine D, Patterson K, Hodges JR, Heard R, Halliday G. Severe anterograde amnesia with extensive hippocampal degeneration in a case of rapidly progressive frontotemporal dementia. *Neurocase* 2001; **7**: 57–64.

Deakin JB, Rahman S, Nestor PJ, Hodges JR, Sahakian BJ. Paroxetine does not improve symptoms and impairs cognition in frontotemporal dementia: a double-blind randomized controlled trial. *Psychopharmacol* 2004; **172**: 400–8.

Doran M, du Plessis DG, Enevoldson TP, *et al.* Pathological heterogeneity of clinically diagnosed corticobasal degeneration. *J Neurol Sci* 2003; **216**: 127–34.

Graham A, Davies R, Xuereb J, *et al.* Pathologically proven frontotemporal dementia presenting with severe amnesia. *Brain* 2005; **128**: 597–605.

Gregory CA, Serra Mestres J, Hodges JR. Early diagnosis of the frontal variant of frontotemporal dementia: how sensitive are standard neuroimaging and neuropsychologic tests? *Neuropsychiatry Neuropsychol Behav Neurol* 1999; **12**: 128–35.

Hodges JR, Davies RR, Xuereb JH, *et al.* Clinicopathological correlates in frontotemporal dementia. *Ann Neurol* 2004; **56**: 399–406.

Larner AJ. 'Dementia unmasked': atypical, acute aphasic, presentations of neurodegenerative dementing disease. *Clin Neurol Neurosurg* 2005; **108**: 8–10.

Lo Coco D, Nacci P. Frontotemporal dementia presenting with pathological gambling. *J Neuropsychiatry Clin Neurosci* 2004; **16**: 117–18.

Miller BL, Cummings J, Mishkin F, *et al.* Emergence of artistic talent in frontotemporal dementia. *Neurology* 1998; **51**: 978–82.

Neary D, Snowden JS, Gustafson L, *et al.* Frontotemporal lobar degeneration: a consensus on clinical diagnostic criteria. *Neurology* 1998; **51**: 1546–54.

Perry RJ, Hodges JR. Differentiating frontal and temporal variant frontotemporal dementia from Alzheimer's disease. *Neurology* 2000; **54**: 2277–84.

Rahman S, Sahakian BJ, Hodges JR, Rogers RD, Robbins TW. Specific cognitive deficits in mild frontal variant frontotemporal dementia. *Brain* 1999; **122**: 1469–93.

Rossor M, Warrington EK, Cipolotti L. The isolation of calculation skills. *J Neurol* 1995; **242**: 78–81.

Snowden JS, Neary D, Mann DMA. *Fronto-Temporal Lobar Degeneration: Fronto-Temporal Dementia, Progressive Aphasia, Semantic Dementia.* New York: Churchill Livingstone, 1996: 9–58.

2.2.2   Semantic dementia (SD), progressive fluent aphasia, temporal variant of frontotemporal dementia (tvFTD)

Warrington (1975) was the first to report patients with selective impairment of semantic memory causing a progressive anomia. The linguistic variant of FTD now generally known as semantic dementia is characterized by a loss of the knowledge about items and their meanings. It affects naming, word comprehension, and object recognition, with relatively stable attention and preserved executive function (Poeck & Luzzatti, 1988; Hodges *et al.*, 1992; Snowden *et al.*, 1996; Garrard & Hodges, 2000; Perry & Hodges, 2000). Activities of daily living are relatively well preserved.

The neuroradiological signature of SD is asymmetric focal atrophy of all anterior temporal lobe structures, especially entorhinal cortex, amygdala, anterior medial and inferior temporal gyri, and anterior fusiform gyrus, with an anteroposterior gradient of atrophy (cf. AD: symmetrical atrophy, especially medial temporal lobe structures including hippocampus, with no anteroposterior gradient; Chan *et al.*, 2001). Left-sided cases of semantic dementia are apparently more common than right-sided (Thompson *et al.*, 2003), but this may be artefactual, the profound anomia drawing attention to the former cases whereas progressive prosopagnosia associated with right-sided cases may not come to clinical attention. The commonest neuropathological substrate is MND-type ubiquitin-positive tau-negative inclusions, although true Pick's disease and Alzheimer's disease may also be seen (Davies *et al.*, 2005; Godbolt *et al.*, 2005).

Neuropsychological profile

The neuropsychological deficits of semantic dementia are shown in Table 2.3.

Attention
In contrast to fvFTD, sustained attention to tasks is good in semantic dementia. Working memory is intact as assessed by digit span and by Corsi span, at least until the very late stages of the disease.

General intelligence, IQ
Performance on the WAIS-R is typically impaired. For patients with a disorder of word meaning, a verbal–performance discrepancy favouring performance is evident, with subtest scores reflecting the semantic component of each task, the most impaired being Vocabulary, Comprehension, Information, Similarities, Picture Completion, and Picture Arrangement, whilst Block Design remains intact.

Memory
Episodic memory is relatively preserved. Patients are not amnesic, since they can relate details about recent activities. However, autobiographical memory for remote events is more impaired (Graham & Hodges, 1997; Larner *et al.*, 2005), a reversal of the temporal gradient effect seen in Alzheimer's disease. Semantic memory is severely impaired; there is a breakdown in factual knowledge. Depending on the lateralization of brain atrophy, this may be more evident for verbal or visual material. Cued recall shows no advantage over free recall, indicating breakdown or impaired access to semantic knowledge.

Language
There is a selective breakdown in the lexicosemantic aspects of language. 'Loss of memory for words' is often the main presenting complaint, with relatives and carers providing examples of the patient's loss of word meaning ('What's Coca-Cola?', 'What's a hobby?'). Marked anomia is evident on testing;

Table 2.3. Neuropsychological deficits in semantic dementia (SD).

Attention	Essentially intact
General intelligence, IQ	↓ FSIQ; VIQ typically more impaired than PIQ due to semantic deficit
Memory	Absence of amnesia for recent events; remote autobiographical memory may be impaired; semantic memory severely impaired
Language	Marked anomia; ↓ verbal fluency (category > letter). Comprehension impaired; syntax, grammar preserved; surface dyslexia (regularization errors)
Perception	Essentially intact
Praxis	Essentially intact
Executive function	↓ Verbal fluency; frontal features may gradually emerge

moreover, unlike the situation in AD, patients are often unable to provide any contextual information about objects they cannot name: a patient with AD unable to name a picture of a kangaroo may nonetheless be able to say that it jumps and is found in Australia, but such details are not available to the patient with SD with degradation of, or loss of access to, semantic memory. Providing semantically related multiple choice alternatives is not helpful. Repetition is common, for example of overlearned words and phrases or of the examiner's questions, although there may be inability to understand what is being repeated. Verbal fluency tasks are severely impaired, letter generally being superior to category since the latter is reliant upon access to semantic knowledge. There may also be difficulty recognizing familiar faces (progressive prosopagnosia: Evans et al., 1995).

Conversational speech is fluent, syntactically and grammatically correct, but may demonstrate anomia, and use of superordinate categories (e.g. all animals are called dogs). Reading often demonstrates regularization errors when reading words with irregular sound–spelling correspondence, for example 'pint' read to rhyme with 'mint', the phenomenon of surface dyslexia. As the disease progresses, utterances may become increasingly brief and stereotyped.

Perception
Visuoperceptual and visuospatial function is preserved. Tests such as Raven's Progressive Matrices, Judgment of Line Orientation, copy of the Rey–Osterrieth Complex Figure, and object matching are intact. Object recognition failure reflects the breakdown in semantics.

Praxis
Praxis is generally intact in semantic dementia, although motor skills with a symbolic basis may be impaired.

Executive function
As previously mentioned, tests of sustained attention are intact but tests thought sensitive in part to frontal lobe function such as verbal fluency are impaired. The Weigl may be completed but patients may fail to understand the instructions for the Wisconsin Card Sorting Test. Behavioural features reminiscent of fvFTD may occasionally be present in semantic dementia, such as apathy, irritability, and disinhibition. However, in contrast to the impulsiveness which compromises fvFTD patients' performance on gambling tasks, we have seen a patient with SD who was still able to bet regularly on horse racing with moderate, better than break-even, success, despite being essentially mute (Larner, 2007).

REFERENCES

Chan D, Fox NC, Scahill RI, et al. Patterns of temporal lobe atrophy in semantic dementia and Alzheimer's disease. Ann Neurol 2001; 49: 433–42.

Davies RR, Hodges JR, Kril JJ, et al. The pathological basis of semantic dementia. Brain 2005; 128: 1984–95.

Evans JJ, Heggs AJ, Antoun N, Hodges JR. Progressive prosopagnosia associated with selective right temporal lobe atrophy: a new syndrome? *Brain* 1995; **118**: 1–13.

Garrard P, Hodges JR. Semantic dementia: clinical, radiological and pathological perspectives. *J Neurol* 2000; **247**: 409–22.

Godbolt AK, Josephs KA, Revesz T, *et al.* Sporadic and familial dementia with ubiquitin-positive tau-negative inclusions: clinical features of one histopathological abnormality underlying frontotemporal lobar degeneration. *Arch Neurol* 2005; **62**: 1097–101.

Graham KS, Hodges JR. Differentiating the roles of the hippocampal complex and the neocortex in long-term memory storage: evidence from the study of semantic dementia and Alzheimer's disease. *Neuropsychology* 1997; **11**: 77–89.

Hodges JR, Patterson K, Oxbury S, Funnell E. Semantic dementia: progressive fluent aphasia with temporal lobe atrophy. *Brain* 1992; **115**: 1783–806.

Larner AJ. Gambling. *Adv Clin Neurosci Rehabil* 2007; **7** (1): 26.

Larner AJ, Brookfield K, Flynn A, *et al.* The cerebral metabolic topography of semantic dementia. *J Neurol* 2005; **252** (suppl 2): II106 (abstract P399).

Perry RJ, Hodges JR. Differentiating frontal and temporal variant frontotemporal dementia from Alzheimer's disease. *Neurology* 2000; **54**: 2277–84.

Poeck K, Luzzatti C. Slowly progressive aphasia in three patients: the problem of accompanying neuropsychological deficit. *Brain* 1988; **111**: 151–68.

Snowden JS, Neary D, Mann DMA. *Fronto-Temporal Lobar Degeneration: Fronto-Temporal Dementia, Progressive Aphasia, Semantic Dementia*. New York: Churchill Livingstone, 1996: 91–114.

Thompson SA, Patterson K, Hodges JR. Left/right asymmetry of atrophy in semantic dementia: behavioural–cognitive implications. *Neurology* 2003; **61**: 1196–203.

Warrington EK. The selective impairment of semantic memory. *Q J Exp Psychol* 1975; **27**: 635–57.

2.2.3   Progressive non-fluent aphasia (PNFA), primary progressive aphasia (PPA)

This syndrome was first described as such by Mesulam (1982). It is characterized by progressive non-fluent aphasia with relative preservation of other cognitive functions and activities of daily living until late in the illness. It is probably the rarest of the FTLD syndromes.

Diagnostic criteria have been suggested (Mesulam, 2001), in part to exclude cases of AD with linguistic presentation. Clinical heterogeneity is apparent (Duffy & Petersen, 1992; Mesulam & Weintraub, 1992; Snowden *et al.*, 1996; Westbury & Bub, 1997; Kertesz, 1998; Amici *et al.*, 2006), as is also the case for the pathological substrate, although non-fluent aphasia more reliably predicts Pick body pathology (Hodges *et al.*, 2004). Most cases are sporadic; although some familial cases have been reported (Krefft *et al.*, 2003), discordance in monozygotic twins has also been recorded (Doran & Larner, 2004), suggesting genetic heterogeneity. Cases of primary progressive aphasia which evolve over time to the phenotype of corticobasal degeneration (Sakurai *et al.*, 1996; Mimura *et al.*, 2001; Ferrer *et al.*, 2003; Le Rhun *et al.*, 2005) or progressive supranuclear palsy (Boeve *et al.*, 2003; Mochizuki *et al.*, 2003) have been reported.

Neuropsychological profile

The description (Table 2.4) is for a 'pure' case, without features of any other underlying neuropathological entity such as AD, corticobasal degeneration, or progressive supranuclear palsy.

Attention
Attentional functions are preserved in progressive non-fluent aphasia.

General intelligence, IQ
A verbal–performance discrepancy on the WAIS-R in favour of non-verbal tasks is found.

Memory
Functional memory skills appear intact, although scores on memory tests may be impaired because of the language disorder, especially for verbal tests. Recognition memory for faces is typically well preserved. Likewise, impaired category verbal fluency is due to language deficits rather than impaired semantic memory.

Table 2.4. Neuropsychological deficits in progressive non-fluent aphasia (PNFA).

Attention	Essentially intact
General Intelligence, IQ	↓ FSIQ; VIQ typically more impaired than PIQ due to linguistic impairment
Memory	Essentially intact; impaired scores may reflect linguistic impairment
Language	Phonological and syntactic breakdown; comprehension preserved; ↓ verbal fluency (letter > category)
Perception	Essentially intact
Praxis	Essentially intact
Executive Function	↓ Verbal fluency, otherwise intact

Language

There is progressive breakdown of phonological and syntactic processes resulting in progressive non-fluent aphasia. Speech output is hesitant and effortful, with phonemic paraphasias and transpositional errors ('Spoonerisms'). Comprehension is largely intact, at least initially, for example in word–picture matching tasks, although complex syntax may prove difficult. Increasing comprehension problems develop with disease progression. Repetition is severely impaired, as is naming to confrontation or description, although semantic information about the item which cannot be named may be provided and the correct word can be selected from alternatives: hence this is a problem of lexical access or phonological selection. Verbal fluency is typically better for category than for letter. Reading and writing deficits mirror those in spoken language. Loss of prosody, a telegraphic quality to speech output, and diminution to the point of mutism occur over time.

Perception

Visuoperceptual and visuospatial function is essentially preserved, any errors resulting from linguistic rather than perceptual dysfunction.

Praxis

Praxis is generally intact. Apraxia for symbolic action may emerge in the later stages.

Executive function

Any deficits on tests of executive function may be explicable in terms of language deficits.

REFERENCES

Amici S, Gorno-Tempini ML, Ogar JM, Dronkers NF, Miller BL. An overview on primary progressive aphasia and its variants. *Behav Neurol* 2006; **17**: 77–87.

Boeve BF, Dickson D, Duffy J, *et al*. Progressive nonfluent aphasia and subsequent aphasic dementia associated with atypical progressive supranuclear palsy pathology. *Eur Neurol* 2003; **49**: 72–8.

Doran M, Larner AJ. Monozygotic twins discordant for primary progressive aphasia. *Alzheimer Dis Assoc Disord* 2004; **18**: 48–9.

Duffy JR, Petersen RC. Primary progressive aphasia. *Aphasiology* 1992; **6**: 1–15.

Ferrer I, Hernandez I, Boada M, *et al*. Primary progressive aphasia as the initial manifestation of corticobasal degeneration and unusual tauopathies. *Acta Neuropathol (Berl)* 2003; **106**: 419–35.

Hodges JR, Davies RR, Xuereb JH, *et al*. Clinicopathological correlates in frontotemporal dementia. *Ann Neurol* 2004; **56**: 399–406.

Kertesz A. Primary progressive aphasia. In: Kertesz A, Munoz DG (eds.), *Pick's Disease and Pick Complex*. New York: Wiley-Liss, 1998: 69–81.

Krefft TA, Graff-Radford NR, Dickson DW, Baker M, Castellani RJ. Familial primary progressive aphasia. *Alzheimer Dis Assoc Disord* 2003; **17**: 106–12.

Le Rhun E, Richard F, Pasquier F. Natural history of primary progressive aphasia. *Neurology* 2005; **65**: 887–91.

Mesulam MM. Slowly progressive aphasia without generalized dementia. *Ann Neurol* 1982; **11**: 592–8.

Mesulam MM. Primary progressive aphasia. *Ann Neurol* 2001; **49**: 425–32.

Mesulam MM, Weintraub S. Spectrum of primary progressive aphasia. In: Rossor MN (ed.), *Unusual Dementias*. London: Bailliere Tindall, 1992: 583–609.

Mimura M, Oda T, Tsuchiya K, *et al.* Corticobasal degeneration presenting with nonfluent primary progressive aphasia: a clinicopathological study. *J Neurol Sci* 2001; **183**: 19–26.

Mochizuki A, Ueda Y, Komatsuzaki Y, *et al.* Progressive supranuclear palsy presenting with primary progressive aphasia: clinicopathological report of an autopsy case. *Acta Neuropathol (Berl)* 2003; **105**: 610–14.

Sakurai Y, Hashida H, Uesugi H, *et al.* A clinical profile of corticobasal degeneration presenting as primary progressive aphasia. *Eur Neurol* 1996; **36**: 134–7.

Snowden JS, Neary D, Mann DMA. *Fronto-Temporal Lobar Degeneration: Fronto-Temporal Dementia, Progressive Aphasia, Semantic Dementia.* New York: Churchill Livingstone, 1996: 73–90.

Westbury C, Bub D. Primary progressive aphasia: a review of 112 cases. *Brain Lang* 1997; **60**: 381–406.

2.2.4   Frontotemporal dementia with parkinsonism linked to chromosome 17 (FTDP-17)

Frontotemporal dementia with parkinsonism linked to chromosome 17 (FTDP-17) was the umbrella term coined by Foster *et al.* (1997) to describe autosomal dominant kindreds linked to chromosome 17q21–22 with a highly penetrant clinical phenotype of frontotemporal dementia and parkinsonism (Wilhelmsen *et al.*, 1994). Prior to this, various clinical and clinicopathological labels had been used, including disinhibition–dementia–parkinsonism–amyotrophy complex (DDPAC: Lynch *et al.*, 1994), hereditary dysphasic disinhibition dementia (HDDD: Lendon *et al.*, 1998), pallido-ponto-nigral degeneration (PPND: Wszolek *et al.*, 1992), progressive subcortical gliosis (Lanska *et al.*, 1994), and multiple system tauopathy with presenile dementia (MSTD: Spillantini *et al.*, 1997). Pathogenic mutations in the gene encoding the microtubule-associated protein tau deterministic for FTDP-17 were first described in 1998 (Hutton *et al.*, 1998; Poorkaj *et al.*, 1998; Spillantini *et al.*, 1998), since when around 30 different mutations have been described (Forman *et al.*, 2004; Mann, 2005; see also the Alzheimer Disease and Frontotemporal Dementia Mutation Database,

www.molgen.ua.ac.be/Admutations). More recently, a further genetic mutation has been defined in FTDP families linked to chromosome 17q21 but with normal tau gene sequence, in the gene encoding progranulin (Baker *et al.*, 2006; Cruts *et al.*, 2006)

Clinical and pathological heterogeneity of FTDP-17 cases has become increasingly apparent: in addition to the prototypical behavioural FTD phenotype, cases are also described with the clinical features of progressive supranuclear palsy (PSP: Delisle *et al.*, 1999; Pastor *et al.*, 2001; Wszolek *et al.*, 2001; Morris *et al.*, 2003; Ros *et al.*, 2005), corticobasal degeneration (CBD: Bugiani *et al.*, 1999), idiopathic Parkinson's disease (Pastor *et al.*, 2001), Alzheimer's disease (van Swieten *et al.*, 1999; Mirra *et al.*, 1999; Doran *et al.*, 2007), and respiratory failure (Nicholl *et al.*, 2003), and with the neuropathological features of PSP and CBD (Bird *et al.*, 1999; Nasreddine *et al.*, 1999). Clinical heterogeneity may be observed with the same tau mutation, with presentation as prototypical FTD or with memory deficits mistaken for AD reported with the R406W (van Swieten *et al.*, 1999; Saito *et al.*, 2002) and 10+16 (Janssen *et al.*, 2002; Pickering-Brown *et al.*, 2002; Doran *et al.*, 2007) mutations.

Identification of tau mutation carriers has permitted presymptomatic testing of neuropsychological function, many years before expected disease onset. Asymptomatic members of a large French-Canadian kindred known to carry the P301L tau mutation (Nasreddine *et al.*, 1999) underwent neuropsychological evaluation and mutation screening. Despite similar mean age, age range, gender, and educational level, mutation carriers were impaired in tasks testing frontal executive and attentional functions, such as verbal fluency, Wisconsin Card Sorting Test categories completed, Stroop interference test, WAIS-R similarities and digit span subtests, and Trails B, compared to those without tau mutations. However, verbal and spatial memory, language, and visuo-motor constructive abilities were preserved in the mutation carriers. Hence the deficits in the mutation carriers mirrored those seen at the onset of clinical disease, but many years before the expected age of onset. This observation has raised the possibility that certain brain areas are more vulnerable due to reduced reserve, hence explaining the focal clinical presentation, perhaps indicating a neurodevelopmental component to disease phenotype (Geschwind *et al.*, 2001).

REFERENCES

Baker M, Mackenzie IR, Pickering-Brown SM, *et al.* Mutations in progranulin cause tau-negative frontotemporal dementia linked to chromosome 17. *Nature* 2006; **442**: 916–19.

Bird TD, Nochlin D, Poorkaj P, *et al.* A clinical pathological comparison of three families with frontotemporal dementia and identical mutations in the tau gene (P301L). *Brain* 1999; **122**: 741–56.

Bugiani O, Murrell JR, Giaccone G, *et al.* Frontotemporal dementia and corticobasal degeneration in a family with a P301S mutation in tau. *J Neuropathol Exp Neurol* 1999; **58**: 667–77.

Cruts M, Gijselinck I, van der Zee J, *et al.* Null mutations in progranulin cause ubiquitin-positive frontotemporal dementia linked to chromosome 17q21. *Nature* 2006; **442**: 920–4.

Delisle MB, Murrell JR, Richardson R, *et al.* A mutation at codon 279 (N279K) in exon 10 of the tau gene causes a tauopathy with dementia and supranuclear palsy. *Acta Neuropathol (Berl)* 1999; **98**: 62–77.

Doran M, du Plessis DG, Ghadiali EJ, *et al.* Familial early-onset dementia with tau intron 10+16 mutation with clinical features similar to those of Alzheimer disease. *Arch Neurol* 2007; **64**: 1535–9.

Forman MS, Trojanowski JQ, Lee VMY. Hereditary tauopathies and idiopathic frontotemporal dementias. In: Esiri MM, Trojanowski JQ, Lee VMY (eds.), *The Neuropathology of Dementia* (2nd edition). Cambridge: Cambridge University Press, 2004: 257–88.

Foster NL, Wilhelmsen K, Sima AAF, *et al.* Frontotemporal dementia and parkinsonism linked to chromosome 17: a consensus conference. *Ann Neurol* 1997; **41**: 706–15.

Geschwind DH, Robidoux J, Alarcón M, *et al.* Dementia and neurodevelopmental predisposition: cognitive dysfunction in presymptomatic subjects precedes dementia by decades in frontotemporal dementia. *Ann Neurol* 2001; **50**: 741–6.

Hutton M, Lendon CL, Rizzu P, *et al.* Association of missense and 5′ splice site mutations in tau with the inherited dementia FTDP-17. *Nature* 1998; **393**: 702–5.

Janssen JC, Warrington EK, Morris HR, *et al.* Clinical features of frontotemporal dementia due to the intronic tau 10^{+16} mutation. *Neurology* 2002; **58**: 1161–8.

Lanska DJ, Currier RD, Cohen M, *et al.* Familial progressive subcortical gliosis. *Neurology* 1994; **44**: 1633–43.

Lendon CL, Lynch T, Norton J, *et al.* Hereditary dysphasic disinhibition dementia: a frontotemporal dementia linked to 17q21–22. *Neurology* 1998; **50**: 1546–55.

Lynch T, Sano M, Marder KS, *et al.* Clinical characteristics of a family with chromosome 17-linked disinhibition–dementia–parkinsonism–amyotrophy complex. *Neurology* 1994; **44**: 1878–84.

Mann DMA. The genetics and molecular pathology of frontotemporal lobar degeneration. In: Burns A, O'Brien J, Ames D (eds.), *Dementia* (3rd edition). London: Hodder Arnold, 2005: 689–701.

Mirra SS, Murrell JR, Gearing M, *et al.* Tau pathology in a family with dementia and a P301L mutation in tau. *J Neuropathol Exp Neurol* 1999; **58**: 335–45.

Morris HR, Osaki Y, Holton J, *et al.* Tau exon 10+16 mutation FTDP-17 presenting clinically as sporadic young onset PSP. *Neurology* 2003; **61**: 102–4.

Nasreddine ZS, Loginov M, Clark LN, *et al.* From genotype to phenotype: a clinical, pathological and biochemical investigation of frontotemporal dementia and parkinsonism (FTDP-17) caused by the P301L tau mutation. *Ann Neurol* 1999; **45**: 704–15.

Nicholl DJ, Greenstone MA, Clarke CE, *et al.* An English kindred with a novel recessive tauopathy and respiratory failure. *Ann Neurol* 2003; **54**: 682–6.

Pastor P, Pastor E, Carnero C, *et al.* Familial atypical progressive supranuclear palsy associated with homozygosity for the delN296 mutation in the tau gene. *Ann Neurol* 2001; **49**: 263–7.

Pickering-Brown SM, Richardson AMT, Snowden JS, *et al.* Inherited frontotemporal dementia in nine British families associated with intronic mutations in the tau gene. *Brain* 2002; **125**: 732–51.

Poorkaj P, Bird T, Wijsman E, *et al.* Tau is a candidate gene for chromosome 17 frontotemporal dementia. *Ann Neurol* 1998; **43**: 815–25.

Ros R, Thobois S, Streichenberger N, *et al.* A new mutation of the τ gene, G303V, in early-onset familial progressive supranuclear palsy. *Arch Neurol* 2005; **62**: 1444–50.

Saito Y, Geyer A, Sasaki R, *et al*. Early-onset, rapidly progressive familial tauopathy with R406W mutation. *Neurology* 2002; **58**: 811–13.

Spillantini MG, Goedert M, Crowther RA, *et al*. Familial multiple system tauopathy with presenile dementia: a disease with abundant neuronal and glial tau filaments. *Proc Natl Acad Sci USA* 1997; **94**: 4113–18.

Spillantini MG, Murrell JR, Goedert M, *et al*. Mutation in the tau gene in familial multiple system tauopathy with presenile dementia. *Proc Natl Acad Sci USA* 1998; **95**: 7737–41.

van Swieten JC, Stevens M, Rosso SM, *et al*. Phenotypic variation in hereditary frontotemporal dementia with tau mutations. *Ann Neurol* 1999; **46**: 617–26.

Wilhelmsen KC, Lynch T, Pavlov E, Higgins M, Nygaard TG. Localization of disinhibition–dementia–parkinsonism–amyotrophy complex to 17q21–22. *Am J Hum Genet* 1994; **55**: 1159–65.

Wszolek ZK, Pfeiffer RF, Bhatt MH, *et al*. Rapidly progressive autosomal dominant parkinsonism and dementia with pallido-ponto-nigral degeneration. *Ann Neurol* 1992; **32**: 312–20.

Wszolek ZK, Tsuboi Y, Uitti RJ, *et al*. Progressive supranuclear palsy as a disease phenotype caused by the S305S tau gene mutation. *Brain* 2001; **124**: 1666–70.

2.2.5 Progressive subcortical gliosis (of Neumann)

The term progressive subcortical gliosis (PSG) was first suggested by Neumann and Cohn (1967) to describe a rare dementing disorder with typical histopathological findings, namely frontotemporal atrophy with a distinctive distribution of fibrillary astrogliosis in the superficial and deep cerebral cortical layers, as well as in the subcortical white matter, the latter sometimes extending to the basal ganglia, thalamus, brainstem, and even to the ventral horns of the spinal cord. Amyloid plaques, neurofibrillary tangles, Pick cells, and Pick bodies were not seen. The clinical correlate of these neuropathological findings is variable. Some reported cases have the clinical features of prototypical FTD (Neumann & Cohn, 1967; Vermersch *et al*., 1994; Larner *et al*., 2003), including one family with an underlying tau gene mutation (Petersen *et al*., 1995; Goedert *et al*., 1999) which would now

be classified as FTDP-17. Cases with the phenotype of Alzheimer's disease (Neumann & Cohn, 1967; Lanska *et al*., 1994, 1998), Creutzfeldt–Jakob disease (Seitelberger, 1968; Bergmann *et al*., 1991), and progressive supranuclear palsy (Will *et al*., 1988) have also been reported. The profile of neuropsychological deficits might be anticipated to vary accordingly. Two reports have appeared claiming that PSG is a prion disorder (Petersen *et al*., 1995; Revesz *et al*., 1995), one later retracted (Gambetti, 1997).

REFERENCES

Bergmann M, Gullotta F, Weitbrecht WU. Progressive subkortikale Gliose. *Fortschr Neurol Psychiatr* 1991; **59**: 328–34.

Gambetti P. Prion in progressive subcortical gliosis revisited. *Neurology* 1997; **49**: 309–10.

Goedert M, Spillantini MG, Crowther RA, *et al*. Tau gene mutation in familial progressive subcortical gliosis. *Nature Med* 1999; **5**: 454–7.

Lanska DJ, Currier RD, Cohen M, *et al*. Familial progressive subcortical gliosis. *Neurology* 1994; **44**: 1633–43.

Lanska DJ, Markesbery WR, Cochran E, *et al*. Late-onset sporadic progressive subcortical gliosis. *J Neurol Sci* 1998; **157**: 143–7.

Larner AJ, Smith ETS, Doran M. Does MRI/MRS permit ante mortem diagnosis of progressive subcortical gliosis of Neumann? *J Neurol Neurosurg Psychiatry* 2003; **74**: 404 (abstract 29).

Neumann MA, Cohn R. Progressive subcortical gliosis, a rare form of presenile dementia. *Brain* 1967; **90**: 405–18.

Petersen RB, Tabaton M, Chen SG, *et al*. Familial progressive subcortical gliosis: presence of prions and linkage to chromosome 17. *Neurology* 1995; **45**: 1062–7.

Revesz T, Daniel SE, Lees AJ, Will RG. A case of progressive subcortical gliosis associated with deposition of abnormal prion protein (PrP). *J Neurol Neurosurg Psychiatry* 1995; **58**: 759–60.

Seitelberger F. Präsenile gliale Dystrophie. *Acta Neuropathol (Berl)* 1968; **Suppl 4**: 109–18.

Vermersch P, Daems-Monpeurt C, Parent M, *et al*. Démence sous-corticale type Neumann. Apport de l'imagérie morphologique et fonctionnelle. *Rev Neurol (Paris)* 1994; **150**: 354–8.

Will RG, Lees AJ, Gibb W, Barnard RO. A case of progressive subcortical gliosis presenting clinically as Steele–Richardson–Olszewski syndrome. *J Neurol Neurosurg Psychiatry* 1988; **51**: 1224–7.

2.2.6 Argyrophilic grain disease (AGD)

This condition is defined neuropathologically (Braak & Braak, 1998) by the presence of spindle-shaped argyrophilic grains in neuronal processes and coiled bodies in oligodendrocytes composed of tau protein, mainly in limbic regions (hippocampus, entorhinal and transentorhinal cortices, amygdala). Immunohistochemical and biochemical studies have shown AGD to be a four-repeat (4R) tauopathy, like PSP and CBD and unlike AD (Togo *et al.*, 2002). Macroscopically there is atrophy of frontal and temporal lobes with little or no atrophy of the hippocampus and amygdala, but the clinical phenotype is similar to the limbic dementias such as AD (Tolnay & Clavaguera, 2004). AGD is said to affect 5% of all patients with dementia, particularly the elderly. No, or only sparse, AD pathology is the norm, but concurrence of AD and AGD may lower the threshold for AD-related cognitive deficits (Thal *et al.*, 2005). Because of the tau inclusions and frontotemporal atrophy, AGD may be classified with the FTLDs with tau inclusions.

REFERENCES

Braak H, Braak E. Argyrophilic grain disease: frequency of occurrence in different age categories and neuropathological diagnostic criteria. *J Neural Transm* 1998; **105**: 801–19.

Thal DR, Schultz C, Botez G, *et al.* The impact of argyrophilic grain disease on the development of dementia and its relationship to concurrent Alzheimer's disease-related pathology. *Neuropath Appl Neurobiol* 2005; **31**: 270–9.

Togo T, Sahara N, Yen SH, *et al.* Argyrophilic grain disease is a sporadic 4-repeat tauopathy. *J Neuropathol Exp Neurol* 2002; **61**: 547–56.

Tolnay M, Clavaguera F. Argyrophilic grain disease: a late-onset dementia with distinctive features among tauopathies. *Neuropathology* 2004; **24**: 269–83.

2.2.7 Neurofibrillary tangle dementia (NTD), diffuse neurofibrillary tangles with calcification (DNTC, Kosaka–Shibayama disease)

Neurofibrillary tangle dementia (NTD; senile dementia with tangles) is a form of late-life dementia characterized by medial temporal lobe neurofibrillary tangles and neuropil threads but without amyloid deposits. The clinical correlate is Alzheimer's disease (Ulrich *et al.*, 1992; Bancher & Jellinger, 1994) or frontotemporal dementia (McKhann *et al.*, 2001).

Diffuse neurofibrillary tangles with calcification (DNTC; Kosaka–Shibayama disease), a condition which pathologically resembles NTD, is mostly reported from Japan. It is characterized radiologically by temporal or temporofrontal atrophy, with pallidal and cerebellar calcification typical of that seen in Fahr's syndrome (see Section 5.1.7), and pathologically by neuronal loss, astrocytosis, and neurofibrillary tangles but without senile plaques, features which may be attended by the clinical correlate of a presenile, cortical, dementia (Kosaka, 1994). Cases without dementia have also been reported (Langlois *et al.*, 1995; Kosaka & Ikeda, 1996). The tau pathology seems to comprise a mixture of 3 and 4 repeat isoforms as in AD (Tanabe *et al.*, 2000). Increased brain lead content has also been noted, suggesting the possibility of lead neurotoxicity (Haraguchi *et al.*, 2001). Neuropsychological assessments show decline in memory retention and intelligence, and anomic aphasia (Ito *et al.*, 2003). Reduced blood flow and metabolism in the temporal lobes has been observed on functional imaging, without change in the basal ganglia or cerebellum, suggesting that the calcification and neurodegeneration occur independently (Ito *et al.*, 2003). However, Fahr's syndrome presenting with a pure and progressive dementia has been reported (Modrego *et al.*,

2005), suggesting that brain calcification per se may not be innocuous to cognitive function.

REFERENCES

Bancher C, Jellinger KA. Neurofibrillary tangle predominant form of senile dementia of Alzheimer type: a rare subtype in very old subjects. *Acta Neuropathol (Berl)* 1994; **88**: 565–70.

Haraguchi T, Ishizu H, Takehisa Y, *et al.* Lead content of brain tissue in diffuse neurofibrillary tangles with calcification (DNTC): the possibility of lead neurotoxicity. *Neuroreport* 2001; **12**: 3887–90.

Ito Y, Kato T, Suzuki T, *et al.* Neuroradiologic and clinical abnormalities in dementia of diffuse neurofibrillary tangles with calcification (Kosaka–Shibayama disease). *J Neurol Sci* 2003; **209**: 105–9.

Kosaka K. Diffuse neurofibrillary tangles with calcification: a new presenile dementia. *J Neurol Neurosurg Psychiatry* 1994; **57**: 594–6.

Kosaka K, Ikeda K. Diffuse neurofibrillary tangles with calcification in a non-demented woman. *J Neurol Neurosurg Psychiatry* 1996; **61**: 116.

Langlois NEI, Grieve JHK, Best PV. Changes of diffuse neurofibrillary tangles with calcification (DNTC) in a woman without evidence of dementia. *J Neurol Neurosurg Psychiatry* 1995; **59**: 103.

McKhann GM, Albert MS, Grossman M, *et al.* Clinical and pathological diagnosis of frontotemporal dementia. Report of the Work Group on Frontotemporal Dementia and Pick's disease. *Arch Neurol* 2001; **58**: 1803–9.

Modrego PJ, Mojonero J, Serrano M, Fayed N. Fahr's syndrome presenting with pure and progressive presenile dementia. *Neurol Sci* 2005; **26**: 367–9.

Tanabe Y, Ishizu H, Ishiguro K, *et al.* Tau pathology in diffuse neurofibrillary tangles with calcification (DNTC): biochemical and immunohistochemical investigation. *Neuroreport* 2000; **11**: 2473–7.

Ulrich J, Spillantini MG, Goedert M, *et al.* Abundant neurofibrillary tangles without senile plaques in a subset of patients with senile dementia. *Neurodegeneration* 1992; **1**: 257–84.

2.2.8   Neuronal intermediate filament inclusion disease (NIFID)

This young-onset dementia has a heterogeneous phenotype including features resembling FTD, such as personality change, apathy, disinhibition, blunted affect, memory and language impairments. Neurological features may also be present, including extrapyramidal signs, hyperreflexia, orofacial apraxia, and supranuclear ophthalmoplegia. Neuroimaging and macroscopic pathological examination show frontotemporal atrophy, also involving the caudate nucleus. Neuropathology is typical of FTLDs, with neuronal loss, status spongiosus and gliosis in frontal and temporal cortex, but in addition there are neuronal inclusions of variable morphology containing intermediate filament (IF) proteins, specifically the neurofilament (NF) proteins NF-H, NF-M, and NF-L, and a-internexin, which may also stain with ubiquitin (Bigio *et al.*, 2003; Josephs *et al.*, 2003; Cairns *et al.*, 2004).

REFERENCES

Bigio EH, Lipton AM, White CL III, *et al.* Frontotemporal and motor neurone degeneration with neurofilament inclusion bodies: additional evidence for overlap between FTD and ALS. *Neuropath Appl Neurobiol* 2003; **29**: 239–53.

Cairns NJ, Grossman M, Arnold SE, *et al.* Clinical and neuropathologic variation in neuronal intermediate filament inclusion disease. *Neurology* 2004; **63**: 1376–84.

Josephs KA, Holton JL, Rossor MN, *et al.* Neurofilament inclusion body disease: a new proteinopathy? *Brain* 2003; **126**: 2291–303.

2.2.9   Basophilic inclusion body disease (BIBD)

Cases with basophilic inclusion bodies may present as juvenile or adult cases of FTD or MND or a combination of both. There is frontotemporal atrophy, with otherwise typical histopathological findings of FTLDs (neuronal loss, status spongiosus, gliosis). The inclusions, which do not stain for tau, a-synuclein, or neuronal intermediate filament proteins, involve not only the superficial laminae of the neocortex but also subcortical nuclei and anterior horns of the spinal cord, but with sparing of the hippocampus and dentate gyrus. Typical pathological findings of MND are not seen (Hamada *et al.*, 1995).

REFERENCES

Hamada K, Fukuzawa T, Yanagihara T, *et al.* Dementia with ALS features and diffuse Pick body-like inclusions (atypical Pick's disease?). *Clin Neuropathol* 1995; **14**: 1–6.

2.3 Motor neurone disease (MND), amyotrophic lateral sclerosis (ALS)

Traditionally it was taught that motor neurone disease (MND) or amyotrophic lateral sclerosis (ALS) was a disorder confined to the motor system, in which the intellect was preserved, and hence patients were all too horribly aware of their progressive neurological predicament. Certainly the earliest description, by Charcot and Joffroy (1869), has no mention of cognitive changes. Alzheimer may have reported a case of MND with dementia in 1891, but it was not until the later part of the twentieth century that definitive cases of MND with concurrent dementia of frontal type were presented (Hudson, 1981; Mitsuyama, 1984; Neary *et al.*, 1990; Snowden *et al.*, 1996).

The view of MND as an exclusively motor disorder has been increasingly eroded, initially by occasional clinical reports both of cognitive impairment in MND patients and of frontotemporal dementia (FTD) complicated by the development of MND, and latterly by more systematic studies suggesting that significant numbers of MND patients, up to 50%, have cognitive deficits when tested, sometimes sufficient to meet diagnostic criteria for FTD (Strong *et al.*, 1999; Lomen-Hoerth *et al.*, 2003; Ringholz *et al.*, 2005), whilst neurophysiological investigation of FTD patients has found evidence for subclinical anterior horn cell disease in some (Lomen-Hoerth *et al.*, 2002). Now FTD and MND are thought to represent a spectrum condition, with pure cognitive and pure motor cases at the boundaries but with

extensive overlap (Bak & Hodges, 2001; Yoshida, 2004; Mackenzie & Feldman, 2005; Strong, 2006).

Clinical diagnostic criteria (McKhann *et al.*, 2001) recognize a syndrome of frontotemporal lobar degeneration with motor neurone disease (FTLD-MND), also known as FTD-MND, MND dementia, or ALS dementia, defined by the neuropathological appearances of frontotemporal neuronal loss and gliosis with ubiquitin-positive tau-negative (MND-type) inclusions without detectable amounts of insoluble tau and with the clinical correlate of MND. Similar neuropathological findings may occur without the clinical correlate of MND, a syndrome known as frontotemporal lobar degeneration with MND-type inclusions but without MND (McKhann *et al.*, 2001) or motor neurone disease inclusion dementia (MNDID: Jackson *et al.*, 1995), or FTD-U. This may be the commonest neuropathological correlate of FTD, accounting for 38% of cases (25/76) in the largest consecutive series of pathologically confirmed FTD cases reported to date (Lipton *et al.*, 2004). Alzheimer type pathology, principally plaques, has been reported in some cases of MND both with and without dementia (Hamilton & Bowser, 2004), whilst both neuritic plaques and neurofibrillary tangles typical of AD but sparing the hippocampus and entorhinal cortex were found in one patient with a clinical presentation of bulbar MND with rapidly progressive aphasia, another patient having numerous cortical Lewy bodies in addition to frontotemporal neuronal loss and spongiosus (Doran *et al.*, 1995).

Clinical heterogeneity is noted in these cases, with presentations encompassing isolated cognitive disorder, contemporaneous cognitive and motor disorder, and isolated motor disorder. In series reported from cognitive neurology clinics, cognitive impairment is noted to precede or coincide with the onset of motor symptoms, but this may of course reflect selection bias (Bak & Hodges, 2001; Sathasivam *et al.*, 2007). Dementia preceding motor disorder has been reported (Vercelletto *et al.*, 1999). The clinical phenotype may also encompass cases fulfilling diagnostic criteria for frontal variant FTD (Godbolt *et al.*, 2005), semantic dementia (Davies *et al.*, 2005; Godbolt *et al.*, 2005), corticobasal degeneration (Grimes *et al.*, 1999), and progressive supranuclear palsy (Morris *et al.*, 2005; Sathasivam *et al.*, 2007), diagnosis only becoming apparent at postmortem in some of these cases. Thalamic dementia complicating MND has been reported (Deymeer *et al.*, 1989).

Genetic linkage of familial FTD-MND to chromosome 9q21–22 has been reported (Hosler *et al.*, 2000), and in one family with cases of both FTD and MND a missense mutation has been identified in the dynactin gene located on chromosome 9q (Munch *et al.*, 2005), although other families are described without linkage to this locus (Ostojic *et al.*, 2003). Pathogenetic mechanisms remain uncertain, but a role for apoptosis, as suggested in MND (Sathasivam & Shaw, 2005), is possible.

Other conditions potentially relevant to the cognitive disorder of MND/ALS include the amyotrophic lateral sclerosis/parkinsonism–dementia complex of Guam (see Section 2.4.6).

Neuropsychological profile

The neuropsychological deficits of MND are summarized in Table 2.5.

Attention
As in fvFTD, economy of effort, impulsiveness, and distractibility may characterize test performance, poor sustained attention compromising test results (Neary *et al.*, 1990; Snowden *et al.*, 1996).

General intelligence, IQ
Performance may be impaired on the WAIS-R, sometimes in all areas, due to underlying executive dysfunction.

Memory
Formal tests of memory, both verbal and visual, may show impaired scores but patients are not amnesic, as reflected in their knowledge of autobiographical events and orientation in time and place, as in FTD.

Language
The frequency of language disorder in MND is uncertain, since concurrent dysarthria may mask language dysfunction unless appropriate tests are used. Bulbar MND with rapidly progressive aphasia has been reported (Kirshner *et al.*, 1987; Caselli *et al.*, 1993; Doran *et al.*, 1995). Marked anomia on picture naming, naming from verbal descriptions, and letter and category verbal fluency may be observed, indicating a disorder of language production, but with additional impairments on syntactically based tasks of language comprehension (Token Test, Test for the Reception of Grammar) and picture–word matching tests of semantic comprehension (Doran *et al.*, 1995). Rakowicz & Hodges (1998) found a subgroup of MND patients with language dysfunction characterized by word-finding difficulties and decreased verbal fluency, and Bak and Hodges (1997) found greater difficulty in confrontation naming of verbs than nouns.

Perception
As in FTD, there is no evidence for visual perceptual disorder in MND, with preserved spatial navigational skills, spatial localization, and orientation, which may be confirmed on tests such as dot counting and maze tracking. Poor performance on tests of drawing may result from lack of planning or strategy or motor deficits rather than from visual perceptual impairment.

Praxis
Impaired temporal sequencing of motor skills may be apparent, reflecting executive dysfunction.

Executive function
Frontal lobe dysfunction is evident on neuropsychological testing, without which it may be overlooked clinically (David & Gillham, 1986; Gallassi *et al.*, 1989; Ludolph *et al.*, 1992; Kew *et al.*, 1993; Talbot *et al.*, 1995; Abrahams *et al.*, 1997; Evdokimidis *et al.*, 2002), in between one-fifth and one-third of non-demented MND patients (Massman *et al.*, 1996; Lomen-Hoerth *et al.*, 2003; Ringholz *et al.*, 2005). There are

Table 2.5. Neuropsychological deficits in motor neurone disease (MND).

Attention	↓ Sustained attention; economy of effort, impulsiveness, distractibility
General intelligence, IQ	FSIQ may be normal or ↓ due to executive dysfunction
Memory	Not amnesic, but scores may be down due to executive dysfunction
Language	+/− aphasia (may be masked by dysarthria); anomia, ↓ verbal fluency
Perception	Essentially intact
Praxis	Impaired temporal sequencing secondary to executive dysfunction
Executive function	Impaired; ↓ verbal fluency, card sorting

impairments on the Wisconsin Card Sorting Test with perseverations, Weigl's Block Test, verbal and design fluency, and WAIS-R Picture Arrangement. These deficits may be more common in patients with predominantly upper motor neurone signs (Iwasaki *et al.*, 1990), including primary lateral sclerosis (see Section 2.3.1), and in patients with predominantly bulbar involvement (Talbot *et al.*, 1995; Abrahams *et al.*, 1997; Schreiber *et al.*, 2005).

REFERENCES

Abrahams S, Goldstein LH, Al-Chalabi A, *et al.* Relation between cognitive dysfunction and pseudobulbar palsy in amyotrophic lateral sclerosis. *J Neurol Neurosurg Psychiatry* 1997; **62**: 464–72.

Alzheimer A. On a case of spinal progressive muscle atrophy with accessory disease of bulbar nuclei and the cortex [in German]. *Arch Psychiatr* 1891; **23**: 459–85.

Bak T, Hodges JR. Noun–verb dissociation in three patients with motor neurone disease and aphasia. *Brain Lang* 1997; **60**: 38–41.

Bak TH, Hodges JR. Motor neurone disease, dementia and aphasia: coincidence, co-occurrence or continuum? *J Neurol* 2001; **248**: 260–70.

Caselli RJ, Windebank AJ, Petersen RC, *et al.* Rapidly progressive aphasic dementia and motor neuron disease. *Ann Neurol* 1993; **33**: 200–7.

Charcot JM, Joffroy A. Deux cas d'atrophie musculaire progressive avec lésions de la substance grise et des faisceaux antérolatéraux de la moelle épinière. *Arch Physiol Norm* 1869; **2**: 354–67.

David AS, Gillham RA. Neuropsychological study of motor neuron disease. *Psychosomatics* 1986; **27**: 441–5.

Davies RR, Hodges JR, Kril JJ, *et al.* The pathological basis of semantic dementia. *Brain* 2005; **128**: 1984–95.

Deymeer F, Smith TW, De Girolami U, Drachman DA. Thalamic dementia and motor neuron disease. *Neurology* 1989; **39**: 58–61.

Doran M, Xuereb J, Hodges JR. Rapidly progressive aphasia with bulbar motor neurone disease: a clinical and neuropsychological study. *Behav Neurol* 1995; **9**: 169–80.

Evdokimidis I, Constantinidis TS, Gourtzelidis P, *et al.* Frontal lobe dysfunction in amyotrophic lateral sclerosis. *J Neurol Sci* 2002; **195**: 25–33.

Gallassi R, Montagna P, Morreale A, *et al.* Neuropsychological, electroencephalogram and brain computed tomography findings in motor neuron disease. *Eur Neurol* 1989; **29**: 115–20.

Godbolt AK, Josephs KA, Revesz T, *et al.* Sporadic and familial dementia with ubiquitin-positive tau-negative inclusions: clinical features of one histopathological abnormality underlying frontotemporal lobar degeneration. *Arch Neurol* 2005; **62**: 1097–101.

Grimes DA, Bergeron CB, Lang AE. Motor neuron disease-inclusion dementia presenting as cortical-basal ganglionic degeneration. *Mov Disord* 1999; **14**: 674–80.

Hamilton RL, Bowser R. Alzheimer disease pathology in amyotrophic lateral sclerosis. *Acta Neuropathol* 2004; **107**: 515–22.

Hosler BA, Siddique T, Sapp PC, *et al.* Linkage of familial amyotrophic lateral sclerosis with frontotemporal dementia to chromosome 9q21–q22. *JAMA* 2000; **284**: 1664–9.

Hudson AJ. Amyotrophic lateral sclerosis and its association with dementia, parkinsonism and other neurological disorders: a review. *Brain* 1981; **104**: 217–47.

Iwasaki K, Kinoshita M, Ikeda K, *et al.* Cognitive impairment in amyotrophic lateral sclerosis and its relation to motor disabilities. *Acta Neurol Scand* 1990; **81**: 141–3.

Jackson M, Lennox G, Lowe J. Motor neurone disease-inclusion dementia. *Neurodegeneration* 1995; **5**: 339–50.

Kew JJM, Goldstein LH, Leigh PN, *et al*. The relationship between abnormalities of cognitive function and cerebral activation in amyotrophic lateral sclerosis: a neuropsychological and positron emission tomography study. *Brain* 1993; **116**: 1399–423.

Kirshner HS, Tanridag O, Thurman L, Whetsell WO. Progressive aphasia without dementia: two cases with focal spongiform degeneration. *Ann Neurol* 1987; **22**: 527–32.

Lipton AM, White CL III, Bigio EH. Frontotemporal lobar degeneration with motor neuron disease-type inclusions predominates in 76 cases of frontotemporal degeneration. *Acta Neuropathol (Berl)* 2004; **108**: 379–85.

Lomen-Hoerth C, Anderson T, Miller B. The overlap of amyotrophic lateral sclerosis and frontotemporal dementia. *Neurology* 2002; **59**: 1077–9.

Lomen-Hoerth C, Murphy J, Langmore S, *et al*. Are amyotrophic lateral sclerosis patients cognitively normal? *Neurology* 2003; **60**: 1094–7.

Ludolph AC, Langen KJ, Regard M, *et al*. Frontal lobe function in amyotrophic lateral sclerosis: a neuropsychologic and positron emission tomography study. *Acta Neurol Scand* 1992; **85**: 81–9.

McKhann GM, Albert MS, Grossman M, *et al*. Clinical and pathological diagnosis of frontotemporal dementia. Report of the Work Group on Frontotemporal Dementia and Pick's disease. *Arch Neurol* 2001; **58**: 1803–9.

Mackenzie IRA, Feldman HH. Ubiquitin immunohistochemistry suggests classic motor neuron disease, motor neuron disease with dementia, and frontotemporal dementia of the motor neuron disease type represent a clinicopathologic spectrum. *J Neuropathol Exp Neurol* 2005; **64**: 730–9.

Massman PJ, Sims J, Cooke N, *et al*. Prevalence and correlates of neuropsychological deficits in amyotrophic lateral sclerosis. *J Neurol Neurosurg Psychiatry* 1996; **61**: 450–5.

Mitsuyama Y. Presenile dementia with motor neuron disease in Japan: a clinico-pathological review of 26 cases. *J Neurol Neurosurg Psychiatry* 1984; **47**: 953–9.

Morris HR, Bronstein AM, Shaw CE, Lees AJ, Love S. Clinical grand round: a rapidly progressive pyramidal and extrapyramidal syndrome with a supranuclear gaze palsy. *Mov Disord* 2005; **20**: 826–31.

Munch C, Rosenbohm A, Sperfeld AD, *et al*. Heterozygous R1101K mutation of the DCTN1 gene in a family with ALS and FTD. *Ann Neurol* 2005; **58**: 777–80.

Neary D, Snowden JS, Mann DMA, *et al*. Frontal lobe dementia and motor neuron disease. *J Neurol Neurosurg Psychiatry* 1990; **53**: 23–32.

Ostojic J, Axelman K, Lannfelt L, Froelich-Fabre S. No evidence of linkage to chromosome 9q21–22 in a Swedish family with frontotemporal dementia and amyotrophic lateral sclerosis. *Neurosci Lett* 2003; **340**: 245–7.

Rakowicz WP, Hodges JR. Dementia and aphasia in motor neuron disease: an underrecognised association? *J Neurol Neurosurg Psychiatry* 1998; **65**: 881–9.

Ringholz GM, Appel SH, Bradshaw M, *et al*. Prevalence and patterns of cognitive impairment in sporadic ALS. *Neurology* 2005; **65**: 586–90.

Sathasivam S, Doran M, Hancock P, Larner AJ. Frontotemporal lobar degeneration with motor neuron disease (FTLD/MND): experience at a cognitive function clinic. *J Neurol Neurosurg Psychiatry* 2007; **78**: 211 (abstract 027).

Sathasivam S, Shaw PJ. Apoptosis in amyotrophic lateral sclerosis: what is the evidence? *Lancet Neurol* 2005; **4**: 500–9.

Schreiber H, Gaigalat T, Wiedemuth-Catrinescu U, *et al*. Cognitive function in bulbar- and spinal-onset amyotrophic lateral sclerosis: a longitudinal study in 52 patients. *J Neurol* 2005; **252**: 772–81.

Snowden JS, Neary D, Mann DMA. *Fronto-Temporal Lobar Degeneration: Fronto-Temporal Dementia, Progressive Aphasia, Semantic Dementia*. New York: Churchill Livingstone, 1996: 59–72.

Strong MJ (ed.). *Dementia and Motor Neuron Disease*. Abingdon: Informa Healthcare, 2006.

Strong MJ, Grace GM, Orange JB, *et al*. A prospective study of cognitive impairment in ALS. *Neurology* 1999; **53**: 1665–70.

Talbot PR, Goulding PJ, Lloyd JJ, *et al*. Interrelation between 'classic' motor neuron disease and frontotemporal dementia: neuropsychological and single photon emission computed tomography study. *J Neurol Neurosurg Psychiatry* 1995; **58**: 541–7.

Vercelletto M, Ronin M, Huvet M, Magne C, Feve JR. Frontal type dementia preceding amyotrophic lateral sclerosis: a neuropsychological and SPECT study of five clinical cases. *Eur J Neurol* 1999; **6**: 295–9.

Yoshida M. Amyotrophic lateral sclerosis with dementia: the clinicopathological spectrum. *Neuropathology* 2004; **24**: 87–102.

2.3.1 Primary lateral sclerosis (PLS), progressive symmetric spinobulbar spasticity

Primary lateral sclerosis (PLS) is a rare variant of MND characterized by progressive spinobulbar spasticity. This is thought to result from isolated involvement of upper motor neurones in the precentral gyrus with secondary pyramidal tract degeneration, without either clinical or neurophysiological evidence of lower motor neurone involvement (Pringle *et al.*, 1992; Grace *et al.*, 2006). Suggested diagnostic criteria require such isolated involvement to persist over a period of at least 3 years (Pringle *et al.*, 1992), PLS tending to pursue a more benign course than typical MND.

Studies of PLS in which cognitive testing was not undertaken concluded that the intellect was preserved (Pringle *et al.*, 1992). However more systematic, albeit retrospective, studies in small cohorts have suggested that mild cognitive dysfunction of frontal lobe type is present in PLS, with deficits in executive function, psychomotor speed, and memory, but with normal orientation, spatial skills, and language (Caselli *et al.*, 1995; Le Forestier *et al.*, 2001; Piquard *et al.*, 2006). A prospective study of neuropsychological function using a broad battery of tests in 18 PLS patients found heterogeneity, but cognitive impairment according to the definitions of the study was present in 11 patients (61%). Verbal fluency was the most sensitive test, but impairment was also noted on tests of auditory verbal learning, visual (but not verbal) recognition memory, and the Wisconsin Card Sorting Test. Language testing showed impaired category verbal fluency, specifically for non-living as opposed to living items. These findings overlap with those documented in MND, whereas others do not, such as the finding that confrontation naming of nouns and verbs was relatively intact (Grace *et al.*, 2006).

REFERENCES

Caselli RJ, Smith BE, Osborne D. Primary lateral sclerosis: a neuropsychological study. *Neurology* 1995; **45**: 2005–9.

Grace GM, Orange JB, Murphy MJ, *et al.* Primary lateral sclerosis: cognitive, language, and cerebral hemodynamic findings. In: Strong MJ (ed.), *Dementia and Motor Neuron Disease*. Abingdon: Informa Healthcare, 2006: 87–97.

Le Forestier N, Maisonobe T, Piquard A, *et al.* Does primary lateral sclerosis exist? A study of 20 patients and a review of the literature. *Brain* 2001; **124**: 1989–99.

Piquard A, Le Forestier N, Baudoin-Madec V, *et al.* Neuropsychological changes in patients with primary lateral sclerosis. *Amyotroph Lateral Scler* 2006; **7**: 150–60.

Pringle CE, Hudson AJ, Munoz DG, *et al.* Primary lateral sclerosis: clinical features, neuropathology and diagnostic criteria. *Brain* 1992; **115**: 495–520.

2.3.2 Mills' syndrome

A syndrome of progressive ascending or descending hemiplegia without significant sensory involvement was first reported by Mills (1900). Its nosological status has been uncertain, but some cases may be hemiplegic forms of motor neurone disease with exclusively upper motor neurone signs (Malin *et al.*, 1986; Gastaut & Bartolomei, 1994), although this clinical picture falls outwith proposed diagnostic criteria for primary lateral sclerosis (Pringle *et al.*, 1992). A case of progressive spastic hemiplegia conforming to the description of Mills' syndrome with concurrent dementia of frontotemporal type, with pathological confirmation of ubiquitin-positive motor neurone disease type inclusions in layer II cortical neurones, hippocampal dentate granule cells, and hypoglossal nerve nucleus neurones, has been reported (Doran *et al.*, 2005).

REFERENCES

Doran M, Enevoldson TP, Ghadiali EJ, Larner AJ. Mills syndrome with dementia: broadening the phenotype of FTD/MND. *J Neurol* 2005; **252**: 846–7.

Gastaut JL, Bartolomei F. Mills' syndrome: ascending (or descending) progressive hemiplegia. A hemiplegic form of primary lateral sclerosis? *J Neurol Neurosurg Psychiatry* 1994; **57**: 1280–1.

Malin JP, Poburski R, Reusche E. Clinical variants of amyotrophic lateral sclerosis: hemiplegic type of ALS and Mills syndrome. A critical review [in German]. *Fortschr Neurol Psychiatr* 1986; **54**: 101–5.

Mills CK. A case of unilateral progressive ascending paralysis probably presenting a new form of degenerative disease. *J Nerv Ment Dis* 1900; **27**: 195–200.

Pringle CE, Hudson AJ, Munoz DG, *et al.* Primary lateral sclerosis: clinical features, neuropathology and diagnostic criteria. *Brain* 1992; **115**: 495–520.

2.3.3 Hippocampal sclerosis, pure hippocampal sclerosis

This condition was initially defined on neuropathological grounds, specifically by neuronal loss in the CA1 region of the hippocampus, in association with the neuroradiological signature of hippocampal atrophy and the clinical correlate of dementia (Corey-Bloom *et al.*, 1997; Ala *et al.*, 2000; Leverenz *et al.*, 2002). Clinical overlap with AD was initially emphasized, but more recently many cases have been reclassified as a subtype of FTD based on the neuropathological finding of tau-negative ubiquitin-positive inclusions typical of MND-inclusion dementia (Hatanpaa *et al.*, 2004), and the overlap of clinical and neuropsychological features with FTD (Blass *et al.*, 2004). Specifically, decreased grooming, inappropriate behaviour, decreased interest, and hyperorality were observed, with most patients meeting diagnostic criteria (McKhann *et al.*, 2001) for FTD. However, other authors have not found the core neuropathological features of FTD (prefrontal neuronal loss, microvacuolation, gliosis) in hippocampal sclerosis brains (McKeel *et al.*, 2007).

REFERENCES

Ala T, Beh GO, Frey WM II. Pure hippocampal sclerosis: a rare cause of dementia mimicking Alzheimer's disease. *Neurology* 2000; **54**: 843–8.

Blass DM, Hatanpaa KJ, Brandt J, *et al.* Dementia in hippocampal sclerosis resembles frontotemporal dementia more than Alzheimer disease. *Neurology* 2004; **63**: 492–7.

Corey-Bloom J, Sabbagh MN, Bondi MW, *et al.* Hippocampal sclerosis contributes to dementia in the elderly. *Neurology* 1997; **48**: 154–60.

Hatanpaa KJ, Blass DM, Pletnikova O, *et al.* Most cases of dementia with hippocampal sclerosis may represent frontotemporal dementia. *Neurology* 2004; **63**: 538–42.

Leverenz JB, Agustin CM, Tsuang D, *et al.* Clinical and neuropathological characteristics of hippocampal sclerosis: a community-based study. *Arch Neurol* 2002; **59**: 1099–106.

McKeel DW Jr, Burns JM, Meuser TM, Morris JC. *An Atlas of Investigation and Diagnosis: Dementia*. Oxford: Clinical Publishing, 2007: 172.

McKhann GM, Albert MS, Grossman M, *et al.* Clinical and pathological diagnosis of frontotemporal dementia. Report of the Work Group on Frontotemporal Dementia and Pick's disease. *Arch Neurol* 2001; **58**: 1803–9.

2.3.4 Progressive muscular atrophy (PMA)

Variants of MND with a clinical phenotype of exclusively lower motor neurone involvement, progressive muscular atrophy (PMA), are rare, and may be even rarer if neuropathological findings are taken into account. One study of 12 PMA patients found no significant difference between subjects and healthy controls on any measure of cognitive, behavioural, or emotional function (Wicks *et al.*, 2006). Further support for the contention that exclusively or predominantly lower motor neurone involvement is not associated with cognitive decline comes from a patient with the flail arm syndrome, symmetrical wasting and weakness of the arms with minimal leg or bulbar involvement at clinical presentation (Hu *et al.*, 1998), also known as the Vulpian–Bernhardt syndrome. A 73-year-old man with flail arm syndrome had no complaints of memory problems 4 years into his illness, and scored 79 on the ACE-R (see Section 1.8.4) out of a possible 88, omitting those sections dependent on upper limb function (90%), above the test cutoff excluding dementia (Larner, unpublished observations).

REFERENCES

Hu MTM, Ellis CM, Al-Chalabi A, Leigh PN, Shaw CE. Flail arm syndrome: a distinctive variant of amyotrophic lateral sclerosis. *J Neurol Neurosurg Psychiatry* 1998; **65**: 950–1.

Wicks P, Abrahams S, Leigh PN, Williams T, Goldstein LH. Absence of cognitive, behavioural, or emotional dysfunction in progressive muscular atrophy. *Neurology* 2006; **67**: 1718–19.

2.4 Parkinson's disease dementia (PDD) and dementia with Lewy bodies (DLB)

In his 1817 account of the disease which later, courtesy of Charcot, would bear his name, James Parkinson stated that intellect was uninjured (a facsimile of Parkinson's book on the shaking palsy is included in Gardner-Thorpe, 1987). Charcot (1875) pointed out that this was not, in fact, the case, and that 'psychic faculties are definitely impaired' and that 'the mind becomes clouded and the memory is lost.'

It is now generally recognized that Parkinson's disease (PD) is more than simply a motor disorder, and that cognitive impairments are common, progressing in some patients to dementia (Starkstein & Merello, 2002). Although this was not reflected in the staging scale for PD developed by Hoehn and Yahr (1967), which referred to motor symptoms only, the broader Unified Parkinson's Disease Rating Scale (UPDRS) does encompass intellectual function. The motor stages of PD do not correlate well with cognitive symptoms (Mortimer *et al.*, 1982).

The exact frequency of Parkinson's disease dementia (PDD) is still debated, with widely divergent figures being reported in different populations and using different criteria for dementia diagnosis (Brown & Marsden, 1984). (There is a possibility that other parkinsonian disorders, which may also be accompanied by cognitive decline, may be mistaken for PD: Stocchi & Brusa, 2000; see Section 2.4.1.) As the prevalence of PD increases with age, the possibility that cognitive impairment reflects concurrent Alzheimer's disease (AD) must also be taken into account, as must concurrent depression and the effects of drugs used in PD treatment (dopaminergic agonists, anticholinergic medications). Furthermore, performance on cognitive tests which are

time-limited or which require motor skills may be impaired in PD because of the motor disorder rather than cognitive impairment per se.

Age, rather than age at onset, is a risk factor for PDD, and symptoms such as rigidity, speech, gait, and postural disorders are related to subsequent development of dementia whereas tremor-dominant disease is not (Starkstein & Merello, 2002; Emre, 2003; Aarsland, 2006). Classically, PDD has been labelled as a subcortical dementia in distinction to the cortical dementia of AD. Cognitive deficits may be found in non-demented PD patients, intermediate between normal and PDD (Goldman *et al.*, 1998), and indeed these may be present in as many as one-third of newly diagnosed PD patients (Foltynie *et al.*, 2004).

The pathological hallmark of PD is the finding of Lewy bodies, intracytoplasmic rounded eosinophilic inclusions in brainstem monoaminergic and cholinergic neurones. The finding of similar structures in the neocortex of patients with dementia and parkinsonism, often with concurrent AD-type pathology, led to the delineation of a syndrome under a variety of names, such as cortical Lewy body disease, senile dementia of the Lewy body type, and the Lewy body variant of Alzheimer's disease. All these entities are now subsumed under the rubric of dementia with Lewy bodies (DLB: O'Brien *et al.*, 2006). A distinction is sometimes drawn between cases with pathological evidence of concurrent AD and Lewy body pathology, labelled Lewy body variant (LBV), and those without significant concomitant AD pathology, labelled diffuse Lewy body disease (DLBD: Hansen *et al.*, 1990). The positive immunostaining of Lewy bodies in both PD and DLB with α-synuclein indicates that both disorders fall into the category of synucleinopathies. Lewy body pathology is also common, if sought, in AD caused by mutations in the presenilin-1 gene, suggesting other possible genetic influences on the development of synuclein-related pathology (Leverenz *et al.*, 2006). Lewy body pathology may also be found in some cases of Gaucher's disease (see Section 5.5.3).

Clinical and pathological diagnostic criteria for DLB have been developed and validated (McKeith *et al.*, 1996, 1999, 2000a, 2005). The central clinical feature is progressive cognitive decline with prominent deficits in attention, visuospatial abilities, and executive function, along with a number of other core features which are essential for diagnosis of probable (two features) or possible (one feature) DLB, namely fluctuating cognition with pronounced variations in attention (the 'unstable platform of attention'), recurrent visual hallucinations, and spontaneous motor features of parkinsonism. A number of other features may support the diagnosis, including marked neuroleptic sensitivity (McKeith *et al.*, 1992) and syncopal episodes. Autonomic dysfunction when sought is reported to be common (Horimoto *et al.*, 2003), and cases of DLB 'evolving' from pure autonomic failure have been reported (Larner *et al.*, 2000; Kaufmann *et al.*, 2004). Greater impairment of attentional and visuospatial function and relative preservation of memory function is seen in DLB as compared to AD (Salmon *et al.*, 1996; Downes *et al.*, 1998; Ballard *et al.*, 1999; Calderon *et al.*, 2001).

What is the relationship between PDD and DLB? A number of possibilities exist (Aarsland, 2006), including distinct diseases, part of a spectrum of dementia related to cortical Lewy body disease, or part of a spectrum of Lewy body and AD pathology. Examination of many PD cases has demonstrated a characteristic pattern of topographical progression of Lewy body changes extending from brainstem to cortex (Braak *et al.*, 2003), supporting the notion of a spectrum disorder, which may also extend to Lewy body involvement of spinal autonomic ganglia (Ince *et al.*, 1998). An arbitrary 1-year rule is sometimes used to distinguish PDD from DLB, i.e. onset of dementia within 1 year of parkinsonism is labelled DLB, whilst more than 1 year of parkinsonism before dementia develops equals PDD. Since there is no clear neuropathological distinction between PDD and DLB, and the clinical boundaries may be blurred, both are dealt with here, assuming them to reflect similar biological processes, both being neurodegenerative disorders with diffuse cortical Lewy bodies (Fleisher & Olichney, 2005; Galvin *et al.*, 2006). Cognitive status seems to correlate with neuropathological staging (Braak *et al.*, 2005).

Cases fulfilling diagnostic criteria for DLB have been reported in patients carrying point mutations in the *a*-synuclein gene (E46K: Zarranz *et al.*, 2004), a recognized but rare cause of genetically determined PD, and in some patients with triplication of the *a*-synuclein gene (Singleton *et al.*, 2003). Likewise, DLB has been reported in occasional patients with mutations in the presenilin-1 gene (ΔT440: Ishikawa *et al.*, 2005) and the prion protein gene (PRNP M232R: Koide *et al.*, 2002). Other disorders which may mimic or be confused with DLB, and hence lead to confounding in defining the neuropsychological profile, include CJD (Doran & Larner, 2004; Kraemer *et al.*, 2005; du Plessis & Larner, 2008) and vascular dementia.

Neuropsychological profile

Table 2.6 summarizes the neuropsychological deficits typical of DLB, described in more detail below.

Attention
The basal ganglia are implicated in the regulation of attention (Brown & Marsden, 1998). There is evidence that PD patients disengage from attended locations more readily, have less effective mechanisms for resisting interference, and have difficulties establishing a new target of attention (Dujardin *et al.*, 1999a). Tests of working memory in PD have shown deficits, with spatial working memory apparently more vulnerable than verbal or visual working memory, which are affected later in the disease course (Owen *et al.*, 1997). Bradyphrenia, a slowness of thought or prolonged information processing time, is said to be a cardinal feature of subcortical dementias, in PD perhaps paralleling the motor slowing (bradykinesia). However, if motor slowing is controlled for, then cognitive slowing does not seem to be a feature of PD (Rafal *et al.*, 1984; Smith *et al.*, 1998). Concurrent depression or mild dementia may also account, perhaps in part, for bradyphrenia.

Table 2.6. Neuropsychological deficits in dementia with Lewy bodies (DLB).

Attention	Prominent deficits: 'unstable platform of attention'; difficulty establishing attentional focus, easy disengagement; bradyphrenia; impaired spatial working memory; fluctuating consciousness
General intelligence, IQ	FSIQ ↓, PIQ worse than VIQ, possibly related to executive dysfunction
Memory	Subcortical pattern of impairment, recognition better than recall
Language	Relatively intact; verbal fluency may be impaired (?phonemic > category)
Perception	Prominent deficits of visuoperceptual and visuospatial function
Praxis	Possible ideomotor apraxia
Executive function	Prominent deficits: impaired; ↓ verbal fluency, card sorting

Fluctuating consciousness, clinically distinguishable from delirium, is one of the core features of DLB, as noted in early clinical descriptions (e.g. Gibb *et al.*, 1987; Burkhardt *et al.*, 1988; Byrne *et al.*, 1989) and enshrined in diagnostic criteria (McKeith *et al.*, 1996, 1999). This may lead to marked variability in performance on cognitive testing both within and between testing sessions. The clinical diagnosis of fluctuating consciousness correlates with psychophysiological measures of variable attentional performance (Walker *et al.*, 2000). This 'unstable platform of attention' may account for the observed impairments in attentional, mnemonic, and executive functions. Impairments of attention may be demonstrated using the WAIS-R Digit Span subtest (Hansen *et al.*, 1990) and on complex set-shifting tasks examining shifts of attention (Saghal *et al.*, 1992). Subtypes of fluctuating cognition which differentiate DLB from AD include daytime drowsiness and lethargy, daytime sleep > 2 hours, staring into space for long periods, and episodes of disorganized speech (Ferman *et al.*, 2004).

General intelligence, IQ
Performance may be impaired on the WAIS-R, for example in Digit Span and Similarities subtests. There may be better verbal IQ than performance IQ. On the MMSE, visuospatial and attentional tests may be more impaired and memory relatively preserved (Ala *et al.*, 2002).

Memory
There is relatively less impairment of memory in PD/PDD/DLB than of visuospatial and executive functions (Ala *et al.*, 2002), but nonetheless memory is not normal. There is impairment of both recent and remote memory in PD, with recognition better than recall consistent with a retrieval deficit typical of impaired subcortical processes. Retrieval difficulties may reflect the prominent executive dysfunction, with impaired allocation of attentional resources for effortful free recall tasks and the formulation of retrieval strategies (Ivory *et al.*, 1999). Registration, storage, and consolidation of memory may be intact (Pillon *et al.*, 1993). Semantic memory is also impaired (Portin *et al.*, 2000).

In DLB, episodic memory deficits are less severe than those of AD patients with an equal degree of dementia (Salmon *et al.*, 1996; Downes *et al.*, 1998; Ballard *et al.*, 1999; Calderon *et al.*, 2001) due to better retention and recognition memory, although learning and delayed recall in the free recall paradigm showed similarly severe impairment. The differences are even more apparent when patients with DLBD (i.e. without concomitant AD pathology) are compared to LBV and AD patients (Hamilton *et al.*, 2004). Semantic memory is impaired (Lambon Ralph *et al.*, 2001).

Language
There is relatively less impairment of language in PD/PDD/DLB than of visuospatial and executive

functions. There is no aphasia, and naming remains intact until late stages, but hypophonia, monotonia, and aprosodia may be evident. Some groups have found reduced information content of spontaneous speech, and impaired comprehension of complex commands and verbal reasoning skills (Cummings *et al.*, 1988; Lewis *et al.*, 1998). Poor verbal fluency is evident, perhaps more so for phonemic than category fluency (Troyer *et al.*, 1998), and this may be an early indicator of developing dementia.

Perception

Visuoperceptual and visuospatial deficits are reported in PD, PDD, and DLB, those in DLB being disproportionate to AD. Recorded deficits in PD include prism adaptation (Canavan *et al.*, 1990), facial recognition (Levin *et al.*, 1991), and complex figure drawing. In DLB, visuoperceptual and visuospatial impairment is evident in tests of fragmented letter identification and overlapping figures (Calderon *et al.*, 2001; Lambon Ralph *et al.*, 2001), the Judgment of Line Orientation (Simard *et al.*, 2003), drawing simple and complex figures (Hansen *et al.*, 1990; Gnanalingham *et al.*, 1996; Salmon *et al.*, 1996; Cormack *et al.*, 2004a), and in tests of visual search (Cormack *et al.*, 2004b). These deficits may reflect the underlying attentional problems and/or executive dysfunction, affecting planning and strategy formation, and/or may be related to occipital cortical hypoperfusion observed in functional imaging studies (Lobotesis *et al.*, 2001). Pentagon drawing in DLB and PDD is worse than in AD or PD, apparently related in DLB to deficits in perception and praxis (Cormack *et al.*, 2004a).

Praxis

Praxis may be difficult to evaluate meaningfully in the context of the motor disorder of PD. However, ideomotor apraxia for transitive movements has been documented in some PD patients, correlating with deficits in tests sensitive to frontal lobe function (verbal fluency, Trail Making, Tower of Hanoi) and suggesting corticostriatal dysfunction (Leiguarda *et al.*, 1997; Zadikoff & Lang, 2005).

Executive function

As with attention, executive function impairments are prominent in PD, PDD, and DLB, those disproportionately affected in DLB being mildly impaired in non-demented PD patients.

Executive dysfunction in PD may be manifest as psychomotor slowing, impairments in abstract reasoning on WAIS-R Similarities subtest and Raven's Progressive Matrices, and impaired performance on the Stroop Test and Wisconsin Card Sorting Test (Lees & Smith, 1983; Brown & Marsden, 1991; Graham & Sagar, 1999). Executive dysfunction has also been reported in some first-degree relatives of patients with familial PD, possibly representing a preclinical form of disease (Dujardin *et al.*, 1999b). Pathological gambling, an executive dysfunction or impulse control disorder, has been reported in some PD patients following treatment with dopamine agonist drugs (Dodd *et al.*, 2005; Larner, 2006).

A study of the qualitative performance characteristics of DLB patients on neuropsychological testing as compared to AD found evidence of inattention, visual distractibility, and perseveration. Externally cued intrusions from the visual environment were common in DLB but never seen in AD (Doubleday *et al.*, 2002).

Treatment of neuropsychological deficits

Since the cholinergic deficit in DLB is greater than that observed in AD, a possible role for cholinesterase inhibitors (ChEIs) was anticipated in DLB. An international randomized double-blind placebo-controlled trial demonstrated efficacy of rivastigmine for both cognitive and psychiatric features (McKeith *et al.* 2000b), benefits maintained apparently up to 2 years (Grace *et al.*, 2001). ChEIs have also been reported beneficial for cognitive impairment in PD (Aarsland *et al.*, 2002; Leroi *et al.*, 2004) and in PDD (Emre *et al.*, 2004; Emre, 2006). However, clinical guidelines have suggested that further research is required to identify those patients who will benefit from ChEIs (National Collaborating Centre for Chronic Conditions, 2006).

The importance of dopaminergic mechanisms in cognition may be demonstrated by the impairments in working memory and attentional set-shifting tasks seen in PD patients off their regular dopaminergic therapy (Lange *et al.*, 1992).

REFERENCES

Aarsland D. Dementia in Parkinson's disease. In: O'Brien J, McKeith I, Ames D, Chiu E (eds.), *Dementia with Lewy Bodies and Parkinson's Disease Dementia*. London: Taylor & Francis, 2006: 221–39.

Aarsland D, Laake K, Larsen JP, *et al.* Donepezil for cognitive impairment in Parkinson's disease: a randomised controlled study. *J Neurol Neurosurg Psychiatry* 2002; **72**: 708–12.

Ala T, Hughes LF, Kyrouac GA, Ghobrial MW, Elble RJ. The Mini-Mental State exam may help in the differentiation of dementia with Lewy bodies and Alzheimer's disease. *Int J Geriatr Psychiatry* 2002; **17**: 503–9.

Ballard CG, Ayre G, O'Brien J, *et al.* Simple standardised neuropsychological assessments aid in the differential diagnosis of dementia with Lewy bodies from Alzheimer's disease and vascular dementia. *Dement Geriatr Cogn Disord* 1999; **10**: 104–8.

Braak H, Del Tredici K, Rüb U, *et al.* Staging of brain pathology related to sporadic Parkinson's disease. *Neurobiol Aging* 2003; **24**: 197–211.

Braak H, Rüb U, Jansen-Steur ENH, Del Tredici K, de Vos RAI. Cognitive status correlates with neuropathologic stage in Parkinson disease. *Neurology* 2005; **64**: 1404–10.

Brown P, Marsden CD. What do the basal ganglia do? *Lancet* 1998; **351**: 1801–4.

Brown RG, Marsden CD. How common is dementia in Parkinson's disease? *Lancet* 1984; **2**: 1262–5.

Brown RG, Marsden CD. Dual task performance and processing resources in normal subjects and patients with Parkinson's disease. *Brain* 1991; **114**: 215–31.

Burkhardt CR, Filley CM, Kleinschmidt-DeMasters BK, *et al.* Diffuse Lewy body disease and progressive dementia. *Neurology* 1988; **38**: 1520–8.

Byrne EJ, Lennox G, Lowe J, Godwin-Austen RB. Diffuse Lewy body disease: clinical features in 15 cases. *J Neurol Neurosurg Psychiatry* 1989; **52**: 709–17.

Calderon J, Perry R, Erzinclioglu S, *et al.* Perception, attention and working memory are disproportionately impaired in dementia with Lewy body (LBD) compared to Alzheimer's disease (AD). *J Neurol Neurosurg Psychiatry* 2001; **70**: 157–64.

Canavan AGM, Passingham RE, Marsden CD. Prism adaptation and other tasks involving spatial abilities in patients with Parkinson's disease, patients with frontal lobe lesions and patients with unilateral temporal lobectomies. *Neuropsychologia* 1990; **28**: 969–84.

Charcot JM. *Leçons sur les maladies du système nerveux*. Paris: Delahaye, 1985 [1875]: 179.

Cormack F, Aarsland D, Ballard C, Tovée MJ. Pentagon drawing and neuropsychological performance in dementia with Lewy bodies, Alzheimer's disease, Parkinson's disease and Parkinson's disease with dementia. *Int J Geriatr Psychiatry* 2004a; **19**: 371–7.

Cormack F, Gray A, Ballard C, Tovée MJ. A failure of 'pop-out' in visual search tasks in dementia with Lewy bodies as compared to Alzheimer's and Parkinson's disease. *Int J Geriatr Psychiatry* 2004b; **19**: 763–72.

Cummings JL, Darkins A, Mendez M, Hill MA, Benson DF. Alzheimer's disease and Parkinson's disease: comparison of speech and language alterations. *Neurology* 1988; **38**: 680–4.

Dodd ML, Klos KJ, Bower JH, *et al.* Pathological gambling caused by drugs used to treat Parkinson disease. *Arch Neurol* 2005; **62**: 1377–81.

Doran M, Larner AJ. EEG findings in dementia with Lewy bodies causing diagnostic confusion with sporadic Creutzfeldt–Jakob disease. *Eur J Neurol* 2004; **11**: 838–41.

Doubleday EK, Snowden JS, Varma A, Neary D. Qualitative performance characteristics differentiate dementia with Lewy bodies and Alzheimer's disease. *J Neurol Neurosurg Psychiatry* 2002; **72**: 602–7.

Downes JJ, Priestley NM, Doran M, *et al.* Intellectual, mnemonic and frontal functions in dementia with Lewy bodies: a comparison with early and advanced Parkinson's disease. *Behav Neurol* 1998; **11**: 173–83.

Dujardin K, Degreef JF, Rogelet P, Defebvre L, Destee A. Impairment of the supervisory attentional system in early untreated patients with Parkinson's disease. *J Neurol* 1999a; **246**: 783–8.

Dujardin K, Duhamel A, Becquet E, *et al.* Neuropsychological abnormalities in first degree relatives of patients with familial Parkinson's disease. *J Neurol Neurosurg Psychiatry* 1999b; **67**: 323–8.

du Plessis DG, Larner AJ. Phenotypic similarities causing clinical misdiagnosis of pathologically confirmed sporadic Creutzfeldt–Jakob disease as dementia with Lewy bodies. *Clin Neurol Neurosurg* 2008; **110**: 194–7.

Emre M. Dementia associated with Parkinson's disease. *Lancet Neurol* 2003; **2**: 229–37.

Emre M. Cholinesterase inhibitors in the treatment of dementia associated with Parkinson's disease. In: Gauthier S, Scheltens P, Cummings JL (eds.), *Alzheimer's Disease and Related Disorders Annual 5*. London: Taylor & Francis, 2006: 181–90.

Emre M, Aarsland D, Albanese A, *et al*. Rivastigmine for dementia associated with Parkinson's disease. *N Engl J Med* 2004; **351**: 2509–18.

Ferman TJ, Smith GE, Boeve BF, *et al*. DLB fluctuations: specific features that reliably differentiate DLB from AD and normal aging. *Neurology* 2004; **62**: 181–7.

Fleisher AS, Olichney JM. Neurodegenerative disorders with diffuse cortical Lewy bodies. *Adv Neurol* 2005; **96**: 148–65.

Foltynie T, Brayne CEG, Robbins TW, Barker RA. The cognitive ability of an incident cohort of Parkinson's patients in the UK. The CamPaIGN study. *Brain* 2004; **127**: 550–60.

Galvin JE, Pollack J, Morris JC. Clinical phenotype of Parkinson disease dementia. *Neurology* 2006; **67**: 1605–11.

Gardner-Thorpe C. *James Parkinson 1755–1824*. Exeter: Wheaton, 1987.

Gibb WR, Esiri MM, Lees AJ. Clinical and pathological features of diffuse Lewy body disease (Lewy body dementia). *Brain* 1987; **110**: 1131–53.

Gnanalingham KK, Byrne EJ, Thornton A. Clock-face drawing to differentiate Lewy body and Alzheimer type dementia syndromes. *Lancet* 1996; **347**: 696–7.

Goldman WP, Baty JD, Buckles VD, Sahrmann S, Morris JC. Cognitive and motor functioning in Parkinson disease. *Arch Neurol* 1998; **55**: 674–80.

Grace J, Daniel S, Stevens T, *et al*. Long-term use of rivastigmine in patients with dementia with Lewy bodies: an open-label trial. *Int Psychogeriatrics* 2001; **13**: 199–205.

Graham JM, Sagar HJ. A data-driven approach to the study of heterogeneity in idiopathic Parkinson's disease: identification of three distinct subtypes. *Mov Disord* 1999; **14**: 10–20.

Hamilton JM, Salmon DP, Galasko D, *et al*. A comparison of episodic memory deficits in neuropathologically-confirmed dementia with Lewy bodies and Alzheimer's disease. *J Int Neuropsychol Soc* 2004; **10**: 689–97.

Hansen L, Salmon D, Galasko D, *et al*. The Lewy body variant of Alzheimer's disease: a clinical and pathologic entity. *Neurology* 1990; **40**: 1–8.

Hoehn MM, Yahr MD. Parkinsonism: onset, progression, and mortality. *Neurology* 1967; **17**: 427–42.

Horimoto Y, Matsumoto M, Akatsu H, *et al*. Autonomic dysfunctions in dementia with Lewy bodies. *J Neurol* 2003; **250**: 530–3.

Ince PG, Perry EK, Morris CM. Dementia with Lewy bodies: a distinct non-Alzheimer dementia syndrome? *Brain Pathol* 1998; **8**: 299–324.

Ishikawa A, Piao YS, Miyashita A, *et al*. A mutant PSEN1 causes dementia with Lewy bodies and variant Alzheimer's disease. *Ann Neurol*, 2005; **57**: 429–34.

Ivory SJ, Knight RG, Longmore BE, Caradoc-Davies T. Verbal memory in non-demented patients with idiopathic Parkinson's disease. *Neuropsychologia* 1999; **37**: 817–28.

Kaufmann H, Nahm K, Purohit D, Wolfe D. Autonomic failure as the initial presentation of Parkinson disease and dementia with Lewy bodies. *Neurology* 2004; **63**: 1093–5.

Koide T, Ohtake H, Nakajima T, *et al*. A patient with dementia with Lewy bodies and codon 232 mutation of PRNP. *Neurology* 2002; **59**: 1619–21.

Kraemer C, Lang K, Weckesser M, Evers S. Creutzfeldt–Jacob [*sic*] disease misdiagnosed as dementia with Lewy bodies. *J Neurol* 2005; **252**: 861–2.

Lambon Ralph MA, Powell J, Howard D, *et al*. Semantic memory is impaired in both dementia with Lewy bodies and dementia of Alzheimer's type: a comparative neuropsychological study and literature review. *J Neurol Neurosurg Psychiatry* 2001; **70**: 149–56.

Lange KW, Robbins TW, Marsden CD, *et al*. L-dopa withdrawal in Parkinson's disease selectively impairs cognitive performance in tests sensitive to frontal lobe dysfunction. *Psychopharmacol (Berl)* 1992; **107**: 394–404.

Larner AJ. Medical hazards of the internet: gambling in Parkinson's disease. *Mov Disord* 2006; **21**: 1789.

Larner AJ, Mathias CJ, Rossor MN. Autonomic failure preceding dementia with Lewy bodies. *J Neurol* 2000; **247**: 229–31.

Lees AJ, Smith E. Cognitive deficits in the early stages of Parkinson's disease. *Brain* 1983; **106**: 257–70.

Leiguarda RC, Pramstaller PP, Merello M, *et al*. Apraxia in Parkinson's disease, progressive supranuclear palsy, multiple system atrophy and neuroleptic-induced parkinsonism. *Brain* 1997; **120**: 75–90.

Leroi I, Brandt J, Reich SG, *et al*. Randomized placebo-controlled trial of donepezil in cognitive impairment in

Parkinson's disease. *Int J Geriatr Psychiatry* 2004; **19**: 1–8.

Leverenz JB, Fishel MA, Peskind ER, *et al.* Lewy body pathology in familial Alzheimer disease: evidence for disease- and mutation-specific pathologic phenotype. *Arch Neurol* 2006; **63**: 370–6.

Levin BE, Llabre MM, Reisman S, *et al.* Visuospatial impairment in Parkinson's disease. *Neurology* 1991; **41**: 365–9.

Lewis FM, Lapointe L, Murdoch BE, Chenery HJ. Language impairment in Parkinson's disease. *Aphasiology* 1998; **12**: 193–206.

Lobotesis K, Fenwick JD, Phipps A, *et al.* Occipital hypoperfusion on SPECT in dementia with Lewy bodies but not AD. *Neurology* 2001; **56**: 643–9.

McKeith IG, Ballard CG, Perry RH, *et al.* Prospective validation of consensus criteria for the diagnosis of dementia with Lewy bodies. *Neurology* 2000a; **54**: 1050–8.

McKeith I, Del Ser T, Spano P, *et al.* Efficacy of rivastigmine in dementia with Lewy bodies: a randomised, double-blind, placebo-controlled international study. *Lancet* 2000b; **356**: 2031–6.

McKeith IG, Dickson DW, Lowe J, *et al.* Diagnosis and management of dementia with Lewy bodies: third report of the DLB Consortium. *Neurology* 2005; **65**: 1863–72.

McKeith I, Fairbairn A, Perry R, Thompson P, Perry E. Neuroleptic sensitivity in patients with senile dementia of Lewy body type. *BMJ* 1992; **305**: 673–8.

McKeith IG, Galasko D, Kosaka K, *et al.* Consensus guidelines for the clinical and pathologic diagnosis of dementia with Lewy bodies (DLB): report of the consortium on DLB international workshop. *Neurology* 1996; **47**: 1113–24.

McKeith IG, Perry EK, Perry RH, for the Consortium on Dementia with Lewy Bodies. Report of the second dementia with Lewy body international workshop. *Neurology* 1999; **53**: 902–5.

Mortimer JA, Pirozzola FJ, Hansch EC, Webster DD. Relationship of motor symptoms to intellectual deficits in Parkinson's disease. *Neurology* 1982; **32**: 133–7.

National Collaborating Centre for Chronic Conditions. *Parkinson's Disease: National Clinical Guideline for Diagnosis and Management in Primary and Secondary Care.* London: Royal College of Physicians, 2006: 121–4.

O'Brien J, McKeith I, Ames D, Chiu E (eds.). *Dementia with Lewy Bodies and Parkinson's Disease Dementia.* London: Taylor & Francis, 2006.

Owen AM, Iddon JL, Hodges JR, Summers BA, Robbins TW. Spatial and non-spatial working memory at different stages of Parkinson's disease. *Neuropsychologia* 1997; **35**: 519–32.

Pillon B, Deweer B, Agid Y, Dubois B. Explicit memory in Alzheimer's, Huntington's, and Parkinson's diseases. *Arch Neurol* 1993; **50**: 374–9.

Portin R, Laatu S, Revonsuo A, Rinne UK. Impairment of semantic knowledge in Parkinson disease. *Arch Neurol* 2000; **57**: 1338–43.

Rafal RD, Posner MJ, Walker JA, Friedrich FJ. Cognition and the basal ganglia: separating mental and motor components of performance in Parkinson's disease. *Brain* 1984; **107**: 1083–94.

Saghal A, Galloway PH, McKeith IG, *et al.* A comparative study of attentional deficits in senile dementias of Alzheimer and Lewy body types. *Dementia* 1992; **3**: 350–4.

Salmon DP, Galasko D, Hansen LA, *et al.* Neuropsychological deficits associated with diffuse Lewy body disease. *Brain Cogn* 1996; **31**: 148–65.

Simard M, van Reekum R, Myran D. Visuospatial impairment in dementia with Lewy bodies and Alzheimer's disease: a process analysis approach. *Int J Geriatr Psychiatry* 2003; **18**: 387–91.

Singleton AB, Farrer M, Johnson J, *et al.* Alpha-synuclein locus triplication causes Parkinson's disease. *Science* 2003; **302**: 841.

Smith MC, Goldman WP, Janer KW, Baty JD, Morris JC. Cognitive speed in nondemented Parkinson's disease. *J Int Neuropsychol Soc* 1998; **4**: 584–92.

Starkstein SE, Merello M. *Psychiatric and Cognitive Disorders in Parkinson's Disease.* Cambridge: Cambridge University Press, 2002: 55–87, 100–103.

Stocchi F, Brusa L. Cognition and emotion in different stages and subtypes of Parkinson's disease. *J Neurol* 2000; **247** (suppl 2): II/114–21.

Troyer AK, Moscovitch M, Winocur G, Leach L, Freedman M. Clustering and switching on verbal fluency tests in Alzheimer's and Parkinson's disease. *J Int Neuropsychol Soc* 1998; **4**: 137–43.

Walker MP, Ayre GA, Cummings JL, *et al.* The clinical assessment of fluctuation and the one day fluctuation assessment scale: two methods to assess fluctuating confusion in dementia. *Br J Psychiatry* 2000; **177**: 252–6.

Zadikoff C, Lang AE. Apraxia in movement disorders. *Brain* 2005; **128**: 1480–97.

Zarranz JJ, Alegre J, Gomez-Esteban JC, *et al.* The new mutation, E46K, of alpha-synuclein causes Parkinson and Lewy body dementia. *Ann Neurol* 2004; **55**: 164–73.

2.4.1 Other ('atypical') parkinsonian syndromes

Disorders which clinically may superficially resemble idiopathic Parkinson's disease (PD) but which in fact have different clinical features, course, and pathogenesis have sometimes been labelled as 'atypical' parkinsonian syndromes, or sometimes as 'parkinsonism plus'. The most common of these syndromes are progressive supranuclear palsy (PSP), corticobasal degeneration (CBD), and multiple system atrophy (MSA). The terminology raises the question as to what is 'atypical' for PD, but features which should dissuade one from a diagnosis of idiopathic PD include early freezing and falls, rapid disease progression, early dysautonomia, early speech or swallowing problems, levodopa unresponsiveness, and early dementia (Quinn, 2006a, b). It is reported that simple bedside cognitive screening tests such as the Dementia Rating Scale and the Addenbrooke's Cognitive Examination can differentiate the commonest 'atypical' parkinsonian disorders (Bak *et al.*, 2005)

The disorders considered here include progressive supranuclear palsy and corticobasal degeneration, tauopathies which some authorities regard as falling within the rubric of frontotemporal lobar degenerations; multiple system atrophy, a synucleinopathy; dementia pugilistica; and the parkinsonism–dementia complex of Guam. Other disorders with clinical features that might cause them to be regarded as 'atypical' parkinsonian syndromes but which are covered elsewhere include frontotemporal dementia with parkinsonism linked to chromosome 17 (FTDP-17: Section 2.2.4), Huntington's disease (Section 5.1.1), Wilson's disease (Section 5.4.1), neurodegeneration with brain iron accumulation (Hallervorden–Spatz disease: Section 5.4.2), neuroacanthocytosis (Section 5.4.3), Fahr's disease (Section 5.1.7), normal pressure hydrocephalus (Section 7.2.1), post-encephalitic parkinsonism (encephalitis lethargica: Section 9.1.10), and some cases of Creutzfeldt–Jakob disease (Section 2.5).

REFERENCES

Bak TH, Crawford LM, Hearn VC, Mathuranath PS, Hodges JR. Subcortical dementia revisited: similarities and differences in cognitive function between progressive supranuclear palsy (PSP), corticobasal degeneration (CBD) and multiple system atrophy (MSA). *Neurocase* 2005; **11**: 268–73.

Quinn N. Other atypical parkinsonian disorders and their differentiation from dementia with Lewy bodies. In: O'Brien J, McKeith I, Ames D, Chiu E (eds.), *Dementia with Lewy Bodies and Parkinson's Disease Dementia.* London: Taylor & Francis, 2006a: 241–53.

Quinn NP. Atypical parkinsonian syndromes. *Eur J Neurol* 2006b; **13** (suppl2): 3 (abstract MT 4–1).

2.4.2 Progressive supranuclear palsy (PSP), Steele–Richardson–Olszewski (SRO) syndrome

Progressive supranuclear palsy (PSP) is an akinetic-rigid syndrome, the clinical phenotype of which was first described as such by Steele and colleagues (1964), although possible earlier cases, even dating to the nineteenth century, have been noted retrospectively (Larner, 2002). Bradykinesia and axial rigidity without tremor, postural instability with early falls, supranuclear gaze palsy, and bulbar symptoms are typical of PSP (Rehman, 2000), although the characteristic eye movement disorder is not always present, since cases with the typical pathological findings but without supranuclear gaze palsy are described. It has been suggested that the typical phenotype be called 'Richardson's syndrome', and the atypical form, which is often confused with idiopathic Parkinson's disease because of asymmetric onset, tremor, and modest response to levodopa, be called 'PSP-P' (Williams *et al.*, 2005). Pathologically, neurofibrillary tangles and neuropil threads are seen using tau immunohistochemistry.

White matter astrocytes containing tangles ('tufted astrocytes') may be seen, an appearance which may be unique to PSP. Cases with tau gene mutations have been reported (i.e. FTDP-17: see Section 2.2.4), as have cases with ubiquitin-positive inclusions typical of the MND type (Paviour *et al.*, 2004), observations which prompt some authors to categorize PSP as a frontotemporal lobar degeneration (FTLD: Section 2.2). Clinical diagnostic criteria for PSP have been published (Litvan *et al.*, 1996).

Dementia as a component of PSP was explicit in the first descriptions (Richardson *et al.*, 1963; Steele *et al.*, 1964). The term 'subcortical dementia' was first used to describe the neuropsychological deficits observed in PSP: forgetfulness, slowing of thought processes, emotional or personality change (apathy, depression with outbursts of irritability), and impaired ability to manipulate acquired knowledge (Albert *et al.*, 1974). Notwithstanding the controversies engendered by the term 'subcortical' (Section 1.11), cognitive deficits are common in PSP (Bak & Hodges, 1998; Brown *et al.*, 2002). Cases of PSP presenting with isolated dementia have been reported (Davis *et al.*, 1985; Masliah *et al.*, 1991).

Cognitive slowing and executive dysfunction are the key findings, with relative preservation of instrumental functions (Robbins *et al.*, 1994). This is manifested as slowed responses to questions or problem solving, impaired verbal fluency, more so for phonological than for semantic categories (Rosser & Hodges, 1994a; Bak *et al.*, 2005), and perseveration, as in the 'applause test' or 'clapping test' (asked to clap three times, the patient often claps more than three times). On the Dementia Rating Scale, PSP patients are more impaired on the initiation/perseveration subtest and less impaired on the memory subtest than AD patients (Rosser & Hodges, 1994b). Nonetheless, memory for long- and short-term material is also impaired, for both immediate and delayed recall, but unlike the situation in AD or other 'cortical dementias' memory performance is significantly improved by cueing and recognition, methods believed to facilitate the retrieval process, itself thought to be related to the frontostriatal system (Pillon *et al.*,

1994). Ideomotor apraxia may occur, which may cause clinical confusion with corticobasal degeneration, but it is usually bilateral (Leiguarda *et al.*, 1997).

REFERENCES

Albert ML, Feldman RG, Willis AL. The 'subcortical dementia' of progressive supranuclear palsy. *J Neurol Neurosurg Psychiatry* 1974; **37**: 121–30.

Bak TH, Crawford LM, Hearn VC, Mathuranath PS, Hodges JR. Subcortical dementia revisited: similarities and differences in cognitive function between progressive supranuclear palsy (PSP), corticobasal degeneration (CBD) and multiple system atrophy (MSA). *Neurocase* 2005; **11**: 268–73.

Bak TH, Hodges JR. The neuropsychology of progressive supranuclear palsy. *Neurocase* 1998; **4**: 89–98.

Brown RG, Pillon B, Uttner I, Payan C, Lacomblez L, Members of the Neuropsychology Working Group and NNIPPS Consortium. Cognitive function in patients with progressive supranuclear palsy (PSP) and multiple system atrophy (MSA). *Mov Disord* 2002; **17** (suppl 5): S221 (abstract P706).

Davis PH, Bergeron C, McLachlan DR. Atypical presentation of progressive supranuclear palsy. *Ann Neurol* 1985; **17**: 337–43.

Larner AJ. Did Charles Dickens describe progressive supranuclear palsy in 1857? *Mov Disord* 2002; **17**: 832–3.

Leiguarda RC, Pramstaller PP, Merello M, *et al.* Apraxia in Parkinson's disease, progressive supranuclear palsy, multiple system atrophy and neuroleptic-induced parkinsonism. *Brain* 1997; **120**: 75–90.

Litvan I, Agid Y, Calne D, *et al.* Clinical research criteria for the diagnosis of progressive supranuclear palsy (Steele–Richardson–Olszewski syndrome): report of the NINDS-SPSP International Workshop. *Neurology* 1996; **47**: 1–9.

Masliah E, Hansen LA, Quijada S, *et al.* Late onset dementia with argyrophilic grains and subcortical tangles or atypical progressive supranuclear palsy? *Ann Neurol* 1991; **29**: 389–96.

Paviour DC, Lees AJ, Josephs KA, *et al.* Frontotemporal lobar degeneration with ubiquitin-only-immunoreactive neuronal changes: broadening the clinical picture to include progressive supranuclear palsy. *Brain* 2004; **127**: 2441–51.

Pillon B, Deweer B, Michon A, *et al.* Are explicit memory disorders of progressive supranuclear palsy related to damage to striatofrontal circuits? Comparison with Alzheimer's, Parkinson's and Huntington's diseases. *Neurology* 1994; **44**: 1264–70.

Rehman HU. Progressive supranuclear palsy. *Postgrad Med J* 2000; **76**: 333–6.

Richardson JC, Steele J, Olszewski J. Supranuclear ophthalmoplegia, pseudobulbar palsy, nuchal dystonia and dementia: a clinical report on eight cases of heterogeneous system degeneration. *Trans Am Neurol Assoc* 1963; **88**: 25–9.

Robbins TW, James M, Lange KW, *et al.* Cognitive deficits in progressive supranuclear palsy, Parkinson's disease, and multiple system atrophy in tests sensitive to frontal lobe dysfunction. *J Neurol Neurosurg Psychiatry* 1994; **57**: 79–88.

Rosser AE, Hodges JR. Initial letter and semantic category fluency in Alzheimer's disease, Huntington's disease and progressive supranuclear palsy. *J Neurol Neurosurg Psychiatry* 1994a; **57**: 1389–94.

Rosser AE, Hodges JR. The Dementia Rating Scale in Alzheimer's disease, Huntington's disease and progressive supranuclear palsy. *J Neurol* 1994b; **241**: 531–6.

Steele JC, Richardson JC, Olszewski J. Progressive supranuclear palsy: a heterogeneous degeneration involving the brainstem, basal ganglia and cerebellum with vertical gaze and pseudobulbar palsy, nuchal dystonia and dementia. *Arch Neurol* 1964; **10**: 333–58.

Williams DR, de Silva R, Paviour DC, *et al.* Characteristics of two distinct clinical phenotypes in pathologically proven progressive supranuclear palsy: Richardson's syndrome and PSP-parkinsonism. *Brain* 2005; **128**: 1247–58.

2.4.3   Corticobasal degeneration (CBD)

Corticobasal degeneration (CBD), also known as cortical-basal ganglionic degeneration, was first defined neuropathologically (Rebeiz *et al.*, 1967). It is characterized by nerve cell loss and gliosis in the cortex, especially frontal and anterior parietal lobes, underlying white matter, thalamus, lentiform nucleus, subthalamic nucleus, substantia nigra, and locus caeruleus, with swollen and chromatolysed residual nerve cells with eccentric nuclei (achromasia). Neuronal inclusions resembling the globose neurofibrillary tangles (NFTs) of

PSP are present in the substantia nigra. There are no cortical NFTs, Pick bodies or Pick cells, senile plaques, Lewy bodies, granulovacuolar change, or amyloid deposits (Mahapatra *et al.*, 2004). Neuropathological diagnostic criteria for CBD have been published (Dickson *et al.*, 2002).

The clinical phenotype is variable: initial reports emphasized a movement disorder, chronic progressive akinetic-rigid syndrome with asymmetric onset, limb apraxia sometimes with the alien limb phenomenon, cortical sensory dysfunction, dystonia, and myoclonus, sometimes with eye movement disorder (Thompson & Marsden, 1992). However, increasingly it has been recognized that CBD is also a cognitive disorder (Grimes *et al.*, 1999b; Graham *et al.*, 2003a). Initial clinicopathological diagnostic criteria for CBD (Lang *et al.*, 1994) did not include cognitive decline, but this has been rectified in more recently proposed criteria, which include variable degrees of focal or lateralized cognitive dysfunction, with relative preservation of learning and memory, on neuropsychometric testing as a supportive investigation (Boeve *et al.*, 2003). Brief 'bedside' neuropsychological tests such as the Addenbrooke's Cognitive Examination are reported to be able to detect cognitive deficits in CBD (Bak *et al.*, 2005b).

Care needs to be taken in defining the cognitive profile of CBD since phenocopies are relatively common (Boeve *et al.*, 1999), with AD and Pick's disease being the commonest neuropathological substrates of 'corticobasal degeneration syndrome' (CBDS: Doran *et al.*, 2003; Larner & Doran, 2004). Motor neurone disease inclusion dementia has also been reported to present as 'CBD' (Grimes *et al.*, 1999a). Hence studies without neuropathological confirmation remain open to possible confounding with CBDS phenocopies.

Neuropsychological studies in CBD have reported deficits of sustained attention and verbal fluency as in AD (but more so for letter than for category fluency: Bak *et al.*, 2005a), and deficits of praxis, finger tapping and motor programming not seen in AD. These latter changes are thought to reflect basal ganglia and posterior frontal lobe involvement in CBD (Pillon *et al.*, 1995; Massman *et al.*, 1996). Apraxia affecting limb function is one of the most typical features of CBD, which may be ideomotor and limb-kinetic (Zadikoff & Lang, 2005). Early and prominent language impairments have also been noted (Lippa *et al.*, 1991), specifically phonological impairments overlapping with those observed in the progressive non-fluent aphasia variant of FTD (Graham *et al.*, 2003b; see Section 2.2.3). Learning and episodic memory are mildly impaired, if at all, particularly in the early stages.

Cases presenting with features of frontotemporal dementia (FTD) without a motor disorder have also been reported (Lennox *et al.*, 1994; Kertesz & Martinez-Lange, 1998; Kertesz & Munoz, 1998; Mathuranath *et al.*, 2000), as have occasional patients with parieto-occipital, Balint-like, cortical dysfunction (Tang-Wai *et al.*, 2003), and a combination of dementia, parkinsonism, and motor neurone disease (Boeve *et al.*, 2002). These findings presumably reflect the regional distribution of pathological change. Some authors categorize CBD as a frontotemporal lobar degeneration (FTLD) with tau inclusions (e.g. Kertesz & Martinez-Lage, 1998), and this phenotype may on occasion be seen in patients harbouring mutations in the tau gene (see Section 2.2.4).

REFERENCES

Bak TH, Crawford LM, Hearn VC, Mathuranath PS, Hodges JR. Subcortical dementia revisited: similarities and differences in cognitive function between progressive supranuclear palsy (PSP), corticobasal degeneration (CBD) and multiple system atrophy (MSA). *Neurocase* 2005a; **11**: 268–73.

Bak TH, Rogers TT, Crawford LM, *et al.* Cognitive bedside assessment in atypical parkinsonian syndromes. *J Neurol Neurosurg Psychiatry* 2005b; **76**: 420–2.

Boeve BF, Lang AE, Litvan I. Corticobasal degeneration and its relationship to progressive supranuclear palsy and frontotemporal dementia. *Ann Neurol* 2003; **54** (suppl 5): S15–19.

Boeve BF, Maraganore MD, Parisi JE, *et al.* Pathologic heterogeneity in clinically diagnosed corticobasal degeneration. *Neurology* 1999; **53**: 795–800.

Boeve B, Parisi J, Petersen R, *et al.* Familial dementia/parkinsonism/motor neuron disease with corticobasal degeneration pathology but absence of a tau mutation. *Neurobiol Aging* 2002; **23** (1S): S269 (abstract 1008).

Dickson DW, Bergeron C, Chin SS, *et al.* Office of Rare Diseases neuropathologic criteria for corticobasal degeneration. *J Neuropathol Exp Neurol* 2002; **61**: 935–46.

Doran M, du Plessis DG, Enevoldson TP, *et al.* Pathological heterogeneity of clinically diagnosed corticobasal degeneration. *J Neurol Sci* 2003; **216**: 127–34.

Graham NL, Bak TH, Hodges JR. Corticobasal degeneration as a cognitive disorder. *Mov Disord* 2003a; **18**: 1224–32.

Graham NL, Bak T, Patterson K, Hodges JR. Language function and dysfunction in corticobasal degeneration. *Neurology* 2003b; **61**: 493–9.

Grimes DA, Bergeron CB, Lang AE. Motor neuron disease-inclusion dementia presenting as cortical-basal ganglionic degeneration. *Mov Disord* 1999a; **14**: 674–80.

Grimes DA, Lang AE, Bergeron CB. Dementia as the most common presentation of cortical-basal ganglionic degeneration. *Neurology* 1999b; **53**: 1969–74.

Kertesz A, Martinez-Lange P. Cognitive changes in corticobasal degeneration. In: Kertesz A, Munoz DG (eds.), *Pick's Disease and Pick Complex*. New York: Wiley-Liss, 1998: 121–8.

Kertesz A, Munoz DG. Clinical and pathological overlap in Pick complex. In: Kertesz A, Munoz DG (eds.), *Pick's Disease and Pick Complex*. New York: Wiley-Liss, 1998: 281–6.

Lang AE, Riley DE, Bergeron C. Cortical-basal ganglionic degeneration. In: Calne DB (ed.), *Neurodegenerative Diseases*. Philadelphia: Saunders, 1994: 877–94.

Larner AJ, Doran M. Language function and dysfunction in corticobasal degeneration. *Neurology* 2004; **62**: 1238.

Lennox G, Jackson M, Lowe J. Corticobasal degeneration manifesting as a frontal lobe dementia. *Ann Neurol* 1994; **36**: 273–4 (abstract P52).

Lippa CF, Cohen R, Smith TW, Drachman DA. Primary progressive aphasia with focal neuronal achromasia. *Neurology* 1991; **41**: 882–6.

Mahapatra RK, Edwards MJ, Schott JM, Bhatia KP. Corticobasal degeneration. *Lancet Neurol* 2004; **3**: 736–43.

Massman PJ, Kreiter KT, Jankovic J, Doody RS. Neuropsychological functioning in cortical-basal ganglionic degeneration: differentiation from Alzheimer's disease. *Neurology* 1996; **46**: 720–6.

Mathuranath PS, Xuereb JH, Bak T, Hodges JR. Corticobasal ganglionic degeneration and/or frontotemporal dementia? A report of two overlap cases and review of literature. *J Neurol Neurosurg Psychiatry* 2000; **68**: 304–12.

Pillon B, Blin J, Vidailhet M, *et al*. The neuropsychological pattern of corticobasal degeneration: comparison with progressive supranuclear palsy and Alzheimer's disease. *Neurology* 1995; **45**: 1477–83.

Rebeiz JJ, Kolodny EH, Richardson EP. Corticodentatonigral degeneration with neuronal achromasia: a progressive disorder of late adult life. *Trans Am Neurol Assoc* 1967; **92**: 23–6.

Tang-Wai DF, Josephs KA, Boeve BF, *et al*. Pathologically confirmed corticobasal degeneration presenting with visuospatial dysfunction. *Neurology* 2003; **61**: 1134–5.

Thompson PD, Marsden CD. Corticobasal degeneration. In: Rossor MN (ed.), *Unusual Dementias*. London: Bailliere Tindall, 1992: 677–86.

Zadikoff C, Lang AE. Apraxia in movement disorders. *Brain* 2005; **128**: 1480–97.

2.4.4   Multiple system atrophy (MSA)

Multiple system atrophy (MSA) is a neurodegenerative disorder characterized as a synucleinopathy on the basis of the signature neuropathological finding of glial cytoplasmic inclusions in basal ganglia, substantia nigra, pontine nuclei, medulla, cerebellum, and white matter, composed of fibrils of polymerized α-synuclein. The clinical phenotype is variable. Initially three syndromes were defined – olivopontocerebellar atrophy (OPCA), striatonigral degeneration (SND), and Shy–Drager syndrome (Graham & Oppenheimer, 1969) – but the current classification, based on the relative predominance of clinical (and pathological) changes, encompasses MSA-C (cerebellar ataxia), roughly equivalent to OPCA, and MSA-P (parkinsonism), roughly equivalent to SND. All cases have autonomic dysfunction, which was the prominent feature of Shy–Drager syndrome. The phenotype of MSA is broad, with many other neurological features sometimes encountered (Geser *et al.*, 2005). Clinicopathological diagnostic criteria for MSA have been proposed (Gilman *et al.*, 1999).

Of the various parkinsonian syndromes, MSA is probably the one least associated with cognitive impairments (Bak *et al.*, 2005a, b). Intelligence is generally normal, but there may be neuropsychological impairments. Frontal lobe dysfunction has been a fairly consistent finding when sought, with difficulties in attentional mechanisms and set-shifting, impinging on working memory and speed of thinking (Sullivan *et al.*, 1991; Robbins *et al.*, 1992, 1994; Meco *et al.*, 1996; Brown *et al.*, 2002). In MSA-P, verbal fluency (phonemic and category) deficits have been noted despite normality on the WAIS, Wisconsin Card Sorting Test, and Stroop Test (Pillon *et al.*, 1995). Apraxia is not a feature of MSA (Leiguarda *et al.*, 1997).

REFERENCES

Bak TH, Crawford LM, Hearn VC, Mathuranath PS, Hodges JR. Subcortical dementia revisited: similarities and differences in cognitive function between progressive supranuclear palsy (PSP), corticobasal degeneration (CBD) and multiple system atrophy (MSA). *Neurocase* 2005a; **11**: 268–73.

Bak TH, Rogers TT, Crawford LM, *et al*. Cognitive bedside assessment in atypical parkinsonian syndromes. *J Neurol Neurosurg Psychiatry* 2005b; **76**: 420–2.

Brown RG, Pillon B, Uttner I, Payan C, Lacomblez L, Members of the Neuropsychology Working Group and NNIPPS Consortium. Cognitive function in patients with progressive supranuclear palsy (PSP) and multiple system atrophy (MSA). *Mov Disord* 2002; **17** (suppl 5): S221 (abstract P706).

Geser F, Colosimo C, Wenning GK. Multiple system atrophy. In: Beal MF, Lang AE, Ludolph A (eds.), *Neurodegenerative Diseases: Neurobiology, Pathogenesis and Therapeutics*. Cambridge: Cambridge University Press, 2005: 623–62.

Gilman S, Low PA, Quinn N, *et al*. Consensus statement on the diagnosis of multiple system atrophy. *J Neurol Sci* 1999; **163**: 94–8.

Graham JG, Oppenheimer DR. Orthostatic hypotension and nicotine sensitivity in a case of multiple system atrophy. *J Neurol Neurosurg Psychiatry* 1969; **32**: 28–34.

Leiguarda RC, Pramstaller PP, Merello M, *et al*. Apraxia in Parkinson's disease, progressive supranuclear palsy, multiple system atrophy and neuroleptic-induced parkinsonism. *Brain* 1997; **120**: 75–90.

Meco G, Gasparini M, Doricchi F. Attentional functions in multiple system atrophy and Parkinson's disease. *J Neurol Neurosurg Psychiatry* 1996; **60**: 393–8.

Pillon B, Gouider-Khouja N, Deweer B, *et al.* Neuropsychological pattern of striatonigral degeneration: comparison with Parkinson's disease and progressive supranuclear palsy. *J Neurol Neurosurg Psychiatry* 1995; **58**: 174–9.

Robbins TW, James M, Lange KW, *et al.* Cognitive performance in multiple system atrophy. *Brain* 1992; **115**: 271–91.

Robbins TW, James M, Lange KW, *et al.* Cognitive deficits in progressive supranuclear palsy, Parkinson's disease, and multiple system atrophy in tests sensitive to frontal lobe dysfunction. *J Neurol Neurosurg Psychiatry* 1994; **57**: 79–88.

Sullivan EV, De La Paz R, Zipursky RB, Pfefferbaum A. Neuropsychological deficits accompanying striatonigral degeneration. *J Clin Exp Neuropsychol* 1991; **13**: 773–88.

2.4.5 Dementia pugilistica

A syndrome of cognitive impairment following repeated blunt head trauma has been described, originally in boxers (hence dementia pugilistica, boxer's dementia, or 'punch drunk syndrome': Corsellis *et al.*, 1973), although other professions may also be at risk of sports-related head injury (e.g. steeplechase jockeys after repeated falls). In addition to cognitive impairment, there may be a parkinsonian syndrome dominated by akinesia and variably responsive to levodopa, as well as dysarthria. Brain imaging may show ventricular dilatation and a cavum septum pellucidum. Pathologically the condition is reminiscent of Alzheimer's disease, with neurofibrillary tangles, deposition of amyloid β-peptide and diffuse neuronal loss. Brain trauma is known to increase expression of amyloid β (Roberts *et al.*, 1994) and epidemiological studies have suggested head injury may be a risk factor for Alzheimer's disease, particularly in the presence of the ApoE ε4 genotype (Nicoll *et al.*, 1995).

Dementia pugilistica lies at one end of a spectrum of neuropsychological deficits following head injury (Erlanger *et al.*, 1999). In assessing these impairments, allowance may need to be made for premorbid intellectual level and for concurrent alcohol misuse. The neuropsychological sequelae of mild traumatic brain injury have been reviewed (Kapur, 1994; Echemendia & Julian, 2001).

REFERENCES

Corsellis JAN, Bruton CJ, Freeman-Browne D. The aftermath of boxing. *Psychol Med* 1973; **3**: 270–303.

Echemendia RJ, Julian LJ. Mild traumatic brain injury in sports: neuropsychology's contribution to a developing field. *Neuropsychol Rev* 2001; **11**: 69–88.

Erlanger DM, Kutner KC, Barth JT, Barnes R. Neuropsychology of sports-related head injury: dementia pugilistica to post concussion syndrome. *Clin Neuropsychol* 1999; **13**: 193–209.

Kapur N. *Memory Disorders in Clinical Practice.* Hove: Lawrence Erlbaum, 1994: 97–113.

Nicoll JAR, Roberts GW, Graham DI. Apolipoprotein E epsilon-4 allele is associated with deposition of amyloid beta-protein following head injury. *Nat Med* 1995; **1**: 135–7.

Roberts GW, Gentleman SM, Lynch A, *et al.* β-amyloid protein deposition in the brain following severe head injury: implications for the pathogenesis of Alzheimer's disease. *J Neurol Neurosurg Psychiatry* 1994; **57**: 419–25.

2.4.6 Amyotrophic lateral sclerosis/ parkinsonism–dementia complex (ALS/PDC) of Guam, Lytico-Bodig, Marianas dementia

The Chamorro people of the island of Guam have been recognized to suffer a high prevalence of neurodegenerative disorders, known locally as Lytico-Bodig, encompassing varying degrees of the clinical features of MND/ALS, Parkinson's disease, and Alzheimer's disease (Perl, 2006). The ALS and parkinsonism–dementia complex (PDC) were initially described separately, but few pure cases of either condition exist, and both have severe neurofibrillary neuropathology with little amyloid, suggesting that there may be shared pathogenetic mechanisms, for which various aetiological concepts have been suggested (Perl, 2006).

The neuropsychological impairments of PDC encompass recent memory loss, disorientation, and impairments of language, visuospatial, and executive function (Galasko *et al.*, 2002), a global pattern similar to that seen in Alzheimer's disease. Very occasionally Chamorros may present with a pure dementing illness without extrapyramidal symptoms or signs, referred to as 'Marianas dementia' (Perl *et al.*, 1994).

REFERENCES

Galasko D, Salmon DP, Craig UK, *et al.* Clinical features and changing patterns of neurodegenerative disorders on Guam, 1997–2000. *Neurology* 2002; **58**: 90–7.

Perl DP. Amyotrophic lateral sclerosis/parkinsonism–dementia complex of Guam. In: Strong MJ (ed.), *Dementia and Motor Neuron Disease*. Abingdon: Informa Healthcare, 2006: 177–91.

Perl DP, Hof PR, Steele JC, *et al.* Neuropathologic studies of a pure dementing syndrome (Marianas dementia) among the inhabitants of Guam, a form of ALS/parkinsonism dementia complex. *Brain Pathol* 1994; **4**: 529 (abstract P31-13).

2.5   Prion diseases

The aetiological agents for the prion group of disorders are conformationally altered proteins, or prions, which autocatalytically convert normal cellular prion protein (PrP), encoded by the *PRNP* gene on chromosome 20, to an abnormal form that is highly resistant to degradation (Prusiner, 1982, 2001; Collinge, 2001).

Prion diseases (or prionoses) may afflict both humans and animals (Collinge & Palmer, 1997; Prusiner, 1999). Human disease takes a number of clinicopathological forms, namely sporadic, genetic, or iatrogenic. Sporadic Creutzfeldt–Jakob disease (sCJD) is the commonest prion disease, occurring with an incidence of around one case per million population throughout the world. The older literature defined a number of clinical variants of sCJD, presenting with prominent cerebellar syn-drome (Brownell–Oppenheimer (ataxic) variant), cortical blindness (Heidenhain variant), or encephalopathy (Nevin–Jones syndrome), but these terms are now seldom used, classification being based on *PRNP* codon 129 genotype and PrP isotype as detected by Western blotting, resulting in six variants (Parchi *et al.*, 1999).

Inherited prion disorders, accounting for approximately 10–15% of the total, are associated with mutations in the *PRNP* gene which encodes PrP (Kovacs *et al.*, 2002). These have a broad phenotype, including familial CJD, Gerstmann–Straussler–Scheinker syndrome (GSS), and fatal familial insomnia (FFI).

Acquired, iatrogenic, or transmissible forms of prion disease account for <1% of the total. These include kuru, a disorder of the Fore people of the eastern highlands of New Guinea transmitted by ritual endocannibalism of brain tissue, a practice which is now outlawed. Iatrogenic disease may result from exposure to contaminated instrumentation (depth EEG electrodes), grafts (cornea, dura mater), exogenous human pituitary hormones (growth hormone, gonadotrophins), and possibly blood transfusion (Peden *et al.*, 2004). Variant CJD (vCJD) is caused by the same prion strain responsible for the epidemic of bovine spongiform encephalopathy (BSE) in cattle, presumably reaching humans through the food chain, and hence is sometimes also known as 'human BSE' (Collinge, 1999). Progressive dementia, often rapid, is common to many of these prion disorders. Brain tissue (biopsy, autopsy) typically shows spongiform vacuolation affecting any part of the cerebral grey matter (hence these disorders are sometimes called 'spongiform encephalopathies'), with astrocytic proliferation, gliosis, neuronal loss, synaptic degeneration, and variable frequencies of PrP-immunopositive amyloid plaques (Ironside & Head, 2004). Prion disease cases without spongiform change have also been described (Collinge *et al.*, 1990).

The pathogenesis of neurodegeneration in the various prion disorders is thought to be common to the different aetiologies (Hegde *et al.*, 1999).

Polymorphism at codon 129 of the *PRNP* gene, which may encode either valine or methionine, may have a dramatic effect on disease phenotype, including susceptibility to disease, the incubation period of the disease, and the duration of illness (Palmer *et al.*, 1991; Parchi *et al.*, 1999).

Prion disorders are rare. Only a handful of cases is seen each year in regional neuroscience centres (Larner & Doran, 2004). No treatment, curative, symptomatic, or palliative, is yet described but research into possible therapeutic interventions continues (Larner & Doran, 2003; Trevitt & Collinge, 2006).

REFERENCES

Collinge J. Variant Creutzfeldt–Jakob disease. *Lancet* 1999; **354**: 317–23.

Collinge J. Prion diseases of humans and animals: their causes and molecular basis. *Annu Rev Neurosci* 2001; **24**: 519–50.

Collinge J, Owen F, Poulter M, *et al.* Prion dementia without characteristic pathology. *Lancet* 1990; **336**: 7–9.

Collinge J, Palmer MS (eds.). *Prion diseases*. Oxford: Oxford University Press, 1997.

Hegde RS, Tremblay P, Groth D, *et al.* Transmissible and genetic prion diseases share a common pathway of neurodegeneration. *Nature* 1999; **402**: 822–6.

Ironside JW, Head MW. Human prion diseases. In: Esiri MM, Lee VM-Y, Trojanowski JQ (eds.), *The Neuropathology of Dementia* (2nd edition). Cambridge: Cambridge University Press, 2004: 402–26.

Kovacs GG, Trabattoni G, Hainfellner JA, *et al.* Mutations of the prion protein gene: phenotypic spectrum. *J Neurol* 2002; **249**: 1567–82.

Larner AJ, Doran M. Prion diseases: update on therapeutic patents, 1999–2002. *Exp Opin Ther Patents* 2003; **13**: 67–78.

Larner AJ, Doran M. Prion disease at a regional neuroscience centre: retrospective audit. *J Neurol Neurosurg Psychiatry* 2004; **75**: 1789–90.

Palmer MS, Dryden AJ, Hughes JT, Collinge J. Homozygous prion protein genotype predisposes to sporadic Creutzfeldt–Jakob disease. *Nature* 1991; **352**: 340–2.

Parchi P, Giese A, Capellari S, *et al.* Classification of sporadic Creutzfeldt–Jakob disease based on molecular and phenotypic analysis of 300 subjects. *Ann Neurol* 1999; **46**: 224–33.

Peden AH, Head MW, Ritchie DL, Bell JE, Ironside JW. Preclinical vCJD after blood transfusion in a PRNP codon 129 heterozygous patient. *Lancet* 2004; **364**: 527–9.

Prusiner SB. Novel proteinaceous particles cause scrapie. *Science* 1982; **216**: 136–44.

Prusiner SB (ed.). *Prion Biology and Diseases*. Cold Spring Harbor: Cold Spring Harbor Laboratory Press, 1999.

Prusiner SB. Shattuck lecture: neurodegenerative diseases and prions. *N Engl J Med* 2001; **344**: 1516–26.

Trevitt CR, Collinge J. A systematic review of prion therapeutics in experimental models. *Brain* 2006; **129**: 2241–65.

2.5.1 Sporadic prion disease: sporadic Creutzfeldt–Jakob disease (sCJD)

CJD occurs in sporadic, familial, and iatrogenic forms. CSF proteins which are markers of neuronal injury may be elevated; although these are not disease-specific, estimations of the 14-3-3 protein have a high degree of sensitivity and specificity for the diagnosis of sCJD (Zerr *et al.*, 2000). EEG may show periodic sharp wave complexes (PSWCs) at a frequency of around 2–3 Hz in a markedly abnormal background in sCJD, again a highly specific and sensitive finding (Zerr *et al.*, 2000), especially if strict criteria for the definition of PSWC are used (Steinhoff *et al.*, 2004). Other disorders which may mimic or be clinically confused with CJD, and hence may lead to confounding in defining the neuropsychological profile, include AD (Tschampa *et al.*, 2001; Reinwald *et al.*, 2004), DLB (Tschampa *et al.*, 2001; Doran & Larner 2004; Kraemer *et al.*, 2005), progressive subcortical gliosis of Neumann (Seitelberger, 1968; Bergmann *et al.*, 1991), Wernicke–Korsakoff syndrome (Pietrini, 1992; Monaghan *et al.*, 2006), nonconvulsive status epilepticus (Cohen *et al.*, 2004; Vaz *et al.*, 2005), angioendotheliomatosis (Drlicek *et al.*, 1991), Hashimoto's encephalopathy (Schott *et al.*, 2003), pellagra encephalopathy (Pellisé *et al.*, 2002), and gliomatosis cerebri (Slee *et al.*, 2006).

Because of the rapid progression of the disease, profound cognitive deficits amounting to dementia may be present before clinical presentation. When assessment has been possible, a subcortical pattern has generally been reported in familial CJD, and both sporadic and familial cases have been found to have episodic unresponsiveness, interference effects, and verbal and motor perseverations, perhaps reflecting thalamic involvement (Snowden *et al.*, 2002). Presentation with isolated aphasia has been reported (Mandell *et al.*, 1989). In a patient undergoing neuropsychological testing in a pre-dementia stage, deficits resembling progressive supranuclear palsy were reported (Zarei *et al.*, 2002). A patient with the Heidenhain variant has been reported whose initial symptom was agraphia, followed by hemianopsia and visual hallucinations, and evolving to dementia over a 3-month period (Pachalska *et al.*, 2001).

REFERENCES

Bergmann M, Gullotta F, Weitbrecht WU. Progressive subkortikale Gliose. *Fortschr Neurol Psychiat* 1991; **59**: 328–34.

Cohen D, Kutluay E, Edwards J, Peltier A, Beydoun A. Sporadic Creutzfeldt–Jakob disease presenting with nonconvulsive status epilepticus. *Epilepsy Behav* 2004; **5**: 792–6.

Doran M, Larner AJ. EEG findings in dementia with Lewy bodies causing diagnostic confusion with sporadic Creutzfeldt–Jakob disease. *Eur J Neurol* 2004; **11**: 838–41.

Drlicek M, Grisold W, Liszka U, Hitzenberger P, Machacek E. Angiotropic lymphoma (malignant angioendotheliomatosis) presenting with rapidly progressive dementia. *Acta Neuropathol (Berl)* 1991; **82**: 533–5.

Kraemer C, Lang K, Weckesser M, Evers S. Creutzfeldt–Jacob [*sic*] disease misdiagnosed as dementia with Lewy bodies. *J Neurol* 2005; **252**: 861–2.

Mandell AM, Alexander MP, Carpenter S. Creutzfeldt–Jakob disease presenting as isolated aphasia. *Neurology* 1989; **39**: 55–8.

Monaghan TS, Murphy DT, Tubridy N, Hutchinson M. The woman who mistook the past for the present. *Adv Clin Neurosci Rehabil* 2006; **6** (3); 27–8.

Pachalska M, Kurzbauer H, MacQueen BD, Forminska-Kapuscik M, Herman-Sucharska I. Neuropsychological features of rapidly progressive dementia in a patient with an atypical presentation of Creutzfeldt–Jakob disease. *Med Sci Monit* 2001; **7**: 1307–15.

Pellisé A, Navarro O, Rey M, Cardozo A, Ferrer I. Protein 14-3-3 in pellagra encephalopathy. *Neurologia* 2002; **17**: 655–6.

Pietrini V. Creutzfeldt–Jakob disease presenting as Wernicke–Korsakoff syndrome. *J Neurol Sci* 1992; **108**: 149–53.

Reinwald S, Westner IM, Niedermaier N. Rapidly progressive Alzheimer's disease mimicking Creutzfeldt–Jakob disease. *J Neurol* 2004; **251**: 1020–2.

Schott JM, Warren JD, Rossor MN. The uncertain nosology of Hashimoto encephalopathy. *Arch Neurol* 2003; **60**: 1812.

Seitelberger F. Präsenile gliale Dystrophie. *Acta Neuropathol (Berl)* 1968; **Suppl 4**: 109–18.

Slee M, Pretorius P, Ansorge O, Stacey R, Butterworth R. Parkinsonism and dementia due to gliomatosis cerebri mimicking sporadic Creutzfeldt–Jakob disease (CJD). *J Neurol Neurosurg Psychiatry* 2006; **77**: 283–4.

Snowden JA, Mann DMA, Neary D. Distinct neuropsychological characteristics in Creutzfeldt–Jakob disease. *J Neurol Neurosurg Psychiatry* 2002; **73**: 686–94.

Steinhoff B, Zerr I, Glatting M, *et al.* Diagnostic value of periodic complexes in Creutzfeldt–Jakob disease. *Ann Neurol* 2004; **56**: 702–8.

Tschampa HJ, Neumann M, Zerr I, *et al.* Patients with Alzheimer's disease and dementia with Lewy bodies mistaken for Creutzfeldt–Jakob disease. *J Neurol Neurosurg Psychiatry* 2001; **71**: 33–9.

Vaz J, Sierazdan K, Kane N. Non convulsive status epilepticus in Creutzfeldt–Jakob disease: a short report. *J Neurol Neurosurg Psychiatry* 2005; **76**: 1318 (abstract 030).

Zarei M, Nouraei SA, Caine D, Hodges JR, Carpenter RH. Neuropsychological and quantitative oculometric study of a case of sporadic Creutzfeldt–Jakob disease at predementia stage. *J Neurol Neurosurg Psychiatry* 2002; **73**: 56–8.

Zerr I, Pocchiari M, Collins S, *et al.* Analysis of EEG and CSF 14-3-3 proteins as aids to the diagnosis of Creutzfeldt–Jakob disease. *Neurology* 2000; **55**: 811–5.

2.5.2 Iatrogenic prion disease: variant Creutzfeldt–Jakob disease (vCJD), kuru

Since its first description in 1996, vCJD has attracted much attention despite its clinical rarity because of its probable aetiology, namely transmission of bovine spongiform encephalopathy across the species barrier from cattle to humans through the consumption of infected meat products (Collinge, 1999). Transmission by blood transfusion is also a possibility (Wroe *et al.*, 2006). Unlike sporadic CJD, vCJD tends to affect younger individuals, and the presentation is often with non-specific sensory and psychiatric features (Spencer *et al.*, 2002), although presentation with epilepsy has been reported (Silverdale *et al.*, 2000). Magnetic resonance imaging may show high signal intensity in the posterior thalamus (pulvinar sign) in vCJD (Zeidler *et al.*, 2000), although this is not unique to vCJD (Monaghan *et al.*, 2006). EEG PSWCs are absent in vCJD. PrP-immunopositive staining may be present in lymphoreticular tissues, even pre-symptomatically (Hilton *et al.*, 1998, 2002). In the appropriate clinical setting, tonsil biopsy is helpful in the diagnosis of vCJD (Hill *et al.*, 1999).

Reports of neuropsychological assessment in vCJD are rare. Kapur *et al.* (2001) reported early deficits in episodic memory, semantic memory, retrieval and executive tasks but with relative sparing of recognition memory, autobiographical memory, and face perception. In a larger cohort, findings were of low performance IQ, with impairments on tests of memory, executive function, attention speed, and visuoperceptual reasoning, with relative preservation of digit span, verbal reasoning, long-term autobiographical memory, and face perception. The profile was one of combined cortical and subcortical dementia (Kapur *et al.*, 2003). A study of ten vCJD patients, comparing them with sCJD and inherited prion disease, found evidence for generalized cognitive decline but with the suggestion that visual perception might be spared (Cordery *et al.*, 2005).

In a series of five patients with iatrogenic prion disease resulting from exposure to cadaveric human growth hormone, only one had a complaint of mild memory problems but four had evidence for mild intellectual decline on the WAIS-R and one had selective visual memory and frontal executive impairments (Cordery *et al.*, 2003).

Kuru, an epidemic disorder transmitted by endocannibalism amongst the Fore people of Papua New Guinea, was the first human prion disease to be extensively described (Gajdusek, 1977; Zigas, 1990). It has become less common since the cessation of endocannibalism, although some new cases are still reported, reflecting extremely long incubation periods of 40–50 years (Collinge *et al.*, 2006). The profile of cognitive deficits is not reported, since common neuropsychological testing methods are not culturally appropriate.

REFERENCES

Collinge J. Variant Creutzfeldt–Jakob disease. *Lancet* 1999; **354**: 317–23.

Collinge J, Whitfield J, McKintosh E, *et al.* Kuru in the 21st century: an acquired human prion disease with very long incubation periods. *Lancet* 2006; **367**: 2068–74.

Cordery RJ, Alner K, Cipolotti L, *et al.* The neuropsychology of variant CJD: a comparative study with inherited and sporadic forms of prion disease. *J Neurol Neurosurg Psychiatry* 2005; **76**: 330–6.

Cordery RJ, Hall M, Cipolotti L, *et al.* Early cognitive decline in Creutzfeldt–Jakob disease associated with human growth hormone treatment. *J Neurol Neurosurg Psychiatry* 2003; **74**: 1412–16.

Gajdusek DC. Unconventional viruses and the origin and disappearance of kuru. *Science* 1977; **197**: 943–60.

Hill AF, Butterworth RJ, Joiner S, *et al.* Investigation of variant Creutzfeldt–Jakob disease and other human prion disease with tonsil biopsy samples. *Lancet* 1999; **353**: 183–9.

Hilton DA, Fathers E, Edwards P, Ironside JW, Zajicek J. Prion immunoreactivity in appendix before clinical onset of variant Creutzfeldt–Jakob disease. *Lancet* 1998; **352**: 703–4.

Hilton D, Ghani AC, Conyers L, *et al.* Accumulation of prion protein in tonsil and appendix: review of tissue samples. *BMJ* 2002; **325**: 633–4.

Kapur N, Abbott P, Lowman A, Will RG. The neuropsychological profile associated with variant Creutzfeldt–Jakob disease. *Brain* 2003; **126**: 2693–702.

Kapur N, Ironside J, Abbott P, *et al.* A neuropsychological–neuropathological case study of variant Creutzfeldt–Jakob disease. *Neurocase* 2001; **7**: 261–7.

Monaghan TS, Murphy DT, Tubridy N, Hutchinson M. The woman who mistook the past for the present. *Adv Clin Neurosci Rehabil* 2006; **6** (3); 27–8.

Silverdale M, Leach JP, Chadwick DW. New variant Creutzfeldt–Jakob disease presenting as localization-related epilepsy. *Neurology* 2000; **54**: 2188.

Spencer MS, Knight RSG, Will RG. First hundred cases of variant Creutzfeldt–Jakob disease: retrospective case note review of early psychiatric and neurological features. *BMJ* 2002; **324**: 1479–82.

Wroe SJ, Pal S, Siddique D, *et al.* Clinical presentation and pre-mortem diagnosis of variant Creutzfeldt–Jakob disease associated with blood transfusion: a case report. *Lancet* 2006; **368**: 2061–7.

Zeidler M, Sellar RJ, Collie DA, *et al.* The pulvinar sign on magnetic resonance imaging in variant Creutzfeldt–Jakob disease. *Lancet* 2000; **355**: 1412–8.

Zigas V. *Laughing death: the untold story of kuru.* Clifton NJ: Humana, 1990.

2.5.3 Inherited prion disease: familial CJD, Gerstmann–Straussler–Scheinker disease (GSS), fatal familial insomnia (FFI)

Inherited prion disease results from mutations in the PrP gene on chromosome 20, with various phenotypes (Kovacs *et al.*, 2002), described as familial CJD, Gerstmann–Straussler–Scheinker disease (GSS), and fatal familial insomnia (FFI). One study found generalized cognitive decline in inherited prion disease with relative preservation of nominal function in some cases (Cordery *et al.*, 2005).

In a single case study of familial CJD, verbal memory, word finding, and dominant hand tactual performance were impaired, with other functions relatively intact (Gass *et al.*, 2000). A family with a novel mutation, T183A, in the *PRNP* gene has been reported with clinical features resembling frontotemporal dementia and parkinsonism linked to chromosome 17 (FTDP-17: see Section 2.2.4; Nitrini *et al.*, 1997, 2001).

GSS is an autosomal dominant disorder due to mutations in the PrP gene with cerebellar ataxia as an early feature, along with dysarthria and eye movement disorders. Extrapyramidal signs may evolve. Progressive dementia with behavioural disturbance (depression, psychosis) is also reported. Deficits seem to vary amongst the different reports, including focal abnormalities suggestive of cortical involvement (acalculia, agnosia, apraxia), and more global impairment including attention and executive functions suggesting possible subcortical involvement (Farlow *et al.*, 1989; Unverzagt *et al.*, 1997). This would be in keeping with the multi-focal nature of brain involvement in prion disorders.

FFI, a rare inherited prion disorder linked to mutations of the PrP gene and a particular polymorphism at codon 129, is characterized clinically by sleep, autonomic, and motor disturbances and pathologically by marked atrophy of the anterior and dorsomedial nuclei of the thalamus. A rare sporadic form of the latter has also been described (Scaravilli *et al.*, 2000). Neuropsychological studies (Gallassi *et al.*, 1992, 1996) have shown early impairments of attention and vigilance, working memory deficits with a particular difficulty in the ordering of events, and a progressive confusional state. The pattern seems to be distinct from that of cortical and subcortical dementias and reflective of a thalamic dementia.

REFERENCES

Cordery RJ, Alner K, Cipolotti L, *et al.* The neuropsychology of variant CJD: a comparative study with inherited and sporadic forms of prion disease. *J Neurol Neurosurg Psychiatry* 2005; **76**: 330–6.

Farlow MR, Yee RD, Dlouhy SR, *et al.* Gerstmann–Straussler–Scheinker disease. I. Extending the clinical spectrum. *Neurology* 1989; **39**: 1446–52.

Gallassi R, Morreale A, Montagna P, Gambetti P, Lugaresi E. Fatal familial insomnia: neuropsychological study of a disease with thalamic degeneration. *Cortex* 1992; **28**: 175–87.

Gallassi R, Morreale A, Montagna P, *et al.* Fatal familial insomnia: behavioral and cognitive features. *Neurology* 1996; **46**: 935–9.

Gass CS, Luis CA, Meyers TL, Kuljis RO. Familial Creutzfeldt–Jakob disease: a neuropsychological case study. *Arch Clin Neuropsychol* 2000; **15**: 165–75.

Kovacs GG, Trabattoni G, Hainfellner JA, *et al*. Mutations of the prion protein gene: phenotypic spectrum. *J Neurol* 2002; **249**: 1567–82.

Nitrini R, Rosemberg S, Passos-Bueno MR, *et al*. Familial spongiform encephalopathy associated with a novel prion protein gene mutation. *Ann Neurol* 1997; **42**: 138–46.

Nitrini R, Teixeira-da-Silva LS, Rosemberg S, *et al*. Prion disease resembling frontotemporal dementia and parkinsonism linked to chromosome 17. *Arq Neuropsiquiatr* 2001; **59**: 161–4.

Scaravilli F, Cordery RJ, Kretschmar H, *et al*. Sporadic fatal insomnia: a case study. *Ann Neurol* 2000; **48**: 665–8.

Unverzagt FW, Farlow MR, Norton J, *et al*. Neuropsychological function in patients with Gerstmann–Straussler disease from the Indiana kindred (F198S). *J Int Neuropsychol Soc* 1997; **3**: 169–78.

2.6 Mild cognitive impairment (MCI)

It has been increasingly recognized in recent times that a degree of age-related cognitive decline may exist in individuals who do not fulfil validated criteria for the diagnosis of Alzheimer's disease (AD: McKhann *et al*., 1984). Various terms have been used to describe this state, including benign senescent forgetfulness, age-associated memory impairment (AAMI), age-associated cognitive decline (AACD), cognitive decline no dementia (CIND), and mild cognitive impairment (MCI).

A degree of consensus has developed around the concept of MCI (Golomb *et al*., 2001; Petersen, 2003, 2007; Winblad *et al*., 2004; Petersen & Morris, 2005; Portet *et al*., 2006; Tuokko & Hultsch, 2006), though not unanimity (Ritchie & Touchon, 2000; Gauthier & Touchon, 2005). MCI may be defined by the presence of a subjective memory complaint, preferably corroborated by an informant; evidence of objective memory impairment for age and level of education; largely normal general cognitive function; essentially intact activities of daily living (ADL); and failure to fulfil criteria for dementia (Petersen *et al*., 1999). Global rating scales have been used to define MCI, such as a Clinical Dementia Rating (CDR: Hughes *et al*., 1982; Morris,

1993) score of 0.5 or a Global Deterioration Scale (GDS: Reisberg *et al*., 1982) score of 3, but Petersen has been at pains to point out that MCI remains a clinical diagnosis (Petersen, 2003). A Preclinical AD Scale to identify cases has been published (Visser *et al*., 2002). Complex ADL may be impaired in MCI (Perneczky *et al*., 2006).

MCI may be clinically and aetiologically heterogeneous. At the time of clinical presentation, a memory complaint is the most common feature, so called amnestic MCI. Other variants have been described, specifically single non-memory-domain MCI and multiple-domain MCI. The former may be the harbinger of AD – for example a focal deficit such as visual agnosia may be due to the 'visual variant of Alzheimer's disease' (Levine *et al*., 1993; Larner, 2004a) – but might also reflect the pathology of another disorder such as frontotemporal dementia, dementia with Lewy bodies, or vascular dementia. Multiple-domain MCI might reflect single or multiple aetiologies (Petersen, 2003; Petersen & Morris, 2005). The possibility that 'MCI' may reflect conditions such as dysphoria, vascular disease, and miscellaneous disorders which may cause cognitive impairment such as obstructive sleep apnoea, alcohol misuse, head injury, and metabolic or nutritional deficiencies, some of them treatable, has been emphasized by some authors (Gauthier & Touchon, 2005).

The neuroanatomical and neuropathological substrates for the changes characterized as MCI have been examined. Structural neuroimaging techniques such as computed tomography (CT) and, particularly, magnetic resonance imaging (MRI) have shown reduced volume of brain tissue and an increased volume of cerebrospinal fluid with increasing age, the former consisting predominantly of a decline in white matter (Albert, 1998). Hence, brain atrophy per se is not specific for the diagnosis of pathological change, an assumption which may lead to clinical misdiagnosis of AD if undue weight is placed on imaging findings (Larner, 2004b). In MCI which is destined to become AD, hippocampal and entorhinal cortex volume are reduced and there may be a higher rate of hippocampal volume loss

(Jack *et al.*, 1999; de Leon *et al.*, 2004; Karas *et al.*, 2004; Korf *et al.*, 2004).

Neuropathological studies of the aging brain have examined both positive and negative phenomena (Gómez-Isla & Hyman, 2003; DeKosky *et al.*, 2006). Of the former, neurofibrillary pathology (neurofibrillary tangles, neuropil threads) and senile neuritic plaques, hallmarks of the AD brain, may be seen in cognitively normal older individuals. The development of neurofibrillary pathology follows a relatively stereotyped hierarchical pattern with age, appearing first in the transentorhinal cortex (Arnold *et al.*, 1991; Braak & Braak, 1991). Spread to hippocampal and association cortex is associated with progressive appearance of cognitive decline. Senile plaques have a broader and more variable distribution; a significant burden may be associated with normal cognition. Negative phenomena include neuronal and synaptic loss. In normal aging, there is relative preservation of cortical and hippocampal neuronal populations, although subcortical structures such as the basal forebrain, locus caeruleus, and substantia nigra do show losses. In contrast, marked cell loss has been observed in entorhinal cortex in MCI, followed later by involvement of association cortex, changes which increase in severity with increasing severity of illness. In other words, preclinical AD (MCI) and normal aging may be differentiated on a pathological basis, the changes in the former falling midway between those seen in normal aging and in AD (Kordower *et al.*, 2001; DeKosky *et al.*, 2006; Markesbery *et al.*, 2006).

Longitudinal studies have shown a conversion rate from MCI to AD of around 10–15% per year. Clearly, if some MCI, mostly amnestic MCI, is prodromal AD, or early-stage AD (Morris, 2006), then a disease-modifying therapeutic intervention at this stage might be anticipated to delay progression to, and hence reduce the incidence of, AD. A double-blind placebo-controlled trial of the cholinesterase inhibitor donepezil in MCI suggested initial delay in conversion rate in the treated group but with equalization of conversion rates by 3 years (Petersen *et al.*, 2005), confirming the lack of effect seen in an earlier trial of donepezil of shorter duration (Salloway *et al.*, 2004). In the future, drugs targeting specific pathogenetic processes in AD may find a role in MCI. Since the amyloid hypothesis remains the most tenable explanation of AD pathogenesis, targeting the Aβ protein, by means of immunotherapy ('vaccine': Schenk *et al.*, 1999; Gilman *et al.*, 2005) or secretase inhibitors (Larner, 2004c), and the consequences of its overproduction such as oxidative stress, would seem logical. However, vitamin E (α-tocopherol), which is believed to act as an antioxidant, failed to slow conversion rate of MCI to AD (Petersen *et al.*, 2005).

REFERENCES

Albert MS. Normal and abnormal memory: aging and Alzheimer's disease. In: Wang E, Snyder DS (eds.), *Handbook of the Aging Brain*. San Diego: Academic Press, 1998: 1–17.

Arnold SE, Hyman BT, Flory J, Damasio AR, Van Hoesen GW. The topographical and neuroanatomical distribution of neurofibrillary tangles and neuritic plaques in cerebral cortex of patients with Alzheimer's disease. *Cerebral Cortex* 1991; **1**: 103–16.

Braak H, Braak E. Neuropathological stageing [*sic*] of Alzheimer-related changes. *Acta Neuropathol (Berl)* 1991; **82**: 239–59.

DeKosky ST, Ikonomovic MD, Hamilton RL, Bennett DA, Mufson EJ. Neuropathology of mild cognitive impairment in the elderly. In: Gauthier S, Scheltens P, Cummings JL (eds.), *Alzheimer's Disease and Related Disorders Annual 5*. London: Taylor & Francis, 2006: 1–16.

de leon MJ, Desanti S, Zinkowski R, *et al*. MRI and CSF studies in the early diagnosis of Alzheimer's disease. *J Intern Med* 2004; **256**: 205–23.

Gauthier S, Touchon J. Mild cognitive impairment is not a clinical entity and should not be treated. *Arch Neurol* 2005; **62**: 1164–6.

Gilman S, Koller M, Black RS, *et al*. Clinical effects of Abeta immunization (AN1792) in patients with AD in an interrupted trial. *Neurology* 2005; **64**: 1553–62.

Golomb J, Kluger A, Garrard P, Ferris S. *Clinician's Manual on Mild Cognitive Impairment*. London: Science Press, 2001.

Gómez-Isla T, Hyman BT. Neuropathological changes in normal aging, mild cognitive impairment, and

Alzheimer's disease. In: Petersen RC (ed.), *Mild Cognitive Impairment: Aging to Alzheimer's Disease*. Oxford: Oxford University Press, 2003: 191–204.

Hughes CP, Berg L, Danziger WL, Coben LA, Martin RL. A new clinical scale for the staging of dementia. *Br J Psychiatry* 1982; **140**: 566–72.

Jack CR Jr, Petersen RC, Xu YC, *et al.* Prediction of AD with MRI-based hippocampal volume in mild cognitive impairment. *Neurology* 1999; **52**: 1397–403.

Karas GB, Scheltens P, Rombouts SARB, *et al.* Global and local gray matter loss in mild cognitive impairment and Alzheimer's disease. *Neuroimage* 2004; **23**: 708–16.

Kordower JH, Chu Y, Stebbins GT, *et al.* Loss and atrophy of layer II entorhinal cortex neurons in elderly people with mild cognitive impairment. *Ann Neurol* 2001; **49**: 202–13.

Korf ESC, Wahlund LO, Visser PJ, Scheltens P. Medial temporal lobe atrophy on MRI predicts dementia in patients with mild cognitive impairment. *Neurology* 2004; **63**: 94–100.

Larner AJ. 'Posterior cortical atrophy' or 'focal-onset Alzheimer's disease'? A clinical, neuropsychological and neuroimaging study. *J Neurol* 2004a; **251** (suppl 3): III102 (abstract P385).

Larner AJ. Getting it wrong: the clinical misdiagnosis of Alzheimer's disease. *Int J Clin Pract* 2004b; **58**: 1092–4.

Larner AJ. Secretases as therapeutic targets in Alzheimer's disease: patents 2000–2004. *Exp Opin Therap Patents* 2004c; **14**: 1403–20.

Levine DN, Lee JM, Fisher CM. The visual variant of Alzheimer's disease: a clinicopathologic case study. *Neurology* 1993; **43**: 305–13.

McKhann G, Drachman D, Folstein M, *et al.* Clinical diagnosis of Alzheimer's disease. Report of the NINCDS-ADRDA work group under the auspices of the Department of Health and Human Service Task forces on Alzheimer's disease. *Neurology* 1984; **34**: 939–44.

Markesbery WR, Schmitt FA, Kryscio RJ, *et al.* Neuropathologic substrate of mild cognitive impairment. *Arch Neurol* 2006; **63**: 38–46.

Morris J. The CDR: current version and scoring rules. *Neurology* 1993; **43**: 2412–4.

Morris JC. Mild cognitive impairment is early-stage Alzheimer disease: time to revise diagnostic criteria. *Arch Neurol* 2006; **63**: 15–16.

Perneczky R, Pohl C, Sorg C, *et al.* Impairment of activities of daily living requiring memory of complex reasoning as part of the MCI syndrome. *Int J Geriatr Psychiatry* 2006; **21**: 158–62.

Petersen RC (ed.). *Mild Cognitive Impairment: Aging to Alzheimer's Disease*. Oxford: Oxford University Press, 2003.

Petersen RC. Mild cognitive impairment: current research and clinical implications. *Semin Neurol* 2007; **27**: 22–31.

Petersen RC, Morris JC. Mild cognitive impairment as a clinical entity and treatment target. *Arch Neurol* 2005; **62**: 1160–3.

Petersen RC, Smith GE, Waring SC, *et al.* Mild cognitive impairment: clinical characterization and outcome. *Arch Neurol* 1999; **56**: 303–8.

Petersen RC, Thomas RG, Grundman M, *et al.* Vitamin E and donepezil for the treatment of mild cognitive impairment. *N Engl J Med* 2005; **352**: 2379–88.

Portet F, Ousset PJ, Visser PJ, *et al.* Mild cognitive impairment (MCI) in medical practice: a critical review of the concept and new diagnostic procedure. Report of the MCI Working Group of the European Consortium on Alzheimer's Disease. *J Neurol Neurosurg Psychiatry* 2006; **77**: 714–18.

Reisberg B, Ferris SH, de Leon MJ, Crook T. The Global Deterioration Scale (GDS) for assessment of primary degenerative dementia. *Am J Psych* 1982; **139**: 1136–9.

Ritchie K, Touchon J. Mild cognitive impairment: conceptual basis and current nosological status. *Lancet* 2000; **355**: 225–8.

Salloway S, Ferris S, Kluger A, *et al.* Efficacy of donepezil in mild cognitive impairment: a randomized placebo-controlled trial. *Neurology* 2004; **63**: 651–7.

Schenk D, Barbour R, Dunn W, *et al.* Immunization with amyloid-β attenuates Alzheimer-disease-like pathology in the PDAPP mouse. *Nature* 1999; **400**: 173–7.

Tuokko HA, Hultsch DF (eds.). *Mild Cognitive Impairment: International Perspectives*. London: Taylor & Francis, 2006.

Visser PJ, Verhey FRJ, Scheltens P, *et al.* Diagnostic accuracy of the Preclinical AD Scale (PAS) in cognitively mildly impaired subjects. *J Neurol* 2002; **249**: 312–19.

Winblad B, Palmer K, Kivipelto M, *et al.* Mild cognitive impairment: beyond controversies, towards a consensus. Report of the International Working Group on Mild Cognitive Impairment. *J Int Med* 2004; **256**: 240–6.

Cerebrovascular disease: vascular dementia and vascular cognitive impairment

Cognitive impairment and dementia associated with cerebrovascular disease is not a unitary entity, but one typified by clinical, pathological, and aetiological heterogeneity. Different variants or subtypes have been noted for over a century but still the classification and categorization of vascular dementia (VaD) and vascular cognitive impairment is evolving, current taxonomies incorporating combinations of lesion aetiology, pathological type, neuroanatomical location, and clinical syndrome (e.g. Amar & Wilcock, 1996; Chiu *et al.*, 2000; Erkinjuntti & Gauthier, 2002; Bowler & Hachinski, 2003; De Leeuw & van Gijn, 2003; O'Brien *et al.*, 2003; Rockwood *et al.*, 2003; Godefroy & Bogousslavsky, 2007). Various consensus diagnostic criteria for VaD have been proposed, including the State of California Alzheimer's Disease Diagnostic and Treatment Centers (ADDTC) criteria (Chui *et al.*, 1992) and the National Institute of Neurological Disorders and Stroke and the Association Internationale pour la Recherche et l'Enseignement en Neurosciences (NINDS-AIREN) criteria (Román *et al.*, 1993), as well as the general criteria of DSM and ICD. NINDS-AIREN recognizes the need to establish a causal relationship between cerebrovascular lesions and cognitive deficit both spatially and temporally, emphasizing the importance of neuroimaging to corroborate clinical findings (Román *et al.*, 1993). However, because memory impairment is the most salient feature in Alzheimer's disease (AD), the most common cause of dementia, it has been noted that many of these diagnostic criteria have been inadvertently 'Alzheimerized', with undue emphasis placed on memory loss at the expense of other neuropsychological features (Bowler & Hachinski, 2003). This may account for the low sensitivity, but high specificity, of these criteria (Holmes *et al.*, 1999).

Perhaps one of the reasons for this is that cerebrovascular disease is very common in AD. In one community-based study most patients with dementia coming to autopsy had mixed AD/cerebrovascular disease (MRC CFAS, 2001). Considering the shared vascular risk factors for AD and VaD (Stewart, 2005) this observation is perhaps not surprising. Conversely, there have been reports of series of patients clinically diagnosed as VaD who at postmortem proved to have either AD alone or mixed disease (Nolan *et al.*, 1998). Double pathology may lower the threshold for clinical manifestation of cognitive deficits (Snowdon *et al.*, 1997; Snowdon, 2001). Pure VaD may be a rare cause of dementia (Hulette *et al.*, 1997).

Clinically the distinction between AD and VaD is not always clear-cut. The Hachinski Ischaemic Score (HIS) has been suggested to differentiate patients with VaD from those with AD (Hachinski *et al.*, 1975) but is recognized to have shortcomings. In a neuropathologically confirmed series of dementia patients, items from the HIS showing independent correlation with VaD were stepwise deterioration, fluctuating course, and a history of hypertension, stroke, and focal neurological symptoms (Moroney *et al.*, 1997).

The definition of vascular cognitive impairment (VCI: Bowler & Hachinski, 1995), a new conceptual approach, stemmed in part from the realization that older concepts were unduly influenced by thinking on AD, and in part from the realization that cognitive decline due to vascular disease is amenable to prevention. VCI might be envisaged as one form of mild cognitive impairment (MCI: see Section 2.6). To detect VCI may require new, specifically designed, neuropsychological test instruments, rather than those typically used for AD, for example a vascular equivalent of the ADAS-Cog, 'VaDAS-Cog'.

Attempts to define the neuropsychological profile of VaD have often been undertaken in comparison with AD, but this has proved difficult because of diagnostic and methodological inconsistencies, and no reliable profile has emerged. Nonetheless, reviewing such studies and using strict inclusion and exclusion criteria, such as matching for level of overall cognitive decline, Sachdev and Looi (2003) found relative preservation of long-term memory and greater deficits in executive function in VaD patients, corroborating previous qualitative reviews (e.g. Hodges & Graham, 2001). Cognitive domains not permitting discrimination of VaD from AD included digit span, attention, visuoconstructive, and conceptual tasks, whilst language was thought to be an area in which AD would be predicted to be superior to VaD (Sachdev & Looi, 2003). Verbal fluency for letter is more affected in VaD (Duff Canning *et al.*, 2004) whilst category fluency is equally impaired in VaD and AD (Bentham *et al.*, 1997). The heterogeneity of the VaD group may mandate subdivision in order to find diagnostically meaningful cognitive profiles.

Pending the development of empirically derived, rather than consensus, criteria which are operationalized and have undergone validation, classification of vascular dementia remains somewhat arbitrary. NINDS-AIREN suggested a pathogenetic classification based on hypoxia–ischaemia and infarction (encompassing multi-infarct, small vessel, and strategic infarct dementia), hypoperfusion (incomplete infarctions), and intracerebral haemorrhage dementia (Román *et al.*, 1993). These mechanisms are not necessarily mutually exclusive, and similarly the neuropathological substrates of vascular dementia are heterogeneous and may overlap (Vinters *et al.*, 2000; Morris *et al.*, 2004). For the purposes of this chapter, classification is largely clinical, examining cortical, subcortical, and strategic infarct subtypes. Haemodynamic or hypoperfusion dementia, associated with occlusive carotid artery disease or watershed infarcts (also known as distal field or borderzone infarcts), is included with cortical VaD. The entity of 'cardiogenic dementia' discussed in the older literature (Lane, 1991) is also assumed to fall within this rubric. The category of haemorrhagic dementia is broad,

and may potentially include any cause of intraparenchymal or subarachnoid haemorrhage (see Section 3.4). The hereditary causes of vascular disease are increasingly defined (Markus, 2003), some of which may be associated with dementia such as CADASIL (Section 3.6.2), MELAS and other mitochondrial disorders (Section 5.5.1), and Anderson–Fabry disease (Section 5.5.3). Other brain vascular disorders considered here include arteriovenous malformations, certain vasculopathies (cerebral vasculitides are discussed in the chapter on inflammatory and systemic disorders: Section 6.10), concluding with a miscellaneous group of conditions in which vascular mechanisms may be suspected rather than proved.

REFERENCES

Amar K, Wilcock G. Vascular dementia. *BMJ* 1996; **312**: 227–31.

Bentham PW, Jones S, Hodges JR. A comparison of semantic memory in vascular dementia and dementia of Alzheimer's type. *Int J Geriatr Psychiatry* 1997; **12**: 575–80.

Bowler JV, Hachinski V. Vascular cognitive impairment: a new approach to vascular dementia. In: Hachinski V (ed.), *Cerebrovascular Disease*. London: Bailliere Tindall, 1995: 357–76.

Bowler JV, Hachinski V (eds.). *Vascular Cognitive Impairment: Reversible Dementia*. Oxford: Oxford University Press, 2003.

Chiu E, Gustafson L, Ames D, Folstein MF (eds.). *Cerebrovascular Disease and Dementia: Pathology, Neuropsychiatry and Management*. London: Martin Dunitz, 2000.

Chui HC, Victoroff JI, Margolin D, *et al.* Criteria for the diagnosis of ischemic vascular dementia proposed by the State of California Alzheimer's Disease Diagnostic and Treatment Centers. *Neurology* 1992; **42**: 473–80.

De Leeuw FE, van Gijn J. Vascular dementia. *Pract Neurol* 2003; **3**: 86–91.

Duff Canning SJ, Leach L, Stuss D, Ngo L, Black SE. Diagnostic utility of abbreviated fluency measures in Alzheimer disease and vascular dementia. *Neurology* 2004; **62**: 556–62.

Erkinjuntti T, Gauthier S (eds.). *Vascular Cognitive Impairment*. London: Martin Dunitz, 2002.

Godefroy O, Bogousslavsky J. *The Behavioral and Cognitive Neurology of Stroke.* Cambridge: Cambridge University Press, 2007.

Hachinski VC, Iliff LD, Zilkha E, *et al.* Cerebral blood flow in dementia. *Arch Neurol* 1975; **32**: 632–7.

Hodges JR, Graham NL. Vascular dementias. In: Hodges JR, (ed.), *Early-Onset Dementia: a Multidisciplinary Approach.* Oxford: Oxford University Press, 2001: 319–37.

Holmes C, Cairns N, Lantos P, *et al.* Validity of current clinical criteria for Alzheimer's disease, vascular dementia and dementia with Lewy bodies. *Br J Psychiatry* 1999; **174**: 45–50.

Hulette C, Nochlin D, McKeel DW, *et al.* Clinical–neuropathologic findings in multi-infarct dementia: a report of six autopsied cases. *Neurology* 1997; **48**: 668–72.

Lane RJM. 'Cardiogenic dementia' revisited. *J R Soc Med* 1991; **84**: 577–9.

Markus HS (ed.). *Stroke Genetics.* Oxford: Oxford University Press, 2003.

Moroney JT, Bagiella E, Desmond DW, *et al.* Meta-analysis of the Hachinski Ischemic Score in pathologically verified dementias. *Neurology* 1997; **49**: 1096–105.

Morris JH, Kalimo H, Viitanen M. Vascular dementias. In: Esiri MM, Trojanowski JQ, Lee VMY (eds.), *The Neuropathology of Dementia* (2nd edition). Cambridge; Cambridge University Press, 2004: 289–329.

MRC CFAS. Pathological correlates of late-onset dementia in a multicentre, community-based population in England and Wales. Neuropathology Group of the Medical Research Council Cognitive Function and Ageing Study. *Lancet* 2001; **357**: 169–75.

Nolan KA, Lino MM, Seligmann AW, *et al.* Absence of vascular dementia in an autopsy series from a dementia clinic. *J Am Geriatr Soc* 1998; **46**: 597–604.

O'Brien J, Ames D, Gustafson L, Folstein MF, Chiu E (eds.). *Cerebrovascular Disease, Cognitive Impairment and Dementia.* London: Martin Dunitz, 2003.

Rockwood K, Burns A, Gauthier S, DeKosky ST. Vascular cognitive impairment. *Lancet Neurol* 2003; **2**: 89–98.

Román GC, Tatemichi TK, Erkinjuntti T, *et al.* Vascular dementia: diagnostic criteria for research studies. Report of the NINDS-AIREN international workshop. *Neurology* 1993; **43**: 250–60.

Sachdev PC, Looi JCL. Neuropsychological differentiation of Alzheimer's disease and vascular dementia. In: Bowler JV, Hachinski V (eds.), *Vascular Cognitive Impairment: Reversible Dementia.* Oxford: Oxford University Press, 2003: 153–75.

Snowdon D. *Aging with Grace: the Nun Study and the Science of Old Age. How We Can All Live Longer, Healthier and More Vital Lives.* London: Fourth Estate, 2001.

Snowdon DA, Greiner LH, Mortimer JA, *et al.* Brain infarction and the clinical expression of Alzheimer's disease. The Nun Study. *JAMA* 1997; **277**: 813–17.

Stewart R. Vascular factors in Alzheimer's disease. In: Burns A, O'Brien J, Ames D (eds.), *Dementia* (3rd edition). London: Hodder Arnold, 2005: 436–43.

Vinters HV, Ellis WG, Zarow C, *et al.* Neuropathologic substrates of vascular dementia. *J Neuropath Exp Neurol* 2000; **59**: 931–45.

3.1 Cortical vascular dementia, multi-infarct dementia (MID), post-stroke dementia

Originally conceived of as multi-infarct dementia (MID: Hachinski *et al.*, 1974), cortical vascular dementia refers to cognitive impairment following large vessel disease, cardiac and carotid embolic events, and hence also post-stroke dementia (Leys *et al.*, 2005), resulting in large cortical and corticosubcortical complete infarcts in arterial territory distribution. Within this category may also be included haemodynamic or hypoperfusion dementia, for example related to occlusive carotid artery disease or watershed (distal field, border-zone) infarction between the territories of anterior, middle, and posterior cerebral arteries, and incomplete infarctions related to global cerebral ischaemia following profound and prolonged hypotension, for example associated with cardiac arrest, cardiac arrhythmias, or hypovolaemic shock. The studies of Tomlinson *et al.* (1970) suggested that dementia correlated with increasing volume of infarcted tissue, above a threshold of 100 ml. Classically cortical VaD is characterized as having an abrupt onset and stepwise deterioration, and it is associated with focal neurological signs (e.g. hemiparesis, hemianopia, gait impairment, pseudobulbar palsy), as expected with stroke (Hachinski *et al.*, 1975).

The cognitive profile of cortical VaD is dependent upon the precise arterial territory affected, but is said to include memory impairment, cortical signs such as aphasia, apraxia, or agnosia, visuospatial and/or visuoconstructive difficulties, and executive dysfunction, although the latter is not as marked as in subcortical VaD. The fact that around 10% or more of stroke patients have pre-existing dementia ('pre-stroke dementia': Hénon *et al.*, 1997; Klimkowicz *et al.*, 2002), which may result from vascular lesions and/or concurrent Alzheimer's disease, may potentially confound these observations.

Occlusive carotid artery disease is a well-recognized risk factor for the development of transient ischaemic attacks (TIA) and stroke. Studies have been undertaken to assess whether occlusive carotid artery disease is also associated with cognitive impairment. A systematic review of such studies (Bakker *et al.*, 2000) found marked heterogeneity in terms of study design, neuropsychological assessment procedures, and interpretation, making it difficult to draw meaningful conclusions. Accepting a degree of case selection bias (i.e. those likely to undergo surgery), the majority of studies found evidence of cognitive impairment, generally mild, in both symptomatic and asymptomatic patients. This was associated with either generalized cognitive impairment or with specific deficits in memory, reasoning, and psychomotor skills. Hence, cognitive impairment may be the sole symptom of carotid artery stenosis (Lehrner *et al.*, 2005).

Similarly, the data on the effects on cognition of carotid endarterectomy for carotid artery occlusive disease are difficult to interpret because of methodological issues (Lunn *et al.*, 1999). Although the majority of studies suggest postoperative improvement, for example in verbal memory, constructive abilities, and visual attention (Antonelli Incalzi *et al.*, 1997), others suggest no change, making it impossible to draw clear conclusions about the efficacy of this procedure for the treatment of cognitive problems (Lunn *et al.*, 1999). Cognitive improvement in a patient with bilateral carotid occlusions who underwent extracranial–intracranial bypass surgery has been reported (Tatemichi *et al.*, 1995). Hypoperfusion may be the cause of cognitive impairments sometimes encountered in patients with dural arteriovenous fistulae (see Section 3.5.1),

Watershed infarction has on occasion been reported to be associated with dementia (Hashiguchi *et al.*, 2000).

Cognitive recovery may occur after stroke, for example in aphasia, visual neglect, attention span, and verbal recall, but this is variable (Wade *et al.*, 1988).

REFERENCES

Antonelli Incalzi R, Gemma A, Landi F, *et al.* Neuropsychologic effects of carotid endarterectomy. *J Clin Exp Neuropsychol* 1997; **19**: 785–94.

Bakker FC, Klijn CJM, Jennekens-Schinkel A, Kappelle LJ. Cognitive disorder in patients with occlusive disease of the carotid artery: a systematic review of the literature. *J Neurol* 2000; **247**: 669–76.

Hachinski VC, Iliff LD, Zilkha E, *et al.* Cerebral blood flow in dementia. *Arch Neurol* 1975; **32**: 632–7.

Hachinski VC, Lassen NA, Marshall J. Multi-infarct dementia: a cause of mental deterioration in the elderly. *Lancet* 1974; **2**: 207–10.

Hashiguchi S, Mine H, Ide M, Kawachi Y. Watershed infarction associated with dementia and cerebral atrophy. *Psychiatry Clin Neurosci* 2000; **54**: 163–8.

Hénon H, Pasquier F, Durieu I, *et al.* Preexisting dementia in stroke patients : baseline frequency, associated factors, and outcome. *Stroke* 1997; **28**: 2429–36.

Klimkowicz A, Dziedzic T, Slowik A, *et al.* Incidence of pre- and poststroke dementia: Cracow Stroke Registry. *Dement Geriatr Cogn Disord* 2002; **14**: 137–40.

Lehrner J, Willfort A, Mlekusch I, *et al.* Neuropsychological outcome 6 months after unilateral carotid stenting. *J Clin Exp Neuropsychol* 2005; **27**: 859–66.

Leys D, Henon H, Mackowiak Cordoliani MA, Pasquier F. Poststroke dementia. *Lancet Neurol* 2005; **4**: 752–9.

Lunn S, Crawley F, Harrison MJG, Brown MM, Newman SP. Impact of carotid endarterectomy upon cognitive functioning: a systematic review of the literature. *Cerebrovasc Dis* 1999; **9**: 74–81.

Tatemichi TK, Desmond DW, Prohovnik I, Eidelberg D. Dementia associated with bilateral carotid occlusions: neuropsychological and haemodynamic course after extracranial to intracranial bypass surgery. *J Neurol Neurosurg Psychiatry* 1995; **58**: 633–6.

Tomlinson BE, Blessed G, Roth M. Observations on the brains of demented old people. *J Neurol Sci* 1970; **11**: 205–42.

Wade DT, Wood VA, Hewer RL. Recovery of cognitive function soon after stroke: a study of visual neglect, attention span and verbal recall. *J Neurol Neurosurg Psychiatry* 1988; **51**: 10–13.

3.2 Subcortical vascular dementia, Binswanger's disease, lacunar state, subcortical ischaemic vascular disease (SIVD)

Diffuse damage to subcortical structures is probably the commonest cause of vascular dementia or vascular cognitive impairment, due to small vessel disease in individuals with hypertension. Subcortical forms of VaD and VCI encompass both the leukoencephalopathy originally described by Binswanger and the *état lacunaire* originally described by Marie.

In 1894 Otto Binswanger reported subcortical obliteration of small cerebral arteries and arterioles, often in association with systemic hypertension, leading to pathological periventricular demyelination and the clinical correlate of dementia (translation by Blass *et al.*, 1991). The condition, subsequently known as Binswanger's disease, Binswanger's encephalopathy, or subcortical arteriosclerotic encephalopathy (SAE), was judged relatively rare until the advent of structural neuroimaging showed radiological evidence of basal ganglia infarcts and periventricular white matter disease often with sparing of subcortical U fibres (the white matter changes sometimes known as leukoaraiosis: Hachinski, 1987), sometimes associated with cognitive impairment, leading to increased use of this diagnostic category (Babikian & Ropper, 1987; Fisher, 1989; Bennett *et al.*, 1990; Caplan, 1995). Leukoaraiosis is associated with

cognitive impairment and the risk of cognitive impairment (Pantoni & Inzitari, 2005)

The *état lacunaire*, or lacunar state, as described by Pierre Marie in 1901, comprised small cavitary lesions in the brain parenchyma, particularly in deep grey matter, internal capsule, basis pontis, and deep hemispheric white matter, reflecting small vessel disease, which occurs frequently in patients with hypertension. Lacunar infarcts, also known as small deep infarcts, are readily seen on neuroimaging, and may be associated with a variety of clinical syndromes, originally described by Fisher (1982), such as pure motor stroke, pure sensory stroke, sensorimotor stroke, and ataxic hemiparesis. In addition, lacunar strokes may be associated with cognitive impairment which, in contrast to cortical VaD, is often of insidious, rather than abrupt, onset, and has a progressive, rather than stepwise, course.

In epidemiological studies of independently living elderly individuals, increasing severity of white matter changes and lacunes on MR imaging has been associated with deteriorating cognition, independent of vascular risk factors and stroke, the more so if there is concurrent medial temporal lobe atrophy (van der Flier *et al.*, 2005a,b).

The cognitive profile of subcortical VaD is typically that of executive dysfunction, as may be anticipated with lesions affecting subcortical circuits, with slowed information processing and impairments of initiation, planning, sequencing, and abstracting (Kramer *et al.*, 2002). Certainly MR imaging has indicated that infarcts and white matter lesions increase the risk of executive dysfunction (Vataja *et al.*, 2003). Episodic memory impairment may, or may not, be present, and is typically milder than in AD, with impaired recall but better recognition and with benefit from cueing (Desmond *et al.*, 1999). There may be additional neuropsychiatric signs (depression, inertia, emotional lability) and neurological signs, although the latter are fewer than in cortical VaD, including gait disorder of frontal type (broad-based, short-stepped), subtle upper motor neurone signs, dysarthria, urinary incontinence, and extrapyramidal signs. Although there is overlap, mild subcortical vascular dementia may be differentiated from AD on the basis of greater impairment in tests of semantic memory, executive function, and visuo-spatial and perceptual skills (Graham *et al.*, 2004).

More recently, cases which might previously have been labelled as Binswanger's disease and/or lacunar infarctions have been incorporated under the rubric of subcortical ischaemic vascular disease (SIVD: Román *et al.*, 2002). Research criteria have been suggested (Erkinjuntti *et al.*, 2000), with diagnosis based on the relationship between clinical and radiological findings, specifically the presence of extensive white matter lesions and multiple lacunar infarcts due to small vessel disease. Progressive cognitive decline may be the clinical correlate. In a series of radiologically (MRI) defined cases of SIVD, executive deficits and subtle delayed memory deficits were found, thought to reflect disruption of frontal-subcortical circuits and medial temporal lobe atrophy respectively (Jokinen *et al.*, 2006).

Treatment of neuropsychological deficits in vascular dementia

Since VaD is associated with cholinergic deficits, the use of cholinesterase inhibitors in the treatment of VaD has been explored in a number of studies, overviews of which suggest that modest benefits in cognitive function may accrue (Erkinjuntti *et al.*, 2004). Memantine may also improve cognition in vascular dementia (Orgogozo *et al.*, 2002; Wilcock *et al.*, 2002).

REFERENCES

Babikian V, Ropper AH. Binswanger's disease: a review. *Stroke* 1987; **18**: 2–12.

Bennett DA, Wilson RS, Gilley DW, Fox JH. Clinical diagnosis of Binswanger's disease. *J Neurol Neurosurg Psychiatry* 1990; **53**: 961–5.

Binswanger O. Die Abgrenzung der allgemeinen progressiven paralyse. *Berl Klin Wochenschr* 1894; **31**: 1102–5, 1137–9, 1180–6.

Blass JP, Hoyer S, Nitsch R. A translation of Otto Binswanger's article, 'The delineation of the generalized progressive paralyses', 1894. *Arch Neurol* 1991; **48**: 961–72.

Caplan LR. Binswanger's disease revisited. *Neurology* 1995; **45**: 626–33.

Desmond DW, Erkinjuntti T, Sano M, *et al.* The cognitive syndrome of vascular dementia: implications for clinical trials. *Alzheimer Dis Assoc Disord* 1999; **13** (suppl 3): S21–9.

Erkinjuntti T, Inzitari D, Pantoni L, *et al.* Research criteria for subcortical vascular dementia in clinical trials. *J Neural Transm Suppl* 2000; **59**: 23–30.

Erkinjuntti T, Roman G, Gauthier S, Feldman H, Rockwood K. Emerging therapies for vascular dementia and vascular cognitive impairment. *Stroke* 2004; **35**: 1010–7.

Fisher CM. Lacunar strokes and infarcts: a review. *Neurology* 1982; **32**: 871–6.

Fisher CM. Binswanger's encephalopathy: a review. *J Neurol* 1989; **236**: 65–79.

Graham NL, Emery T, Hodges JR. Distinctive cognitive profiles in Alzheimer's disease and subcortical vascular dementia. *J Neurol Neurosurg Psychiatry* 2004; **75**: 61–71.

Hachinski VC. Leukoaraiosis. *Arch Neurol* 1987; **44**: 21–3.

Jokinen H, Kalska H, Mäntylä R, *et al.* Cognitive profile of subcortical ischaemic vascular disease. *J Neurol Neurosurg Psychiatry* 2006; **77**: 28–33.

Kramer JH, Reed BR, Mungas D, Weiner MW, Chui HC. Executive dysfunction in subcortical ischaemic vascular disease. *J Neurol Neurosurg Psychiatry* 2002; **72**: 217–20.

Marie P. Des foyers lacunaires de désintégration de différents autres états cavitaires du cerveau. *Rev Méd* 1901; **21**: 281–98.

Orgogozo JM, Rigaud AS, Stöffler A, Möbius HJ, Forette F. Efficacy and safety of memantine in patients with mild to moderate vascular dementia: a randomized, placebo-controlled trial (MMM 300). *Stroke* 2002; **33**: 1834–9.

Pantoni L, Inzitari D. Leukoaraiosis and cognitive impairment. In: Burns A, O'Brien J, Ames D (eds.), *Dementia* (3rd edition). London: Hodder Arnold, 2005: 546–64.

Román GC, Erkinjuntti T, Pantoni L, Wallin A, Chui HC. Subcortical ischaemic vascular dementia. *Lancet Neurol* 2002; **1**: 426–36.

van der Flier WM, van Straaten ECW, Barkhof F, *et al.* Small vessel disease and general cognitive function in nondisabled elderly: the LADIS study. *Stroke* 2005a; **36**: 2116–20.

van der Flier WM, van Straaten ECW, Barkhof F *et al.* Medial temporal lobe atrophy and white matter hyperintensities are associated with mild cognitive deficits in non-disabled elderly people: the LADIS study. *J Neurol Neurosurg Psychiatry* 2005b; **76**: 1497–500.

Vataja R, Pohjasvaara T, Mäntylä R, *et al.* MRI correlates of executive dysfunction in patients with ischaemic stroke. *Eur J Neurol* 2003; **10**: 625–31.

Wilcock GK, Möbius HJ, Stöffler A. A double-blind placebo-controlled multicentre study of memantine in mild to moderate vascular dementia (MMM500). *Int Clin Psychopharmacol* 2002; **17**: 297–305.

3.3   Strategic infarct dementia, strategic strokes

Strategic infarct dementia refers to focal ischaemic lesions in regions eloquent for cognitive processes, although they may not cause dementia in the strict sense of the DSM or ICD criteria, and hence strategic strokes may be a better term. The possibility that other subclinical lesions may contribute to the clinical picture cannot be entirely excluded. Nonetheless, a variety of locations have been associated with cognitive deficits (Katz *et al.*, 1987; Tatemichi *et al.*, 1995).

REFERENCES

Katz DI, Alexander MP, Mandell AM. Dementia following strokes in the mesencephalon and diencephalon. *Arch Neurol* 1987; **44**: 1127–33.

Tatemichi TK, Desmond DW, Prohovnik I. Strategic infarcts in vascular dementia: a clinical and brain imaging experience. *Arzneimittelforschung* 1995; **45**: 371–85.

3.3.1   Angular gyrus

Infarction of the angular gyrus in the posterior parietotemporal region of the dominant hemisphere in the territory of the posterior branch of the middle cerebral artery may be associated with combinations of aphasia, alexia with agraphia, and Gerstmann syndrome (acalculia, right–left disorientation, finger agnosia), sometimes in the absence of focal sensorimotor deficit and sometimes simulating Alzheimer's disease (Benson *et al.*, 1982; Roeltgen *et al.*, 1983).

REFERENCES

Benson DF, Cummings JL, Tsai SY. Angular gyrus syndrome simulating Alzheimer's disease. *Arch Neurol* 1982; **39**: 616–20.

Roeltgen DP, Sevush S, Heilman KM. Pure Gerstmann's syndrome from a focal lesion. *Arch Neurol* 1983; **40**: 46–7.

3.3.2   Corpus callosum, fornix

Acute anterograde amnesia following ischaemic infarct of the genu of the corpus callosum and both columns and the body of the fornix has been reported, with subjective improvement in memory on follow-up (Moudgil *et al.*, 2000). Such a strategic infarct must be exceedingly rare. Selective damage to the fornix is more commonly seen after surgery for third ventricle lesions such as colloid cyst (see Section 7.2.3).

REFERENCES

Moudgil SS, Azzouz M, Al-Azzaz A, Haut M, Gutmann L. Amnesia due to fornix infarction. *Stroke* 2000; **31**: 1418–19.

3.3.3   Thalamus

Several types of thalamic infarct have been described, involving differing thalamic vascular territories and damaging differing nuclei (Schmahmann, 2003). Various neuropsychological deficits have been described with thalamic infarctions, particularly paramedian or polar infarcts, including aphasia, hemineglect, amnesia, and dementia (Van Der Werf *et al.*, 2000; de Freitas & Bogousslavsky, 2002).

A single branch of the posterior cerebral artery may supply the medial thalamic nuclei bilaterally. Occlusion of this paramedian thalamic artery may therefore cause bilateral medial thalamic infarction, with acute onset of confusion followed by a persistent amnesia, so-called diencephalic amnesia. This amnesia may be global, or may resemble Wernicke–Korsakoff syndrome (see Section 8.3.1; Parkin *et al.*, 1994), or cause principally autobiographical amnesia (e.g. Graff-Radford *et al.*, 1990; Tatemichi *et al.*, 1992; Hodges & McCarthy, 1993; Crews *et al.*, 1996).

The topographical correlates of amnesia are involvement of either the dorsomedial thalamic nucleus or the mammillothalamic tract and internal medullary lamina. Anterograde memory impairment for verbal material has been reported after left dorsomedial thalamic infarct, and for visuospatial material after right dorsomedial thalamic infarct (Speedie & Heilman, 1982, 1983). Functional imaging may also show frontal cortical hypoperfusion or hypometabolism. Selective verbal memory impairment after a left thalamic infarct involving the mammillothalamic tract has been reported (Schott *et al.*, 2003). Long-lasting amnesia is more often associated with bilateral lesions, as is dementia (see Section 1.11). Associated features include impaired attention, apathy, slow verbal and motor responses, and amnesia, with athymhormia (psychic akinesia) or akinetic mutism (Kalashnikova *et al.*, 1999).

Aphasia, usually of non-fluent type, may occur with left-sided thalamic lesions, and neglect and anosognosia with right-sided lesions, (Karussis *et al.*, 2000). Thalamic involvement may also have contributed to an unusual case of prolonged post-stroke mutism (Larner, 2006). Apraxia has also been reported with thalamic infarction (Nadeau *et al.*, 1994).

Executive impairment and attentional deficit may contribute to cognitive dysfunction after thalamic infarction (Van Der Werf *et al.*, 1999), and utilization behaviour may be seen (Eslinger *et al.*, 1991), although the latter has also been recorded with caudate lesions (Rudd *et al.*, 1998).

REFERENCES

Crews WD, Manning CA, Skalabrin E. Neuropsychological impairments of executive functions and memory in a case of bilateral paramedian thalamic infarction. *Neurocase* 1996; **2**: 405–12.

de Freitas GR, Bogousslavsky J. Thalamic infarcts. In: Donnan G, Norrving B, Bamford J, Bogousslavsky J (eds.), *Subcortical Stroke* (2nd edition). Oxford: Oxford University Press, 2002: 255–85.

Eslinger PJ, Warner GC, Grattan LM, Easton JD. Frontal lobe utilization behavior associated with paramedian thalamic infarction. *Neurology* 1991; **41**: 450–2.

Graff-Radford NR, Tranel D, Van Hoesen GW, Brandt JP. Diencephalic amnesia. *Brain* 1990; **113**: 1–25.

Hodges JR, McCarthy RA. Autobiographical amnesia resulting from bilateral paramedian thalamic infarction. *Brain* 1993; **116**: 921–40.

Kalashnikova LA, Gulevskaya TS, Kashina EM. Disorders of higher mental function due to single infarctions in the thalamus and in the area of the thalamofrontal tracts. *Neurosci Behav Physiol* 1999; **29**: 397–403.

Karussis D, Leker RR, Abramsky O. Cognitive dysfunction following thalamic stroke: a study of 16 cases and review of the literature. *J Neurol Sci* 2000; **172**: 25–9.

Larner AJ. Post-stroke mutism. *Pract Neurol* 2006; **6**: 192–4.

Nadeau SE, Roeltgen DP, Sevush S, Ballinger WE, Watson RT. Apraxia due to a pathologically documented thalamic infarction. *Neurology* 1994; **44**: 2133–7.

Parkin AJ, Rees JE, Hunkin NM, Rose PE. Impairment of memory following discrete thalamic infarction. *Neuropsychologia* 1994; **32**: 39–51.

Rudd R, Maruff P, MacCupsie-Moore C, *et al.* Stimulus relevance in eliciting utilisation behaviour: case study in a patient with a caudate lesion. *Cogn Neuropsychiatry* 1998; **3**: 287–98.

Schmahmann JD. Vascular syndromes of the thalamus. *Stroke* 2003; **34**: 2264–78.

Schott JM, Crutch SJ, Fox NC, Warrington EK. Development of selective verbal memory impairment secondary to a left thalamic infarct: a longitudinal case study. *J Neurol Neurosurg Psychiatry* 2003; **74**: 255–7.

Speedie LJ, Heilman KM. Amnestic disturbance following infarction of the left dorsomedial nucleus of the thalamus. *Neuropsychologia* 1982; **20**: 597–604.

Speedie LJ, Heilman KM. Anterograde memory deficits for visuospatial material after infarction of the right thalamus. *Arch Neurol* 1983; **40**: 183–6.

Tatemichi TK, Steinke W, Duncan C, *et al.* Paramedian thalamopeduncular infarction: clinical syndromes and magnetic resonance imaging. *Ann Neurol* 1992; **32**: 162–71.

Van Der Werf YD, Weerts JGE, Jolles J, *et al.* Neuropsychological correlates of a right unilateral lacunar thalamic infarction. *J Neurol Neurosurg Psychiatry* 1999; **66**: 36–42.

Van Der Werf YD, Witter MP, Uylings HB, Jolles J. Neuropsychology of infarctions in the thalamus: a review. *Neuropsychologia* 2000; **38**: 613–27.

3.3.4 Genu of the internal capsule

Infarction of the inferior genu of the internal capsule may cause an acute confusional state with inattention, memory loss, psychomotor retardation, apathy, and abulia (Tatemichi *et al.*, 1992). Persistent deficits associated with dominant hemisphere lesions include verbal memory, naming, and verbal fluency, reflecting damage to the limbic system (Kooistra & Heilman, 1988; Markowitsch *et al.*, 1990; Schnider *et al.*, 1996; Madureira *et al.*, 1999; van Zandvoort *et al.*, 2000; Pantoni *et al.*, 2001). As with thalamic infarcts, these neuropsychological sequelae may reflect disruption of thalamocortical pathways.

REFERENCES

Kooistra CA, Heilman KM. Memory loss from a subcortical white matter infarct. *J Neurol Neurosurg Psychiatry* 1988; **51**: 866–9.

Madureira S, Guerriero M, Ferro JM. A follow-up study of cognitive impairment due to inferior capsular genu infarction. *J Neurol* 1999; **246**: 764–9.

Markowitsch HJ, von Cramon DY, Hofmann E, Sick CD, Kinzler P. Verbal memory deterioration after unilateral infarct of the internal capsule in an adolescent. *Cortex* 1990; **26**: 597–609.

Pantoni L, Basile AM, Romanelli M, *et al.* Abulia and cognitive impairment in two patients with capsular genu infarct. *Acta Neurol Scand* 2001; **104**: 185–90.

Schnider A, Gutbrod K, Hess CW, Schroth G. Memory without context: amnesia with confabulations after infarction of the right capsular genu. *J Neurol Neurosurg Psychiatry* 1996; **61**: 186–93.

Tatemichi TK, Desmond DW, Prohovnik I, *et al.* Confusion and memory loss from capsular genu infarction: a thalamocortical disconnection syndrome? *Neurology* 1992; **42**: 1966–79.

van Zandvoort MJ, Aleman A, Kappelle LJ, De Haan EH. Cognitive functioning before and after a lacunar infarct. *Cerebrovasc Dis* 2000; **10**: 478–9.

3.3.5 Caudate nucleus, globus pallidus

Cognitive and neurobehavioural problems are common with vascular lesions of the caudate nucleus, which may also extend to involve the anterior limb of the internal capsule and the putamen. Mendez *et al.* (1989) found impaired sustained attention and executive function, and poor recall on tests of immediate and delayed recall in a series of 12 patients with mostly unilateral caudate lesions: some were apathetic or abulic, others disinhibited and impulsive. Similar observations have been made in other series (Caplan *et al.*, 1990; Kumral *et al.*, 1999), with additional aphasia with left-sided lesions and neglect with right-sided lesions. Executive dysfunction has also been noted (Kumral *et al.*, 1999). Poor recall of long-term verbal memory was the principal feature in an adolescent with an isolated infarct of the left caudate, internal capsule, and putamen (Markowitsch et al., 1990). A 2-year study of subcortical strokes found that patients with caudate lesions had lower scores on the MMSE (perhaps not a good test for subcortical deficits) on long-term follow-up than other locations, with evidence of deterioration despite no new strokes (Bokura & Robinson, 1997). These various cognitive changes have been ascribed to interruption of striatal efferents to the cortex.

Isolated athymhormia (psychic akinesia) has been reported with ischaemic pallidal lesions (Mori *et al.*, 1996).

REFERENCES

Bokura H, Robinson RG. Long-term cognitive impairment associated with caudate stroke. *Stroke* 1997; **28**: 970–5.

Caplan LR, Schmahmann JD, Kase CS, *et al.* Caudate infarcts. *Arch Neurol* 1990; **47**: 133–43.

Kumral E, Evyapan D, Balkir K. Acute caudate vascular lesions. *Stroke* 1999; **30**: 100–8.

Markowitsch HJ, von Cramon DY, Hofmann E, Sick CD, Kinzler P. Verbal memory deterioration after unilateral infarct of the internal capsule in an adolescent. *Cortex* 1990; **26**: 597–609.

Mendez MF, Adams NL, Lewandowski KS. Neurobehavioral changes associated with caudate lesions. *Neurology* 1989; **39**: 349–54.

Mori E, Yamashita H, Takauchi S, Kondo K. Isolated athymhormia following hypoxic bilateral pallidal lesions. *Behav Neurol* 1996; **9**: 17–23.

3.3.6 Hippocampus

Stroke limited to the hippocampus is a rare event; first-ever stroke confined to the hippocampus even more so. One patient with possible hippocampal ischaemic infarcts causing bilateral hippocampal volume loss has been extensively studied, showing impaired recall but relatively preserved item recognition memory (e.g. Mayes *et al.*, 2002). In a 41-year old right-handed man with first-ever stroke affecting the left posterior choroidal artery territory and involving the left posterior hippocampus, presentation was with an amnesic syndrome resembling transient global amnesia (see Section 3.7.3) but with additional 'amnestic aphasia.'. Improvement over 24–48 hours was followed by a severe deficit of episodic long-term memory, particularly in the verbal modality, with default of encoding and semantic intrusions. This case suggested specialization of the left hippocampus for encoding of verbal material (Scacchi *et al.*, 2006).

REFERENCES

Mayes AR, Holdstock JS, Isaac CL, Hunkin NM, Roberts N. Relative sparing of item recognition memory in a patient with adult-onset damage limited to the hippocampus. *Hippocampus* 2002; **12**: 325–40.

Scacchi F, Carota A, Morier J, Bogousslavsky J. Predominantly verbal deficit of encoding with stroke limited to the left posterior hippocampus. *J Neurol* 2006; **253** (suppl 2): II137 (abstract P543).

3.3.7 Basal forebrain

'Basal forebrain amnesia' has been reported following surgery for ruptured anterior communicating artery aneurysm (see Section 3.4.1; Damasio *et al.*, 1985; Rajaram, 1997), presumably due to disruption of the basal forebrain cholinergic projection to the hippocampus (which is also a key site of pathology in Alzheimer's disease). Features may be akin to the amnesia seen in Korsakoff syndrome (see Section 8.3.1), although this is not invariably so.

REFERENCES

Damasio AR, Graff-Radford NR, Eslinger PJ, Damasio H, Kassell N. Amnesia following basal forebrain lesions. *Arch Neurol* 1985; **42**: 263–71.

Rajaram S. Basal forebrain amnesia. *Neurocase* 1997; **3**: 405–15.

3.3.8 Brainstem and cerebellum

Can isolated infratentorial ischaemic lesions cause cognitive impairment? Transient amnesia has been reported as a herald of brainstem infarction (Howard *et al.*, 1992) and basilar artery thrombosis (Taylor *et al.*, 2005), but these syndromes may conceivably have involved memory-eloquent structures in the thalamus. The question may be addressed by examining patients with lesions confined to brainstem and cerebellum.

In a series of 17 patients with lacunar infarcts in the brainstem, neuropsychological evaluation showed impairments in naming, category fluency, and trail making, a profile similar to that seen with supratentorial lacunar infarcts, prompting the conclusion that small white matter infarcts affect cognitive function in a non-specific way (van Zandvoort *et al.*, 2003). Occasional cases of cognitive impairment in patients with brainstem vascular events complicated by peduncular hallucinosis have been reported (Benke, 2006).

In a series of 15 patients with isolated cerebellar infarcts, confirmed by MR imaging, neuropsychological testing showed changes consistent with a frontal deficit in comparison with controls (Neau *et al.*, 2000). A study of 26 patients with exclusively cerebellar infarcts found slow performance on visuospatial tasks with left-sided lesions and in verbal memory with right-sided lesions. The subtle deficits were interpreted as being mediated by the contralateral cortical hemisphere (Hokkanen *et al.*, 2006).

Hence, from the limited information currently available, it would seem likely that isolated ischaemic infratentorial lesions may have subtle effects on cognition.

REFERENCES

Benke T. Peduncular hallucinosis: a syndrome of impaired reality monitoring. *J Neurol* 2006; **253**: 1561–71.

Hokkanen LS, Kauranen V, Roine RO, Salonen O, Kotila M. Subtle cognitive deficits after cerebellar infarcts. *Eur J Neurol* 2006; **13**: 161–70.

Howard RS, Festenstein R, Mellers J, Kartsounis LD, Ron M. Transient amnesia heralding brain stem infarction. *J Neurol Neurosurg Psychiatry* 1992; **55**: 977.

Neau JP, Arroyo-Anllo E, Bonnaud V, Ingrand P, Gil R. Neuropsychological disturbances in cerebellar infarcts. *Acta Neurol Scand* 2000; **102**: 363–70.

Taylor RA, Wu GF, Hurst RW, Kasner SE, Cucchiara BL. Transient global amnesia heralding basilar artery thrombosis. *Clin Neurol Neurosurg* 2005; **108**: 60–2.

van Zandvoort M, de Haan E, van Gijn J, Kappelle LJ. Cognitive functioning in patients with a small infarct in the brainstem. *J Int Neuropsychol Soc* 2003; **9**: 490–4.

3.4 Subarachnoid haemorrhage (SAH)

Subarachnoid haemorrhage (SAH), bleeding into the space between pia and arachnoid mater, is the least common form of stroke, accounting for perhaps 5% of the total. Bleeding may originate from a ruptured intracranial aneurysm, or from an arteriovenous malformation (see Section 3.5.1), but in some cases no specific bleeding source is identified (van Gijn & Rinkel, 2001). Unruptured intracranial aneurysms may be discovered as a result of screening in families with a history of SAH (Crawley *et al.*, 1999; Teasdale *et al.*, 2005) or incidentally when neuroimaging is undertaken for other reasons. A careful reckoning of risk–benefit ratio must be undertaken before deciding on treatment of such asymptomatic lesions.

SAH patients are heterogeneous with respect to bleeding source (aneurysms may be on the internal carotid, anterior communicating, middle cerebral, posterior cerebral, or basilar artery), the severity of the initial bleed (which may be graded, for example using the Hunt & Hess classification, or the World Federation of Neurological Surgeons scale based on the Glasgow Coma Scale), degree of brain injury, occurrence of complications such as vasospasm or hydrocephalus, and treatment method used. Ruptured aneurysms may be treated by open surgical clipping or, increasingly frequently, by intravascular embolization ('coiling'), both procedures isolating the aneurysm from the circulation (Molyneux *et al.*, 2002, 2005). Add to this the significant psychological sequelae of SAH, including fatigue and anxiety, and the difficulty of defining the neuropsychological profile associated with SAH becomes apparent.

REFERENCES

Crawley F, Clifton A, Brown MM. Should we screen for familial intracranial aneurysm? *Stroke* 1999; **30**: 312–16.

Molyneux A, Kerr R, Stratton I, *et al.* International Subarachnoid Aneurysm Trial (ISAT) of neurosurgical clipping versus endovascular coiling in 2143 patients with ruptured intracranial aneurysms: a randomised trial. *Lancet* 2002; **360**: 1267–74.

Molyneux A, Kerr R, Yu LM, *et al.* International Subarachnoid Aneurysm Trial (ISAT) of neurosurgical clipping versus endovascular coiling in 2143 patients with ruptured intracranial aneurysms: a randomised comparison of effects on survival, dependency, seizures, rebleeding, subgroups, and aneurysm occlusion. *Lancet* 2005; **366**: 809–17.

Teasdale GM, Wardlaw JM, White PM, *et al.* The familial risk of subarachnoid haemorrhage. *Brain* 2005; **128**: 1677–85.

van Gijn J, Rinkel GJE. Sub-arachnoid haemorrhage: diagnosis, causes and management. *Brain* 2001; **124**: 249–78.

3.4.1 Aneurysmal SAH, unruptured aneurysms

The large literature on the neuropsychological sequelae of subarachnoid haemorrhage (SAH), most often following aneurysm rupture, has been reviewed by Hütter (2000) and DeLuca & Chiaravalloti (2002).

It has become increasingly recognized that patients who survive the acute phase of SAH may be left with significant neuropsychological deficits despite an apparently excellent neurological outcome. For example, in a retrospective survey Hütter et al. (1995) found that significant cognitive performance deficits were present in between one-third and two-thirds of patients adjudged to have a good neurological outcome after SAH. Similar findings are reported from other studies, including those with a prospective design (Ogden et al., 1993; Tidswell et al., 1995).

The pattern of cognitive impairments is global in some patients, even amounting to dementia, whereas in others general intelligence as measured by conventional IQ tests remains intact but there may be specific impairments of psychomotor speed, language function, and verbal memory (DeLuca & Diamond, 1995). Working memory and verbal short-term memory seem most affected, with features sometimes reported to resemble the amnesia of Korsakoff syndrome, with or without confabulation. Basal forebrain injury, damaging the septo-hippocampal system, may be responsible for amnesia (Damasio et al., 1985). Concurrent frontal lobe injury may be required for the presence of confabulation (Downes & Mayes, 1995; DeLuca & Chiaravalloti, 2002). In addition there may be deficits in perceptual speed and accuracy, visuospatial and visuoconstructive function, and abstraction and cognitive flexibility, for example in the Wisconsin Card Sorting Test, the latter suggesting frontocortical cognitive dysfunction (Stenhouse et al., 1991). Executive dysfunction may significantly affect anterograde memory (Diamond et al., 1997). The similarity of this profile to that seen following mild traumatic brain injury has been noted. An apraxic, alien hand, syndrome has on occasion been reported after anterior communicating artery (AcoA) aneurysm rupture (Banks et al., 1989).

Although older studies suggested that cognitive deficits were greatest with ruptured AcoA aneurysms, even suggesting the existence of an 'AcoA syndrome' characterized by severe memory deficit, confabulation, and personality change (Talland et al., 1967), more systematic studies have found the pattern of deficits to be unrelated to the location of the ruptured aneurysm, and to be persistent over time (Maurice-Williams et al., 1991; Ogden et al., 1993; Tidswell et al., 1995). The profile may be aggravated by concurrent infarction in the vascular territory of the ruptured aneurysm. Left-sided infarcts and global cerebral oedema were reported to be predictors of post-SAH cognitive dysfunction in one study (Kreiter et al., 2002).

Cognitive impairments impact on functional status and quality of life (Mayer et al., 2002). Comparison of cognitive outcome between aneurysm coiling and clipping showed a trend toward poorer outcome in the surgical, clipping group, who also had a significantly higher incidence of infarcts in the vascular territory of the aneurysm, suggesting that the complications of SAH are the principal determinants of cognitive outcome (Hadjivassiliou et al., 2001). These findings add to the argument in favour of coiling rather than clipping of aneurysms (Molyneux et al., 2005).

The detection and management of unruptured intracranial aneurysms remains an area of investigation (Wardlaw & White, 2001). Neuropsychological sequelae of treatment of unruptured aneurysms are not unknown, and are an important consideration, since most patients are healthy at the time of treatment (Towgood et al., 2004).

REFERENCES

Banks G, Short P, Martinez J, et al. The alien hand syndrome: clinical and postmortem findings. Arch Neurol 1989; **46**: 456–9.

Damasio AR, Graff-Radford NR, Eslinger PJ, Damasio H, Kassell N. Amnesia following basal forebrain lesions. *Arch Neurol* 1985; **42**: 263–71.

DeLuca J, Chiaravalloti ND. The neuropsychological consequences of ruptured aneurysms of the anterior communicating artery. In: Harrison JE, Owen AM (eds.), *Cognitive Deficits in Brain Disorders*. London: Martin Dunitz, 2002: 17–36.

DeLuca J, Diamond BJ. Aneurysm of the anterior communicating artery: a review of neuroanatomical and neuropsychological sequelae. *J Clin Exp Neuropsychol* 1995; **17**: 100–21.

Diamond BJ, DeLuca J, Kelley SM. Memory and executive functions in amnesic and non-amnesic patients with aneurysms of the anterior communicating artery. *Brain* 1997; **120**: 1015–25.

Downes JJ, Mayes AR. How bad memories can sometimes lead to fantastic beliefs and strange visions. In: Campbell R, Conway MA (eds.), *Broken Memories: Case Studies in Memory Impairment*. Oxford: Blackwell, 1995: 115–23.

Hadjivassiliou M, Tooth CL, Romanowski CA, *et al*. Aneurysmal SAH: cognitive outcome and structural damage after clipping or coiling. *Neurology* 2001; **56**: 1672–7.

Hütter BO. *Neuropsychological Sequelae of Subarachnoid Hemorrhage and its Treatment*. Berlin: Springer, 2000.

Hütter BO, Gilsbach JM, Kreitschmann I. Quality of life and cognitive deficits in patients after subarachnoid haemorrhage. *Br J Neurosurg* 1995; **9**: 465–75.

Kreiter KT, Copeland D, Bernardini GL, *et al*. Predictors of cognitive dysfunction after subarachnoid haemorrhage. *Stroke* 2002; **33**: 200–8.

Maurice-Williams RS, Willison JR, Hatfield R. The cognitive and psychological sequelae of uncomplicated aneurysm surgery. *J Neurol Neurosurg Psychiatry* 1991; **54**: 335–40.

Mayer SA, Kreiter KT, Copeland D, *et al*. Global and domain-specific cognitive impairment and outcome after subarachnoid haemorrhage. *Neurology* 2002; **59**: 1750–8.

Ogden JA, Mee EW, Henning M. A prospective study of impairment of cognition and memory and recovery after subarachnoid haemorrhage. *Neurosurgery* 1993; **33**: 572–87.

Stenhouse LM, Knight RG, Longmore BE, Bishara SN. Long-term cognitive deficits in patients after surgery on aneurysms of the anterior communicating artery. *J Neurol Neurosurg Psychiatry* 1991; **54**: 909–14.

Talland GA, Sweet WH, Ballantine HT Jr. Amnesic syndrome with anterior communicating artery aneurysm. *J Nerv Ment Dis* 1967; **145**: 179–92.

Tidswell P, Dias PS, Sagar HJ, Mayes AR, Battersby RD. Cognitive outcome after aneurysm rupture: relationship to aneurysm site and perioperative complications. *Neurology* 1995; **45**: 875–82.

Towgood K, Ogden JA, Mee E. Neurological, neuropsychological, and psychosocial outcome following treatment of unruptured intracranial aneurysms: a review and commentary. *J Int Neuropsychol Soc* 2004; **10**: 1–21.

Wardlaw JM, White PM. The detection and management of unruptured intracranial aneurysms. *Brain* 2001; **123**: 205–21.

3.4.2   Perimesencephalic (non-aneurysmal) SAH

In perimesencephalic SAH (pSAH), no underlying aneurysm(s) may be identified with conventional angiography in 15–20% of cases. Hence, pSAH differs from other types of SAH in its excellent prognosis, since there is a very low risk of re-bleeding (van Gijn *et al.*, 1985). Only minor cognitive deficits have been identified on follow-up of pSAH patients, but high scores on a depression scale, suggesting that vigorous reassurance and treatment of depression might improve outcome in this subgroup (Madureira *et al.*, 2000).

REFERENCES

Madureira S, Canhao P, Guerreiro M, Ferro JM. Cognitive and emotional consequences of perimesencephalic subarachnoid haemorrhage. *J Neurol* 2000: **247**: 862–7.

van Gijn J, van Dongen KJ, Vermeulen M, Hijdra A. Perimesencephalic hemorrhage: a nonaneurysmal and benign form of subarachnoid hemorrhage. *Neurology* 1985; **35**: 493–7.

3.4.3   Superficial siderosis of the nervous system

Deposition of ferritin in the superficial layers of the CNS as a consequence of repeated or continuous leakage of blood into the CSF is the cause of this unusual condition, with subsequent gliosis and neuronal loss, particularly in the eighth cranial nerve, the cerebellar vermis, and the inferior frontal cerebral cortex. Clinical features include sensorineural hearing loss, cerebellar ataxia, dysarthria, anosmia, and pyramidal signs, with typical appearances of signal void around affected areas of brain on T_2-weighted MR images, corresponding to deposition of haemosiderin (Fearnley *et al.*, 1995).

In a review of the literature, 14 cases with dementia of variable severity were identified, with onset between 1 and more than 30 years after disease onset (Fearnley *et al.*, 1995). Only one systematic study of the cognitive impairments in superficial siderosis has been reported (van Harskamp *et al.*, 2005). In six patients tested, general intellectual function was well preserved, but speech production difficulties, impairment of visual recall, and executive impairments formed the core neuropsychological deficits. Impaired executive function was evident in tests of both initiation (phonemic fluency, Hayling sentence completion part A) and inhibition (Stroop, Hayling sentence completion part B). Naming, literacy, calculation, visual perceptual and visuospatial skills, verbal and visual recognition memory, verbal recall memory, and speed of information processing were all relatively preserved. All patients also failed a theory of mind test, indicating a mentalizing impairment. Overall the deficits were akin to the previously described cerebellar cognitive affective syndrome (Schmahmann & Sherman, 1998).

REFERENCES

Fearnley JM, Stevens JM, Rudge P. Superficial siderosis of the central nervous system. *Brain* 1995; **118**: 1051–66.
Schmahmann JD, Sherman JC. The cerebellar cognitive affective syndrome. *Brain* 1998; **121**: 561–79.
van Harskamp NJ, Rudge P, Cipolotti L. Cognitive and social impairments in patients with superficial siderosis. *Brain* 2005; **128**: 1082–92.

3.5   Intracranial vascular malformations

The classification of intracranial arteriovenous vascular anomalies has been subject to various approaches, lesions not always having been described in a standardized way. Distinction may be made between haemangiomas, in which endothelial hyperplasia occurs, and non-proliferating vascular anomalies in which there is no hyperplasia. These latter include arterial malformations (angiodysplasia, aneurysms) and lesions in which there is arteriovenous shunting of blood, either through a tangled anastomosis of vessels ('arteriovenous malformation', AVM) or a direct high flow connection between artery and vein ('arteriovenous fistula', AVF). AVMs and AVFs may be within the brain parenchyma or in the dura (Chaloupka & Huddle, 1998; Choi & Mohr, 2005).

REFERENCES

Chaloupka JC, Huddle DC. Classification of vascular malformations of the central nervous system. *Neuroimaging Clin North Am* 1998; **8**: 295–321.
Choi JH, Mohr JP. Brain arteriovenous malformations in adults. *Lancet Neurol* 2005; **4**: 299–308.

3.5.1   Arteriovenous malformations (AVMs)

Whether AVMs cause cognitive deficits over and above their haemorrhagic and epileptic complications, which generally are what bring cases to clinical attention, is uncertain (Al-Shahi & Warlow, 2001). Some early studies suggested 'mental changes' in 50% of patients with 'AVMs' (Olivecrona & Reeves, 1948) whereas others found normal fullscale IQ and no lateralizing changes comparable with those seen with acute focal lesions (Waltimo & Putkonen, 1974). Mahalick *et al.* (1991) reported a series of 24 patients, 12 each with right and left AVMs, and found compromised higher cortical function (attention, memory, learning, fluency) both ipsilateral and contralateral to the lesion, more so ipsilateral, prompting them to argue that a vascular 'steal' phenomenon accounted for contralateral deficits. However, there were no concomitant vascular imaging studies. To answer the question of the neuropsychological effects of

AVMs, one ideally would wish to study asymptomatic individuals, perhaps discovered by chance on brain imaging for other reasons.

Cases of higher cortical dysfunction have been reported in association with dural AVFs, sometimes amounting to dementia (Hirono *et al.*, 1993; Nencini *et al.*, 1993). Five out of 40 cases in the series of Hurst *et al.* (1998) had dementia or encephalopathy with remission after embolization. Detailed pre- and post-ablation neuropsychological investigations of such patients have not been identified. In a further example, a man with a 12-month history of progressive cognitive decline, precluding occupational function, who had profound psychomotor slowing, returned to normal after endovascular embolization of a dural AV fistula (Bernstein *et al.*, 2003). Combined embolization/ligation and surgical 'scalping' has also been reported to reverse dementia (Datta *et al.*, 1998).

It is argued that the mechanism of cognitive impairment in these patients is high flow through the AV shunt combined with venous outflow obstruction causing impaired cerebral venous drainage, and hence widespread venous hypertension and diffuse ischaemia (which may be manifest neuroradiologically as a leukoencephalopathy: Waragai *et al.*, 2006), and thus progressive cognitive dysfunction, in the same way that spinal dural AVFs cause a myelopathy in Foix–Alajouanine syndrome (Hurst *et al.*, 1998). Thalamic ischaemia has also been implicated (Tanaka *et al.*, 1999). Hence it is reasoned that dural AVFs are a cause of reversible vascular dementia. Newer neuroimaging modalities (PET, DWI) may help to clarify some of the uncertainty around these issues.

REFERENCES

Al-Shahi R, Warlow CP. A systematic review of the frequency and prognosis of arteriovenous malformations of the brain in adults. *Brain* 2001; **124**: 1900–26 [esp. 1913–14].

Bernstein R, Dowd CF, Gress DR. Rapidly reversible dementia. *Lancet* 2003; **361**: 392.

Datta NN, Rehman SU, Kwok JC, Chan KY, Poon CY. Reversible dementia due to arteriovenous fistula: a simple surgical option. *Neurosurg Rev* 1998; **21**: 174–6.

Hirono N, Yamadori A, Komiyama M. Dural arteriovenous fistula: a cause of hypoperfusion-induced intellectual impairment. *Eur Neurol* 1993; **33**: 5–8.

Hurst RW, Bagley LJ, Galetta S, *et al.* Dementia resulting from dural arteriovenous fistulas: the pathologic findings of venous hypertensive encephalopathy. *AJNR Am J Neuroradiol* 1998; **19**: 1267–73.

Mahalick DM, Ruff RM, U HS. Neuropsychological sequelae of arteriovenous malformations. *Neurosurgery* 1991; **29**: 351–7.

Nencini P, Inzitari D, Gibbs J, Mangiafico S. Dementia with leukoaraiosis and dural arteriovenous malformation: clinical and PET case study. *J Neurol Neurosurg Psychiatry* 1993; **56**: 929–31.

Olivecrona H, Reeves J. Arteriovenous malformations of the brain: their diagnosis and treatment. *Arch Neurol Psychiatr Chicago* 1948; **59**: 567–602.

Tanaka K, Morooka Y, Nakagawa Y, Shimizu S. Dural arteriovenous malformation manifesting as dementia due to ischemia in bilateral thalami. A case report. *Surg Neurol* 1999; **51**: 489–93.

Waltimo O, Putkonen AR. Intellectual performance of patients with intracranial arteriovenous malformations. *Brain* 1974; **97**: 511–20.

Waragai M, Takeuchi H, Fukushima T, Haisa T, Yonemitsu T. MRI and SPECT studies of dural arteriovenous fistulas presenting as pure progressive dementia with leukoencephalopathy: a cause of treatable dementia. *Eur J Neurol* 2006; **13**: 754–9.

3.5.2 Cavernous haemangiomas

Cavernous haemangiomas or cavernomas are thin-walled vascular spaces lacking a shunt, hence not arteriovenous malformations. They may present as space-occupying lesions, with seizures or relapsing–remitting symptoms related to haemorrhage. Multiple cavernous angiomas (cavernomatosis) which undergo multiple and recurrent haemorrhages may rarely be associated with cognitive decline and dementia (Hayman *et al.*, 1982; Gil-Nagel *et al.*, 1995; Kageyama *et al.*, 2000; Kariya *et al.*, 2000).

REFERENCES

Gil-Nagel A, Wilcox KJ, Stewart JM, *et al.* Familial cerebral cavernous angioma: clinical analysis of a family and phenotypic classification. *Epilepsy Res* 1995; **21**: 27–36.

Hayman L, Evans R, Ferrell R, *et al.* Familial cavernous angiomas: natural history and genetic study over a 5-year period. *Am J Med Genet* 1982; **11**: 147–60.

Kageyama Y, Kodama Y, Yamamoto S, *et al.* A case of multiple intracranial cavernous angiomas presented with dementia and parkinsonism: clinical and MRI study for 10 years [in Japanese]. *Rinsho Shinkeigaku* 2000; **40**: 1105–9.

Kariya S, Kawahara M, Suzumura A. A case of multiple cavernous angioma with dementia [in Japanese]. *Rinsho Shinkeigaku* 2000; **40**: 1003–7.

3.6   Vasculopathies

Vasculopathy is a relatively non-specific term for blood vessel abnormalities, which is here interpreted to encompass not only primary abnormalities of blood vessel wall structure predisposing to intraluminal thrombosis, but also rheologic abnormalities promoting a thrombotic tendency. Although there may be overlap at the level of pathophysiology, inflammatory disorders of blood vessels such as the primary and secondary cerebral vasculitides are considered elsewhere (Sections 6.10.1 and 6.10.2, respectively), as are primary metabolic disorders affecting blood vessels such as Anderson–Fabry disease (Section 5.5.3).

3.6.1   Angioendotheliomatosis, intravascular lymphomatosis

Angioendotheliomatosis, also known as intravascular lymphomatosis and neoplastic angioendotheliomatosis, is a malignant intravascular proliferation of endothelial cells or lymphocytes defined as an angiotropic intravascular large-cell lymphoma of B-cell type. The commonest clinical presentation is with multifocal ischaemic events due to vascular occlusion with neoplastic cells, but it may also cause dementia, leading to classification with the vascular dementias (Reinglass *et al.*, 1977; Drlicek *et al.*, 1991; Treves *et al.*, 1995). Brain and/ or meningeal biopsy is usually required for diagnosis. A case associated with a reversible dementia following immunosuppressive treatment in a transplant recipient has been reported (Heafield *et al.*, 1993).

REFERENCES

Drlicek M, Grisold W, Liszka U, Hitzenberger P, Machacek E. Angiotropic lymphoma (malignant angioendotheliomatosis) presenting with rapidly progressive dementia. *Acta Neuropathol* 1991; **82**: 533–5.

Heafield MT, Carey M, Williams AC, Cullen M. Neoplastic angioendotheliomatosis: a treatable 'vascular dementia' occurring in an immunosuppressed transplant recipient. *Clin Neuropathol* 1993; **12**: 102–6.

Reinglass JL, Muller J, Wissman S, Wellman H. Central nervous system angioendotheliosis: a treatable multiple infarct dementia. *Stroke* 1977; **8**: 218–21.

Treves TA, Gadoth N, Blumen S, Korczyn AD. Intravascular malignant lymphomatosis: a cause of subacute dementia. *Dementia* 1995; **6**: 286–93.

3.6.2   CADASIL

Cerebral autosomal dominant arteriopathy with subcortical infarcts and leukoencephalopathy (CADASIL) is an autosomal dominant vasculopathy resulting from mutations within the gene encoding the notch3 protein on chromosome 19q12 (Joutel *et al.*, 1996). It is characterized clinically by recurrent subcortical strokes, both symptomatic and silent, migraine, psychiatric disturbances, with late pseudobulbar palsy, occasionally epilepsy, and a reversible encephalopathy (Schon *et al.*, 2003). Skin biopsy may show granular osmiophilic material adjacent to the basement membrane of smooth muscle cells of dermal arterioles; similar deposits may be observed in the thickened arterial media in vessels on brain biopsy (Lammie *et al.*, 1995). MR brain imaging shows confluent high signal in periventricular and deep white matter, basal ganglia lacunar infarcts, and characteristic high signal in the anterior temporal pole and external capsule. The mechanism(s) by which mutations lead to disease are not currently understood.

A subcortical-type, white matter, vascular dementia may also occur, with both stepwise and progressive course (Martin & Markus, 2001). This dementia may occur in the absence of other neurological features other than migraine (Mellies et al., 1998). The neuropsychological profile is characterized by a deficit in sustained attention, cognitive slowing, impaired learning with intact recognition, and perseveration, in other words a pattern resembling that in other white matter disorders (Filley et al., 1999). Executive and attentional dysfunction has been identified in non-demented patients, some without a history of prior vascular events (Taillia et al., 1998). In a cross-sectional study of 42 patients, Buffon et al. (2006) found a heterogeneous cognitive profile at disease onset, most often affecting executive skills leading to impaired memory and attention, evolving to a more homogeneous pattern affecting all domains with increasing age, including language and visuospatial function, although distinct from Alzheimer's disease. Retrieval was better with cueing, suggesting that encoding was relatively spared, as were recognition and semantic memory. The authors speculated that this pattern resulted from initial damage to frontal–subcortical networks with sparing of the hippocampus, with diffuse cortical dysfunction in later disease reflecting the accumulation of subcortical ischaemic insults, although since history of stroke was not associated with dementia most of these events must have been silent. In one series of 64 patients, not selected for the presence or absence of dementia, a significant inverse correlation was noted between overall cognitive performance, as assessed with the MMSE score, and total MRI lesion volume (Dichgans et al., 1999).

Cholinergic denervation has been shown in one pathologically examined case of CADASIL, despite this being a pure vascular dementia (Mesulam et al., 2003), adding weight to the argument in favour of cholinesterase inhibitors for the treatment of vascular dementia, as well as Alzheimer's disease (Erkinjuntti et al., 2004).

REFERENCES

Buffon F, Porcher R, Hernandez K, et al. Cognitive profile in CADASIL. *J Neurol Neurosurg Psychiatry* 2006; **77**: 175–80.

Dichgans M, Filippi M, Brüning R, et al. Quantitative MRI in CADASIL: correlation with disability and cognitive performance. *Neurology* 1999; **52**: 1361–7.

Erkinjuntti T, Roman G, Gauthier S, Feldman H, Rockwood K. Emerging therapies for vascular dementia and vascular cognitive impairment. *Stroke* 2004; **35**: 1010–17.

Filley CM, Thompson LL, Sze CI, et al. White matter demetia in CADASIL. *J Neurol Sci* 1999; **163**: 163–7.

Joutel A, Corpechot C, Ducros A, et al. Notch3 mutations in CADASIL, a hereditary adult-onset condition causing stroke and dementia. *Nature* 1996; **383**: 707–10.

Lammie GA, Rakshi J, Rossor MN, Harding AE, Scaravilli F. Cerebral autosomal dominant arteriopathy with subcortical infarcts and leukoencephalopathy (CADASIL): confirmation by cerebral biopsy in 2 cases. *Clin Neuropathol* 1995; **14**: 201–6.

Martin R, Markus H. CADASIL: a genetic form of subcortical vascular dementia. *Dementia Rev* 2001; **4** (1): 1–6.

Mellies JK, Bäumer T, Müller JA, et al. SPECT study of a German CADASIL family: a phenotype with migraine and progressive dementia only. *Neurology* 1998; **50**: 1715–21.

Mesulam M, Siddique T, Cohen B. Cholinergic denervation in a pure multi-infarct state: observations in CADASIL. *Neurology* 2003; **60**: 1183–5.

Schon F, Martin RJ, Prevett M, et al. 'CADASIL coma': an underdiagnosed acute encephalopathy. *J Neurol Neurosurg Psychiatry* 2003; **74**: 249–52.

Taillia H, Chabriat H, Kurtz A, et al. Cognitive alterations in non-demented CADASIL patients. *Cerebrovasc Dis* 1998; **8**: 97–101.

3.6.3   Cerebral amyloid angiopathies (CAA)

Cerebral amyloid angiopathy (CAA) refers to the deposition of amyloidogenic peptides in the walls of small parenchymal and leptomeningeal arteries (congophilic angiopathy), sometimes extending from around vessel walls into the brain parenchyma (dyshoric angiopathy) (Vinters, 1987; Coria & Rubio, 1996; Yamada, 2000; Revesz et al., 2003). CAA may be one feature of AD brain pathology, but may also occur in relative isolation as either a sporadic or a familial condition, a classification system for which has been proposed (Greenberg et al., 1996). Cerebral haemorrhage in a lobar distribution is the commonest complication of CAA, although other transient focal neurological features may occur, including transient ischaemic attacks, focal seizures, and multifocal cortical myoclonus (Greenberg et al., 1993; Larner et al., 1998), as well as a leukoencephalopathy (Gray et al., 1985). Dementia without major lobar haemorrhage is also reported (Greenberg et al., 1993).

It has been suggested that CAA may contribute to neurodegeneration in Alzheimer's disease associated with certain presenilin-1 gene mutations (Dermaut et al., 2001). CAA in association with a granulomatous angiitis resembling primary angiitis of the CNS (PACNS), so-called Aβ-related angiitis (ABRA), has been reported to produce prominent cognitive problems (Scolding et al., 2005; see Section 6.10.1).

Of the familial CAAs, hereditary cerebral haemorrhage with amyloidosis Dutch type (HCHWA-D) results from mutations at codon 693 of the amyloid precursor protein (APP) gene; other mutations within this gene are deterministic for autosomal dominant Alzheimer's disease (see Section 2.1). The phenotype is one of cerebral haemorrhages which may result in cognitive impairment of cortical type (Haan et al., 1990), although dementia in the absence of a history of stroke or focal radiological change may occur. Dementia in HCHWA-D is independent of neurofibrillary pathology, plaque density, and age, but related to the CAA load in frontal cortex, as quantified by computerized morphometry, and vessel wall thickening, suggesting that CAA per se may cause dementia (Natté et al., 2001). Hereditary cerebral haemorrhage with amyloidosis Icelandic type (HCHWA-I), resulting from mutations in the cystatin c gene, also causes intracerebral haemorrhages. One family with a late-onset dementia as the only manifestation of HCHWA-I has been reported, with cortical and subcortical infarctions (Sveinbjörnsdóttir et al., 1996).

Autosomal dominant familial CAA causing dementia usually without strokes or haemorrhages, of British and Danish types (Plant et al., 2004), is also described (see Sections 5.1.3 and 5.1.4, respectively).

REFERENCES

Coria F, Rubio I. Cerebral amyloid angiopathies. *Neuropathol Appl Neurobiol* 1996; **22**: 216–27.

Dermaut B, Kumar-Singh S, De Jonghe C, et al. Cerebral amyloid angiopathy is a pathogenic lesion in Alzheimer's disease due to a novel presenilin 1 mutation. *Brain* 2001; **124**: 2383–92.

Gray F, Dubas F, Roullet E, Escourolle R. Leukoencephalopathy in diffuse hemorrhagic cerebral amyloid angiopathy. *Ann Neurol* 1985; **18**: 54–9.

Greenberg SM, Edgar MA, Kunz DP, et al. Cerebral hemorrhage in a 69-year-old woman receiving warfarin: cerebral amyloid angiopathy (MGH Case Records Case 22-1996). *N Engl J Med* 1996; **335**: 189–96.

Greenberg SM, Vonsattel JP, Stekes JW, Gruber M, Finklestein SP. The clinical spectrum of cerebral amyloid angiopathy: presentations without lobar haemorrhage. *Neurology* 1993; **43**: 2073–9.

Haan J, Lanser JB, Zijderveld I, van der Does IG, Roos RA. Dementia in hereditary cerebral haemorrhage with amyloidosis – Dutch type. *Arch Neurol* 1990; **47**: 965–7.

Larner AJ, Elkington P, Mehta H, et al. Multifocal cortical myoclonus and cerebral amyloid β-peptide angiopathy. *J Neurol Neurosurg Psychiatry* 1998; **65**: 951–2.

Natté R, Maat-Schieman MLC, Haan J, et al. Dementia in hereditary cerebral hemorrhage with amyloidosis–Dutch type is associated with cerebral amyloid angiopathy but is independent of plaques and neurofibrillary tangles. *Ann Neurol* 2001; **50**: 765–72.

Plant GT, Ghiso J, Holton JL, Frangione B, Revesz T. Familial and sporadic cerebral amyloid angiopathies associated with dementia and the BRI dementias. In: Esiri MM, Lee VMY, Trojanowski JQ (eds.), *The Neuropathology of Dementia* (2nd edition). Cambridge: Cambridge University Press, 2004: 330–52.

Revesz T, Ghiso J, Lashley T, *et al.* Cerebral amyloid angiopathies: a pathologic, biochemical and genetic view. *J Neuropathol Exp Neurol* 2003; **62**: 885–98.

Scolding NJ, Joseph F, Kirby PA, *et al.* Aβ-related angiitis: primary angiitis of the central nervous system associated with cerebral amyloid angiopathy. *Brain* 2005; **128**: 500–15.

Sveinbjörnsdóttir S, Blöndal H, Gudmundsson G, *et al.* Progressive dementia and leucoencephalopathy as the initial presentation of late onset hereditary cystatin-C amyloidosis: clinicopathological presentation of two cases. *J Neurol Sci* 1996; **140**: 101–8.

Vinters HV. Cerebral amyloid angiopathy: a critical review. *Stroke* 1987; **18**: 311–24.

Yamada M. Cerebral amyloid angiopathy: an overview. *Neuropathology* 2000; **20**: 8–22.

3.6.4 Familial young-adult-onset arteriosclerotic leukoencephalopathy with alopecia and lumbago without arterial hypertension

In this rare syndrome, reported only in Japanese families, progressive subcortical dementia is common, with accompanying pseudobulbar palsy and pyramidal signs. Lacunar strokes occurred in about half of the patients (Fukutake & Hirayama, 1995).

REFERENCES

Fukutake T, Hirayama K. Familial young-adult-onset arteriosclerotic leukoencephalopathy with alopecia and lumbago without arterial hypertension. *Eur Neurol* 1995; **35**: 69–79.

3.6.5 Familial occipital calcifications, haemorrhagic strokes, leukoencephalopathy, dementia and external carotid dysplasia (FOCHS-LADD)

Described in one family of Spanish descent, with presumed autosomal dominant transmission, this syndrome featured dementia and cerebral haemorrhages with radiological evidence of fine tramline occipital calcifications (Iglesias *et al.*, 2000).

The genetic defect remains unknown. Of the six affected individuals in two generations, neuropsychological testing was only reported in one patient, who developed progressive memory decline in the early 60s with additional evidence of visuoconstructional problems, 'ideokinetic' apraxia, calculation and writing errors, and frontal lobe symptoms.

REFERENCES

Iglesias S, Chapon F, Baron JC. Familial occipital calcifications, haemorrhagic strokes, leukoencephalopathy, dementia and external carotid dysplasia. *Neurology* 2000; **55**: 1661–7.

3.6.6 Hereditary endotheliopathy with retinopathy, nephropathy, and stroke (HERNS)

This microangiopathy of the brain and retina, inherited as an autosomal dominant condition linked to chromosome 3p21, is characterized clinically by progressive visual loss, headache, seizures, focal neurological deficits, and progressive cognitive decline (Grand *et al.*, 1988; Jen *et al.*, 1997).

REFERENCES

Grand MG, Kaine J, Fulling K, *et al.* Cerebroretinal vasculopathy: a new hereditary syndrome. *Ophthalmology* 1988; **95**: 649–59.

Jen J, Cohen AH, Yue Q, *et al.* Hereditary endotheliopathy with retinopathy, nephropathy and stroke (HERNS). *Neurology* 1997; **49**: 1322–30.

3.6.7 Hereditary multi-infarct dementia of Swedish type

Sourander and Wålinder (1977) described a Swedish pedigree with a hereditary disorder characterized by multiple infarcts and cognitive decline. When CADASIL was described as such in 1993 (see Section 3.6.2) it was thought that this 'hereditary multi-infarct dementia' was in fact an example of

CADASIL. However, further clinical, neuro-radiological, neuropathological, and neurogenetic examination of the Swedish pedigree refutes this suggestion. Patients from this kindred did not have migraine, MR appearances did not show the typical anterior temporal pole or external capsule hyperintensities seen in CADASIL, skin biopsy did not show granular osmiophilic deposits, and neurogenetic testing found no pathogenic mutation in the *NOTCH3* gene. Hence Swedish multi-infarct dementia is a novel small vessel disease (Low *et al.*, 2007).

REFERENCES

Low WC, Junna M, Borjesson-Hanson A, *et al.* Hereditary multi-infarct dementia of the Swedish type is a novel disorder different from *NOTCH3* causing CADASIL. *Brain* 2007; **130**: 357–67.

Sourander P, Wålinder J. Hereditary multi-infarct dementia. Morphological and clinical studies of a new disease. *Acta Neuropathol (Berl)* 1977; **39**: 247–54.

3.6.8   Hughes' syndrome (primary antiphospholipid antibody syndrome)

Antiphospholipid antibodies (lupus anticoagulant, or anticardiolipin antibodies) may be associated with various neurological features including seizures, chorea, transverse myelitis, depression, psychosis, and cognitive decline. Whether these clinical features are linked to arterial and venous thromboses or to immune-mediated mechanisms, or both, remains uncertain, and hence whether optimal treatment is with antiplatelet and anticoagulant therapy or immunosuppression or both (Brey & Escalante, 1998). Antiphospholipid antibodies may occur in association with conditions such as SLE, rheumatoid arthritis, Sjögren's syndrome, and scleroderma, known as secondary antiphospholipid antibody syndromes; or without evidence of accompanying connective tissue disease, known as primary antiphospholipid antibody syndrome, or Hughes' syndrome. Diagnostic criteria require both clinical (thrombotic) and laboratory features, and a 'probable' category has also been suggested, in which the antibodies occur without a history of large vessel thromboses (Asherson, 2006). There is also overlap between Hughes syndrome and Sneddon's syndrome (see Section 3.6.11).

Cognitive impairment and dementia have been recorded in primary antiphospholipid antibody syndrome. For example, in a young woman not meeting diagnostic criteria for SLE (Tan *et al.*, 1982), decline in intellect and occupational failure were the presenting features, with MMSE score 28/30 (5-minute recall = 1/3), poor right–left orientation, right inattention, reduced motor speed, mild impulsivity, and poor concentration. MR brain imaging showed small high-signal lesions in the right caudate and frontal–subcortical white matter. The patient improved after treatment with corticosteroids, aspirin, and hydroxychloroquine (van Horn *et al.*, 1996). Reviewing the literature over the period 1983–2003 and their own experience, Gómez-Puerta *et al.* (2005) identified 30 cases of dementia associated with antiphospholipid syndrome (primary : secondary = 14 : 16, the latter having SLE or 'lupus-like syndrome'). On brain imaging, cortical infarcts were common (in more than half the cases), subcortical and basal ganglia infarcts less so (in less than one-third). Hence dementia would seem to be an unusual complication of antiphospholipid syndromes.

REFERENCES

Asherson RA. New subsets of the antiphospholipid syndrome in 2006: PRE-APS (probable APS) and microangiopathic antiphospholipid syndromes (MAPS). *Autoimmun Rev* 2006; **6**: 76–80.

Brey RL, Escalante A. Neurological manifestations of antiphospholipid antibody syndrome. *Lupus* 1998; **7** (suppl 2): S67–74.

Gómez-Puerta JA, Cervera R, Calvo LM, *et al.* Dementia associated with the antiphospholipid syndrome: clinical and radiological characteristics of 30 patients. *Rheumatology (Oxford)* 2005; **44**: 95–9.

Tan EM, Cohen AS, Fries JF, *et al.* The 1982 revised criteria for the classification of systemic lupus erythematosus. *Arthritis Rheum* 1982; **25**: 1271–7.

van Horn G, Arnett FC, Dimachkie MM. Reversible dementia and chorea in a young woman with the lupus anticoagulant. *Neurology* 1996; **46**: 1599–603.

3.6.9 Polycythaemia rubra vera

Polycythaemia rubra vera is a myeloproliferative disease characterized by increased red cell mass and blood volume, resulting in erythrocytosis (raised haematocrit) and increased blood viscosity. Associated neurological features include transient ischaemic attacks and thrombotic strokes, less commonly with cerebral haemorrhage, and chorea. Cognitive decline, which partially reversed on reduction of the haematocrit, has been reported (Di Pollina *et al.*, 2000).

REFERENCES

Di Pollina L, Mulligan R, Juillerat van der Linden A, Michel JP, Gold G. Cognitive impairment in polycythaemia rubra vera: partial reversibility upon lowering of the hematocrit. *Eur Neurol* 2000; **44**: 57–9.

3.6.10 Sickle cell disease

Dementia may be a feature of sickle cell disease as a consequence of multiple ischaemic strokes, although diffuse brain injury, perhaps related to hypoxia, may also contribute (Steen *et al.*, 2003). A progressive encephalopathy related to small vessel disease has also been reported (Pavlakis *et al.*, 1989).

REFERENCES

Pavlakis S, Prohovnik I, Piomelli S, DeVivo DC. Neurologic complications of sickle cell disease. *Adv Pediatr* 1989; **36**: 247–76.

Steen RG, Miles MA, Helton KJ, *et al.* Cognitive impairment in children with hemoglobin SS sickle cell disease: relationship to MR imaging findings and hematocrit. *AJNR Am J Neuroradiol* 2003; **24**: 382–9.

3.6.11 Sneddon's syndrome

Sneddon's syndrome is a non-inflammatory, thrombo-occlusive, arteriolar vasculopathy, affecting skin and brain and often, but not invariably, associated with antiphospholipid antibodies. The disorder occurs primarily in young patients, with a female preponderance. Clinical features include livedo reticularis or livedo racemosa, recurrent strokes in the absence of obvious risk factors, focal neurological signs, seizures, and sometimes cognitive decline (Sneddon, 1965; Frances *et al.*, 1999). Cases presenting with cognitive decline or dementia without a clinical history of stroke, but with imaging evidence of cortical and subcortical infarcts with brain atrophy, have been reported (Wright & Kokmen, 1999; Adair *et al.*, 2001). Of 30 patients with dementia and antiphospholipid antibody syndrome reported in a 20-year literature review (Gómez-Puerta *et al.*, 2005), 10 had Sneddon's syndrome.

REFERENCES

Adair JC, Digre KB, Swanda RM, *et al.* Sneddon's syndrome: a cause of cognitive decline in young adults. *Neuropsychiatry Neuropsychol Behav Neurol* 2001; **14**: 197–204.

Frances C, Papo T, Wechsler B, *et al.* Sneddon syndrome with or without antiphospholipid antibodies: a comparative study in 46 patients. *Medicine (Baltimore)* 1999; **78**: 209–19.

Gómez-Puerta JA, Cervera R, Calvo LM, *et al.* Dementia associated with the antiphospholipid syndrome: clinical and radiological characteristics of 30 patients. *Rheumatology (Oxford)* 2005; **44**: 95–9.

Sneddon IB. Cerebrovascular lesions and livedo reticularis. *Br J Dermatol* 1965; **77**: 180–5.

Wright RA, Kokmen E. Gradually progressive dementia without discrete cerebrovascular events in a patient with Sneddon's syndrome. *Mayo Clin Proc* 1999; **74**: 57–61.

3.6.12   Spatz–Lindenberg disease (von Winiwarter–Buerger's disease)

This rarely described condition is characterized pathologically by isolated cerebral non-inflammatory occlusive vasculopathy ('thromboangiitis obliterans'), hence Buerger's disease confined to the brain (Zhan *et al.*, 1993). A vascular dementia with additional upper motor neurone signs (hemiparesis, aphasia) and seizures may result (Larner *et al.*, 1999), but no systematic exploration of the neuropsychological deficits has been reported.

REFERENCES

Larner AJ, Kidd D, Elkington P, Rudge P, Scaravilli F. Spatz–Lindenberg disease: a rare cause of vascular dementia. *Stroke* 1999; **30**: 687–9.

Zhan S-S, Beyreuther K, Schmitt HP. Vascular dementia in Spatz–Lindenberg disease (SLD): cortical synaptophysin immunoreactivity as compared with dementia of Alzheimer type and non-demented controls. *Acta Neuropathol (Berl)* 1993; **86**: 259–64.

3.6.13   Susac syndrome

Susac syndrome, or retinocochleocerebral vasculopathy, is a rare, idiopathic, non-inflammatory vasculopathy affecting principally young women. It usually follows a monophasic but fluctuating course, causing small infarcts in the cochlea, retina, and brain. Characteristic clinical features are sensorineural deafness, branch retinal arteriolar occlusions, encephalopathy, acute psychiatric features, upper motor neurone limb signs, cranial nerve palsies, and seizures. Cognitive dysfunction is reported, specifically impaired short-term memory, and dementia is said to be a rare late sequela (Papo *et al.*, 1998).

REFERENCES

Papo T, Biousse V, Lehoang P, *et al.* Susac syndrome. *Medicine (Baltimore)* 1998; **77**: 3–11.

3.7   Other cerebrovascular disorders

3.7.1   Cortical venous sinus thrombosis (CVST)

Cortical venous sinus thrombosis (CVST) is a rare cause of stroke, with many possible causes (Bousser & Ross Russell, 1997). Studies examining cognitive outcomes have been small. De Bruijn *et al.* (2000) found cognitive impairments in around one-third of survivors at 1 year, suggesting an unfavourable outcome, whereas Buccino *et al.* (2003) found mild non-fluent aphasia in 9% and working memory deficits in 18% of a cohort of 34 patients seen over a 10-year period, suggesting good cognitive long-term outcome. The variable results may relate to case mix and duration of follow-up. In children, lateral and sigmoid sinus involvement was reported to be a predictor of good cognitive outcome (Sébire *et al.*, 2003).

REFERENCES

Bousser MG, Ross Russell RW. *Cerebral Venous Thrombosis*. London: Saunders, 1997.

Buccino G, Scoditti U, Patteri I, Bertolino C, Mancia D. Neurological and cognitive long-term outcome in patients with cerebral venous sinus thrombosis. *Acta Neurol Scand* 2003; **107**: 330–5.

De Bruijn SF, Budde M, Teunisse S, de Haan RJ, Stam J. Long-term outcome of cognition and functional health after cerebral venous sinus thrombosis. *Neurology* 2000; **54**: 1687–9.

Sébire G, Tabarki B, Saunders DE, *et al.* Cerebral venous sinus thrombosis in children: risk factors, presentation, diagnosis and outcome. *Brain* 2005; **128**: 477–89.

3.7.2   Migraine

Migraine may be symptomatic of a neurological disorder that may also cause cognitive impairment, e.g. CADASIL (Section 3.6.2) or mitochondrial disease (Section 5.5.1), but it is more usually a primary or idiopathic headache disorder which occurs with or without aura (MA, MO: International Headache Society Classification Subcommittee, 2004). Whether migraine disorders are associated with cognitive deficits, either between or within attacks, has been a subject of ongoing debate. The rare entity of migraine stroke may be associated with focal deficits, as with strokes of other aetiologies.

Studies have been published showing subtle changes in cognition in migraineurs examined either during or between migraine episodes (O'Bryant *et al.*, 2006). Interictal deficits have been reported, involving certain frontal lobe functions (Mongini *et al.*, 2005), or associated with right-sided pain (Le Pira *et al.*, 2004), or with higher frequency of attacks or length of migraine history (Calandre *et al.*, 2002). Certainly migraine patients show an interictal loss of normal cognitive habituation, although this does not seem to occur in cluster headache (Evers *et al.*, 1999). Conversely, case–control and group studies have been published that do not support a link between migraine and cognitive impairment (Bell *et al.*, 1999; Pearson *et al.*, 2006). A 10-year study suggested impairments of immediate and delayed memory in MA patients at baseline but less decline over time than controls (Kalaydjian *et al.*, 2007).

During migraine attacks, simple reaction time, sustained attention, and visuospatial processing may be adversely affected, changes which may be effectively reversed by triptans (Mulder *et al.*, 1999; Farmer *et al.*, 2000, 2001) or sleep (Meyer *et al.*, 2000). However, some of these studies were performed without control groups, so it is difficult to know whether these problems relate to concurrent pain or the pathophysiology of the headache syndrome per se. Moreover, information processing speed and memory may be influenced by age, independent of migraine (Jelicic *et al.*, 2000).

REFERENCES

Bell BD, Primeau M, Sweet JJ, Lofland KR. Neuropsychological functioning in migraine headache, nonheadache chronic pain, and mild traumatic brain injury patients. *Arch Clin Neuropsychol* 1999; **14**: 389–99.

Calandre EP, Bembibre J, Arnedo ML, Becerra D. Cognitive disturbances and regional cerebral blood flow abnormalities in migraine patients: their relationship with the clinical manifestation of the illness. *Cephalalgia* 2002; **22**: 291–302.

Evers S, Frese A, Sörös P, *et al.* Involvement of cognitive processing in cluster headache. In: Olesen J, Goadsby PJ (eds.), *Cluster Headache and Related Conditions* (Frontiers in headache research, volume 9). Oxford: Oxford University Press, 1999: 201–6.

Farmer K, Cady R, Bleiberg J, Reeves D. A pilot study to measure cognitive efficiency during migraine. *Headache* 2000; **40**: 657–61.

Farmer K, Cady R, Bleiberg J, *et al.* Sumatriptan nasal spray and cognitive function during migraine: results of an open-label study. *Headache* 2001; **41**: 377–84.

International Headache Society Classification Subcommittee. The international classification of headache disorders, second edition. *Cephalalgia* 2004; **24** (suppl 1): 1–160.

Jelicic M, van Boxtel MP, Houx PJ, Jolles J. Does migraine headache affect cognitive function in the elderly? Report from the Maastricht Aging Study (MAAS). *Headache* 2000; **40**: 715–19.

Kalaydjian A, Zandi PP, Swartz KL, Eaton WW, Lyketsos C. How migraines impact cognitive function: findings from the Baltimore ECA. *Neurology* 2007; **68**: 1417–24.

Le Pira F, Lanaia F, Zappala G, *et al.* Relationship between clinical variables and cognitive performances in migraineurs with and without aura. *Funct Neurol* 2004; **19**: 101–5.

Meyer JS, Thornby J, Crawford K, Rauch GM. Reversible cognitive decline accompanies migraine and cluster headaches. *Headache* 2000; **40**: 638–46.

Mongini F, Keller R, Deregibus A, Barbalonga E, Mongini T. Frontal lobe dysfunction in patients with chronic migraine: a clinical–neuropsychological study. *Psychiatry Res* 2005; **133**: 101–6.

Mulder EJ, Linssen WH, Passchier J, Orlebeke JF, de Geus EJ. Interictal and postictal cognitive changes in migraine. *Cephalalgia* 1999; **19**: 557–65.

O'Bryant SE, Marcus DA, Rains JC, Penzien DB. The neuropsychology of recurrent headache. *Headache* 2006; **46**: 1364–76.

Pearson AJ, Chronicle EP, Maylor EA, Bruce LAM. Cognitive function is not impaired in people with a long history of migraine: a blinded study. *Cephalalgia* 2006; **26**: 74–80.

3.7.3   Transient global amnesia (TGA)

The aetiopathogenesis of transient global amnesia (TGA) is imperfectly understood (Quinette *et al.*, 2006). Recent evidence of vascular involvement, specifically from diffusion-weighted MR imaging techniques (Sander & Sander, 2005), and the increased incidence of jugular vein valve insufficiency (Nedelmann *et al.*, 2005), prompt its inclusion in this chapter.

The syndrome of TGA consists of an abrupt attack of impaired anterograde memory, often manifest as repeated questioning, without clouding of consciousness or focal neurological signs (Fisher & Adams, 1964; Caplan, 1985). Episodes are of brief duration (< 24 hours), with no recollection of the amnesic period following resolution. Diagnostic criteria for TGA have been suggested (Caplan 1985; Hodges & Warlow, 1990). Subgroups have been suggested, with the suggestion of different precipitating events in men (physical) and women (emotional), with headache being a risk factor in younger individuals (Quinette *et al.*, 2006).

As expected for an acute and transient syndrome, most cases which come to medical attention are seen by primary care physicians in the community or district general hospitals (Larner, 2007) rather than by neurologists, let alone those with an interest in neuropsychology. Nonetheless, occasionally it has been possible to undertake neuropsychological assessment during an attack. This shows a dense anterograde amnesia, with a variably severe retrograde amnesia, but intact working memory and semantic memory. Implicit memory functions (e.g. for driving) are usually intact (Hodges & Ward, 1989). A variant in which transient impairment of semantic memory was present has been described (Hodges, 1997).

After an attack patients are usually normal, although there may be subtle impairment of anterograde verbal memory on neuropsychological assessment. Prolonged retrograde amnesia after an attack has been reported (Roman-Campos *et al.*, 1980), although it is possible that this patient had epilepsy with a left temporal EEG focus (transient epileptic amnesia should be considered in the differential diagnosis: Section 4.3.1). The majority of attacks of TGA occur in isolation with a low recurrence rate (3% per year). It has been suggested that TGA may be a risk factor for the amnestic variant of mild cognitive impairment (Borroni *et al.*, 2004).

REFERENCES

Borroni B, Agosti C, Brambilla C, *et al.* Is transient global amnesia a risk factor for amnestic mild cognitive impairment? *J Neurol* 2004; **251**: 1125–7.

Caplan LR. *Transient Global Amnesia*. Amsterdam: Elsevier, 1985.

Fisher CM, Adams RD. Transient global amnesia. *Acta Neurol Scand* 1964; **40** (Suppl 9): 1–81.

Hodges JR. Transient semantic amnesia. *J Neurol Neurosurg Psychiatry* 1997; **63**: 548–9.

Hodges JR, Ward CD. Observations during transient global amnesia: a behavioural and neuropsychological study of five cases. *Brain* 1989; **112**: 595–620.

Hodges JR, Warlow CP. Syndromes of transient amnesia: towards a classification. A study of 153 cases. *J Neurol Neurosurg Psychiatry* 1990; **53**: 834–43.

Larner AJ. Transient global amnesia in the district general hospital. *Int J Clin Pract* 2007; **61**: 255–8.

Nedelmann M, Eicke BM, Dieterich M. Increased incidence of jugular valve insufficiency in patients with transient global amnesia. *J Neurol* 2005; **252**: 1482–6.

Quinette P, Guillery-Girard B, Dayan J, *et al.* What does transient global amnesia really mean? Review of the literature and thorough study of 142 cases. *Brain* 2006; **129**: 1640–58.

Roman-Campos G, Poser CM, Wood F. Persistent retrograde memory deficit after transient global amnesia. *Cortex* 1980; **16**: 500–19.

Sander K, Sander D. New insights into transient global amnesia: recent imaging and clinical findings. *Lancet Neurol* 2005; **4**: 437–44.

The epilepsies

4.1 Epilepsy and cognitive impairment

As far back as the seventeenth century, Thomas Willis recognized that long-term epilepsy could bring on 'stupidity', a term roughly corresponding to our notion of dementia (Zimmer, 2004). Nineteenth-century authors such as Henry Maudsley and William Gowers both regarded epileptics as prone to dementia or defective memory; Maudsley thought such decline inevitable (Brown & Vaughan, 1988). Their views may have been determined by clinical practice amongst patients with very severe seizure disorders, and with the advent of effective antiepileptic drugs in the twentieth century a more optimistic outlook generally prevailed. Now, however, cognitive impairment in epilepsy is once again a subject of increasing concern. Rather than an 'epileptic dementia', it is now thought better to consider 'dementia in people with epilepsy', a syndrome with various possible causes.

The marked heterogeneity of epilepsy syndromes, with respect to factors such as site of seizure origin (generalized versus partial, or localization-related), aetiology (idiopathic versus symptomatic), and pathology (Engel & Pedley, 1997; Panayiotopoulos, 2002), means that definition of a specific profile of neuropsychological impairments is as untenable for epilepsy as it is for cerebrovascular disease. Nonetheless certain common patterns may be identified in certain epilepsy syndromes.

Historically, epilepsy surgery provided one of the critical clues to the relevance of certain brain structures in cognitive function through one of the most remarkable cases in the history of neuropsychology, Henry or HM, who developed profound anterograde amnesia following surgical removal of the anterior temporal lobes, including the hippocampus, bilaterally for intractable seizures of temporal lobe origin (Scoville & Milner, 1957; Ogden, 2005). Occasional cases of amnesia following unilateral surgery have also been reported (Kapur & Prevett, 2003).

There are at least three possible reasons for an association between cognitive decline and epileptic seizures (Trimble & Reynolds, 1988; Kwan & Brodie, 2001; Trimble & Schmitz, 2002; Motamedi & Meador, 2003; Elger *et al.*, 2004):

- Cognitive decline and epilepsy may share an underlying aetiology.
- Seizures per se may lead to acquired cognitive impairment.
- Antiepileptic drug therapy may cause cognitive decline.

These variables are not necessarily independent: specific brain diseases or brain injuries may be associated with longer duration of seizure disorder and/or more frequent seizures, requiring polytherapy and/or higher doses of antiepileptic drugs. Because of this potential confounding, it is difficult to dissect the various parameters apart. Indeed, most cognitive problems in patients with epilepsy are of multifactorial origin. Psychiatric comorbidity may also need to be taken into account; depression may contribute more to subjective memory complaints and poor quality of life in epilepsy than seizures. Brain plasticity and epilepsy surgery may also have cognitive consequences, but are not considered further here (Elger *et al.*, 2004).

Memory problems in epilepsy are a subject of increasing concern in the management of epilepsy, over and above simple reduction in seizure frequency and severity (Brookes & Baker, 2006). How appropriate standard neuropsychological tests are in the detection of cognitive impairments in epilepsy patients is open to question (Baker & Marson, 2001), particularly in the assessment of executive functions.

REFERENCES

Baker GA, Marson AG. Cognitive and behavioural assessments in clinical trials: what type of measure? *Epilepsy Res* 2001; **45**: 163–7.

Brookes JA, Baker GA. Epilepsy and memory. *Epilepsy Professional* 2006; **1** (2): 21–3.

Brown SW, Vaughan M. Dementia in epileptic patients. In: Trimble MR, Reynolds EH (eds.), *Epilepsy, Behaviour and Cognitive Function*. Chichester: Wiley, 1988: 177–88.

Elger CE, Helmstaedter C, Kurthen M. Chronic epilepsy and cognition. *Lancet Neurol* 2004; **3**: 663–72.

Engel J, Pedley TA (eds.). *Epilepsy: a Comprehensive Textbook*. Philadelphia: Lippincott-Raven, 1997.

Kapur N, Prevett M. Unexpected amnesia: are there lessons to be learned from cases of amnesia following unilateral temporal lobe surgery? *Brain* 2003; **126**: 2573–85.

Kwan P, Brodie MJ. Neuropsychological effects of epilepsy and antiepileptic drugs. *Lancet* 2001; **357**: 216–22.

Motamedi G, Meador K. Epilepsy and cognition. *Epilepsy Behav* 2003; **4**: S25–38.

Ogden JA. *Fractured Minds: a Case-Study Approach to Clinical Neuropsychology* (2nd edition). Oxford: Oxford University Press, 2005: 46–63.

Panayiotopoulos CP. *A Clinical Guide to Epileptic Syndromes and Their Treatment: Based on the New ILAE Diagnostic Scheme*. Chipping Norton: Bladon, 2002.

Scoville W, Milner B. Loss of recent memory after bilateral hippocampal lesions. *J Neurol Neurosurg Psychiatry* 1957; **20**: 11–21.

Trimble MR, Reynolds EH (eds.). *Epilepsy, Behaviour and Cognitive Function*. Chichester: Wiley, 1988.

Trimble M, Schmitz B (eds.). *The Neuropsychiatry of Epilepsy*. Cambridge: Cambridge University Press, 2002: 135–85.

Zimmer C. *Soul Made Flesh. The Discovery of the Brain – and How it Changed the World*. London: Heinemann, 2004: 226.

4.2 Cognitive decline and epilepsy: shared aetiology

Cognitive decline and epilepsy may both be features of certain brain disorders. The symptomatic epilepsies include those due to brain tumour, stroke (infarct or haemorrhage), demyelination, infection (encephalitis, meningitis), and various dementia syndromes (Larner, 2007). The concurrence of seizures and cognitive impairment does not necessarily imply a causal link (i.e. seizures causing cognitive impairment) in these conditions. For example, seizures may sometimes be a feature of Huntington's disease (HD; see Section 5.1.1), particularly early-onset forms, but there is no suggestion that these seizures are responsible for, or even contribute to, the cognitive deficits of HD. Likewise Alzheimer's disease (AD) is recognized to be a risk factor for the development of late-onset seizures (Hauser *et al.*, 1986; Romanelli *et al.*, 1990), of both partial and generalized onset (Hesdorffer *et al.*, 1996), and seizures become increasingly common with the progression of AD (Mendez & Lim, 2003), but they cannot be held responsible for progression of cognitive impairments, not even when present in the earliest stages of the disease (Lozsadi & Larner, 2006). More likely, cognitive decline and seizures reflect a shared pathogenesis in terms of neuronal disconnection. Seizures may be a symptomatic feature of various other pathologies associated with cognitive decline (e.g. encephalitis, mitochondrial disease, progressive myoclonic epilepsy syndromes). The corollary of this observation is that treatment of the underlying disease, where possible, might ameliorate both cognitive decline and seizures.

In contrast to symptomatic epilepsies, many seizure disorders remain idiopathic despite extensive investigation. These idiopathic epilepsies may be categorized according to whether the seizures are of generalized or partial onset. Group studies have suggested that epilepsy patients have reduced speed of mental processing, reaction and response times (Bruhn & Parsons, 1977), as well as impairments in remembering lists of words and geometric patterns (Loiseau *et al.*, 1980). Attention deficits may be more common in generalized than in focal epilepsy (Mirsky *et al.*, 1960; Kimura, 1964), memory difficulties more common in focal (temporal lobe) epilepsy.

REFERENCES

Bruhn P, Parsons OA. Reaction time variability in epileptic and brain-damaged patients. *Cortex* 1977; **13**: 373–84.

Hauser WA, Morris ML, Heston LL, Anderson VE. Seizures and myoclonus in patients with Alzheimer's disease. *Neurology* 1986; **36**: 1226–30.

Hesdorffer DC, Hauser WA, Annegers JF, Kokmen E, Rocca WA. Dementia and adult-onset unprovoked seizures. *Neurology* 1996; **46**: 727–30.

Kimura D. Cognitive deficit related to seizure patterns in centrencephalic epilepsy. *J Neurol Neurosurg Psychiatry* 1964; **27**: 291–5.

Larner AJ. Epilepsy and dementia: confusion over seizures. *Epilepsy Professional* 2007; Issue **6**: 21–3.

Loiseau P, Strube E, Broustet D, *et al.* Evaluation of memory function in a population of epileptic patients and matched controls. *Acta Neurol Scand Suppl* 1980; **80**: 58–61.

Lozsadi DA, Larner AJ. Prevalence and causes of seizures at time of diagnosis of probable Alzheimer's disease. *Dementia Geriatr Cogn Disord* 2006; **22**: 121–4.

Mendez MF, Lim GTH. Seizures in elderly patients with dementia: epidemiology and management. *Drugs Aging* 2003; **20**: 791–803.

Mirsky AF, Primac DW, Marsan CA, Rosvold HE, Stevens JR. A comparison of the psychological test performance of patients with focal and non-focal epilepsy. *Exp Neurol* 1960; **2**: 75–89.

Romanelli MF, Morris JC, Ashkin K, Coben LA. Advanced Alzheimer's disease is a risk factor for late-onset seizures. *Arch Neurol* 1990; **47**: 847–50.

4.2.1 Localization-related (partial) epilepsies

Partial or focal seizures may be of temporal, frontal, or occipital lobe onset, with or without secondary generalization. Cognitive features have been most extensively investigated in temporal lobe epilepsy. Generally, cognitive deficits are localized to the brain region affected. Thus partial seizures with epileptic foci in the left temporal region have generally been associated with impaired verbal long-term memory, whilst right temporal lobe foci cause greater difficulty with visual long-term memory, whereas early group studies found patients with unilateral frontal lobe foci to be no different from controls (Làdavas *et al.*, 1979; Delaney *et al.*, 1980). These findings may in part explain why even patients with well-controlled partial seizures, doing a regular job or attending a normal school, may be found on neuropsychological testing to have impaired cognition (Engelberts *et al.*, 2002).

Temporal lobe epilepsy

Symptomatic temporal lobe epilepsy (TLE) with the neuroradiological signature of hippocampal sclerosis or mesial temporal sclerosis (MTS) is thought to be the commonest form of localization-related epilepsy (Wieser, 2004). Precipitating incidents such as febrile convulsions, brain trauma, ischaemia, or intracranial infection are common, and most individuals have seizure onset in childhood or adolescence.

Because of the involvement of structures important for memory processes, it has been natural to examine cognitive function in TLE patients. Even at disease onset deficits may be apparent, suggesting that these are symptoms of the disease and not simply consequences of frequent seizures or the effects of antiepileptic drug therapy (Aikia *et al.*, 2001). Left-sided (dominant hemisphere) TLE is characterized by deficits in material-specific verbal memory (Hermann *et al.*, 1997), whereas right TLE is associated with non-verbal/visual memory deficit, albeit less consistently (Gleissner *et al.*, 1998). Other profiles are sometimes encountered, for example relatively selective autobiographical amnesia (Kapur, 1997). Quantitative MR imaging studies suggest that both the hippocampus and other related structures such as the fornix are atrophied in TLE patients (Kuzniecky *et al.*, 1999).

Some studies have indicated that higher seizure frequency and duration of TLE are associated with more severe cognitive decline (Jokheit & Ebner, 1999), but in a report on patients with TLE undergoing temporal lobe resection no correlation was found between disease-related parameters, such as cumulative number of seizures, and neuropsychological deficits, suggesting that factors other than repetitive seizures are responsible for cognitive dysfunction in TLE patients (Kramer *et al.*, 2006). Longitudinal studies have suggested that there is an early epilepsy-related memory deficit which then remains relatively stable over time, with any additional changes typical of those related to aging.

Frontal lobe epilepsy

The frontal lobe epilepsies (FLE), resulting from a primary epileptic focus anywhere within the frontal lobe, have various seizure patterns. Motor manifestations are more common than in seizures arising elsewhere, for example simple focal motor seizures with or without Jacksonian march, and tonic posturing in seizures of supplementary motor-area origin (fencer's posture, *en garde*, salutatory seizures). FLE may be idiopathic or symptomatic.

There is evidence for frontal-type, executive, cognitive dysfunction in FLE, in terms of attention, working memory, planning, and psychomotor speed (Helmstaedter *et al.*, 1996; Upton & Thompson, 1997; Exner *et al.*, 2002). Elements of social cognition, such as humour appreciation and ability to detect emotional expression, but not tests of theory of mind, may also be impaired (Farrant *et al.*, 2005).

A nocturnal variant of FLE may be either sporadic or inherited as an autosomal dominant disorder, the latter (ADNFLE) associated with mutations in at least two genes, *CHRNA4* and *CHRNB2* (Combi *et al.*, 2004). ADNFLE associated with one mutation in *CHRNB2*, I312M, is reported to be associated with distinct memory deficits involving the storage of verbal information (Bertrand *et al.*, 2005).

REFERENCES

Aikia M, Salmenpera T, Partanen K, Kalviainen R. Verbal memory in newly diagnosed patients and patients with chronic left temporal lobe epilepsy. *Epilepsy Behav* 2001; **2**: 20–7.

Bertrand D, Elmslie F, Hughes E, *et al.* The CHRNB2 mutation I312M is associated with epilepsy and distinct memory deficits. *Neurobiol Dis* 2005; **20**: 799–804.

Combi R, Dalpra L, Tenchini ML, Ferini-Strambi L. Autosomal dominant nocturnal frontal lobe epilepsy: a critical review. *J Neurol* 2004; **251**: 923–34.

Delaney RC, Rosen AJ, Mattson RH, Novelly RA. Memory function in focal epilepsy: a comparison of non-surgical, unilateral temporal lobe and frontal lobe samples. *Cortex* 1980; **16**: 103–17.

Engelberts NHJ, Klein M, van der Ploeg HM, *et al.* Cognition and health-related quality of life in a well-defined subgroup of patients with partial epilepsy. *J Neurol* 2002; **249**: 294–9.

Exner C, Boucsein K, Lange C, *et al.* Neuropsychological performance in frontal lobe epilepsy. *Seizure* 2002; **11**: 20–32.

Farrant A, Morris RG, Russell T, *et al.* Social cognition in frontal lobe epilepsy. *Epilepsy Behav* 2005; **7**: 506–16.

Gleissner U, Helmstaedter C, Elger CE. Right hippocampal contribution to visual memory: a presurgical and postsurgical study in patients with temporal lobe epilepsy. *J Neurol Neurosurg Psychiatry* 1998; **65**: 665–9.

Helmstaedter C, Kemper B, Elger CE. Neuropsychological aspects of frontal lobe epilepsy. *Neuropsychologia* 1996; **34**: 399–406.

Hermann BP, Seidenberg M, Schoenfeld J, Davies K. Neuropsychological characteristics of the syndrome of mesial temporal lobe epilepsy. *Arch Neurol* 1997; **54**: 369–76.

Jokheit H, Ebner A. Long term effects of refractory temporal lobe epilepsy on cognitive abilities: a cross sectional study. *J Neurol Neurosurg Psychiatry* 1999; **67**: 44–50.

Kapur N. Autobiographical amnesia and temporal lobe pathology. In: Parkin AJ (ed.), *Case Studies in the Neuropsychology of Memory*. Hove: Psychology Press, 1997: 37–62.

Kramer U, Kipervasser S, Neufeld MY, *et al.* Is there any correlation between severity of epilepsy and cognitive abilities in patients with temporal lobe epilepsy? *Eur J Neurol* 2006; **13**: 130–4.

Kuzniecky R, Bilir E, Gilliam F, *et al.* Quantitative MRI in temporal lobe epilepsy: evidence for fornix atrophy. *Neurology* 1999; **53**: 496–501.

Làdavas E, Umiltà C, Provinciali L. Hemisphere-dependent cognitive performances in epileptic patients. *Epilepsia* 1979; **20**: 493–502.

Upton D, Thompson PJ. Age at onset and neuropsychological function in frontal lobe epilepsy. *Epilepsia* 1997; **38**: 1103–13.

Wieser HG. Mesial temporal lobe epilepsy with hippocampal sclerosis. *Epilepsia* 2004; **45**: 695–714.

4.2.2 Rasmussen's syndrome (chronic encephalitis and epilepsy)

A syndrome of chronic partial, often intractable, epileptic seizures attended by progressive focal sensorimotor neurological deficit and cognitive decline was described by Rasmussen *et al.* (1958); a similar syndrome was described by Kozhevnikov in Russian in 1952. The pathogenesis of Rasmussen's syndrome, also known as chronic encephalitis and epilepsy, remains uncertain: possibilities include viral infection and autoimmune mechanisms (Larner & Anderson, 1995; Bien *et al.*, 2005). Although typically a disorder with childhood onset (Andermann, 1991), cases with adult onset have been described on occasion (e.g. McLachlan *et al.*, 1993; Nicholas *et al.*, 2002). These appear to have a more protracted and milder clinical course with less in the way of residual functional deficits, lesser degrees of brain hemiatrophy, but with identical clinical, EEG, neuroimaging, and histopathology findings (Bien *et al.*, 2002).

Neuropsychological assessment of patients with Rasmussen's syndrome is subject to various biases, such as selected cohorts, ongoing seizures or even epilepsia partialis continua, and surgical interventions. Low IQ is typical in childhood-onset cases, usually with little change after surgery, although exceptionally improvement is noted (Taylor, 1991). In adult-onset cases, McLachlan *et al.* (1993) noted decline in IQ in two of their three patients, with greater left hemisphere dysfunction (PIQ > VIQ), consistent in one patient with exclusively left hemisphere involvement. Over an 8-year period, between the ages of 22 and 30 years, another adult-onset patient developed IQ decline, impaired auditory verbal memory, motor and sensory aphasia in association with left temporo-occipital cortical MR imaging change and EEG multifocal spike discharges in the left posterior quadrant (Larner *et al.*, 1995). However, cases with no recorded cognitive deficit have been presented (Gawler, 2006). Improvements in neuropsychological function, as well as in seizure frequency, have been recorded in adult-onset cases following cycles of treatment with human intravenous immunoglobulin (Leach *et al.*, 1999).

REFERENCES

Andermann F (ed.). *Chronic Encephalitis and Epilepsy: Rasmussen's Syndrome.* Boston: Butterworth-Heinemann, 1991.

Bien CG, Granata T, Antozzi C, *et al.* Pathogenesis, diagnosis and treatment of Rasmussen encephalitis: a

European consensus statement. *Brain* 2005; **128**: 454–71.

Bien CG, Widman G, Urbach H, *et al*. The natural history of Rasmussen's encephalitis. *Brain* 2002; **125**: 1751–9.

Gawler J. A 'glioma' that was cured. *Pract Neurol* 2006; **6**: 117–21.

Larner AJ, Anderson M. Rasmussen's syndrome: pathogenetic theories and therapeutic strategies. *J Neurol* 1995; **242**: 355–8.

Larner AJ, Smith SJM, Duncan JS, Howard RS. Late-onset Rasmussen's syndrome with first seizure during pregnancy. *Eur Neurol* 1995; **35**: 172.

Leach JP, Chadwick DW, Miles JB, Hart IK. Improvement in adult-onset Rasmussen's encephalitis with long-term immunomodulatory therapy. *Neurology* 1999; **52**: 738–42.

McLachlan RS, Girvin JP, Blume WT, Reichman H. Rasmussen's chronic encephalitis in adults. *Arch Neurol* 1993; **50**: 269–74.

Nicholas RS, Scott AC, Hart IK. Two clinical presentations of adult onset Rasmussen's syndrome share common immunological and pathological features. *J Neurol Neurosurg Psychiatry* 2002; **72**: 141 (abstract).

Rasmussen T, Olszewski J, Lloyd-Smith D. Focal seizures due to chronic localized encephalitis. *Neurology* 1958; **8**: 435–45.

Taylor LB. Neuropsychologic assessment of patients with chronic encephalitis. In: Andermann F (ed.), *Chronic Encephalitis and Epilepsy: Rasmussen's Syndrome*. Boston: Butterworth-Heinemann, 1991: 111–21.

4.2.3 Idiopathic generalized epilepsies

Idiopathic generalized epilepsies (IGE) are characterized by primary generalized seizures which, unlike localization-related epilepsies, occur in the absence of any macroscopic brain abnormalities. Hence, IGEs may facilitate the study of the effect of seizures on cognitive function. However, controlled studies in homogeneous groups of IGE patients are in their infancy. IGE patients are reported to perform worse than controls on speed of information processing and in tests of memory encompassing word and face recognition and verbal and visual recall, with MR spectroscopy evidence that this may correlate with neuronal dysfunction secondary to epileptic activity (Dickson *et al.*, 2006). In

juvenile myoclonic epilepsy (JME), abstract reasoning, planning, and mental flexibility are reported to be impaired, suggesting frontal type dysfunction (Devinsky *et al.*, 1997).

REFERENCES

Devinsky O, Gershengorn J, Brown E, *et al*. Frontal functions in juvenile myoclonic epilepsy. *Neuropsychiatry Neuropsychol Behav Neurol* 1997; **10**: 243–6.

Dickson JM, Wilkinson ID, Howell SJL, Griffiths PD, Grünewald RA. Idiopathic generalised epilepsy: a pilot study of memory and neuronal dysfunction in the temporal lobes, assessed by magnetic resonance spectroscopy. *J Neurol Neurosurg Psychiatry* 2006; **77**: 834–40.

4.3 Seizures causing acquired cognitive impairment

Seizures may unequivocally lead to cognitive impairment (Aldenkamp, 1997), as may frequent interictal epileptiform discharges (Aldenkamp & Arends, 2004). Impairments have been noted in psychomotor speed, attention, memory, and visuomotor tasks which cannot be ascribed to the encephalopathy associated with status epilepticus, postictal state, or antiepileptic drug toxicity, and which are reversible with good seizure control. Longitudinal studies suggest a link between adverse cognitive change and number of seizures or presence of tonic–clonic status epilepticus (Dodrill, 2004).

Amnesia is the norm for complex partial seizures, and for primary and secondary generalized seizures. Sometimes the effects of frequent complex partial seizures are sufficient to manifest as a dementia syndrome that may even be confused with Alzheimer's disease (Tatum *et al.*, 1998; Høgh *et al.*, 2002; Sinforiani *et al.*, 2003). The frequency of such 'epileptic pseudodementia' is not known, but clinically it merits consideration in light of the fact that the incidence of complex partial seizures rises sharply after the age of 60 years. However, the classic example of seizures causing cognitive impairment is seen in the syndrome of transient epileptic amnesia.

REFERENCES

Aldenkamp AP. Effect of seizures and epileptiform discharges on cognitive function. *Epilepsia* 1997; **38** (suppl 1): S52–5.

Aldenkamp AP, Arends J. Effects of epileptiform EEG discharges on cognitive function: is the concept of 'transient cognitive impairment' still valid? *Epilepsy Behav* 2004; **5** (suppl 1): S25–34.

Dodrill CB. Neuropsychological effects of seizures. *Epilepsy Behav* 2004; **5** (suppl 1): S21–4.

Høgh P, Smith SJ, Scahill RI, *et al.* Epilepsy presenting as AD: neuroimaging, electroclinical features, and response to treatment. *Neurology* 2002; **58**: 298–301.

Sinforiani E, Manni R, Bernasconi L, Banchieri LM, Zucchella C. Memory disturbances and temporal lobe epilepsy simulating Alzheimer's disease: a case report. *Funct Neurol* 2003; **18**: 39–41.

Tatum WO, Ross J, Cole AJ. Epileptic pseudodementia. *Neurology* 1998; **50**: 1472–5.

4.3.1 Transient epileptic amnesia (TEA)

Attacks of transient amnesia of epileptic origin are usually brief, 1 hour or less in duration, often occur on waking, and may be associated with clear-cut EEG abnormalities. There may be a concurrent history of other seizure types. Clinically this condition resembles transient global amnesia (TGA), but generally responds favourably to standard antiepileptic medications such as sodium valproate or carbamazepine (Pritchard *et al.*, 1985; Gallassi *et al.*, 1992; Kapur, 1993; Zeman *et al.*, 1998). An accelerated loss of new information and impaired remote autobiographical memory has been demonstrated in TEA patients, but the aetiology of these deficits remains uncertain, possibilities including ongoing seizure activity, seizure-induced medial temporal lobe damage, or subtle ischaemic pathology (Manes *et al.*, 2005).

REFERENCES

Gallassi R, Morreale A, Di Sarro R, Lugaresi E. Epileptic amnesic syndrome. *Epilepsia* 1992; **33** (suppl 6): S21–5.

Kapur N. Transient epileptic amnesia: a clinical update and a reformulation. *J Neurol Neurosurg Psychiatry* 1993; **56**: 1184–90.

Manes F, Graham KS, Zeman A, de Luján Calcagno M, Hodges JR. Autobiographical amnesia and accelerated forgetting in transient epileptic amnesia. *J Neurol Neurosurg Psychiatry* 2005; **76**: 1387–91.

Pritchard PB III, Holmstrom VL, Roitzsch JC, Giacinto J. Epileptic amnesic attacks: benefit from antiepileptic drugs. *Neurology* 1985; **35**: 1188–9.

Zeman AZJ, Boniface SJ, Hodges JR. Transient epileptic amnesia: a description of the clinical and neuropsychological features in 10 cases and a review of the literature. *J Neurol Neurosurg Psychiatry* 1998; **64**: 435–43.

4.3.2 Epileptic aphasia, ictal speech arrest

Aphasia is the principal symptom in the childhood epilepsy disorder of Landau–Kleffner syndrome (acquired epileptic aphasia), possibly reflecting a verbal auditory agnosia (Paquier *et al.*, 1992). Isolated epileptic aphasia is uncommon, perhaps obscured in some cases by ictal motor activity (Rosenbaum *et al.*, 1986). Non-convulsive status epilepticus may manifest with aphasia ('status aphasicus'), usually with abrupt onset and rapid resolution with appropriate antiepileptic drug therapy, although persistent aphasia has also been reported (DeToledo *et al.*, 2000; Chung *et al.*, 2002). Aphasic status most often reflects left frontotemporal or temporoparietal pathology (Grimes & Guberman, 1997), although visual stimuli provoking an occipital lobe seizure spreading to the left inferior frontal lobe has been reported (Kobayashi *et al.*, 1999), as has a right-sided focus (DeToledo *et al.*, 2000). Parasagittal lesions confined to the left superior frontal gyrus (supplementary motor area) may be sufficient to cause the syndrome (Wieshmann *et al.*, 1997). Other reported causes include non-ketotic hyperglycaemia (Carril *et al.*, 1992), AIDS–toxoplasmosis (Ozkaya *et al.*, 2006), and multiple sclerosis (Trinka *et al.*, 2002; see Section 6.1).

REFERENCES

Carril JM, Guijarro C, Portocarrero JS, *et al*. Speech arrest as manifestation of seizures in non-ketotic hyperglycaemia. *Lancet* 1992; **340**: 1227.

Chung PW, Seo DW, Kwon JC, Kim H, Na DL. Non-convulsive status epilepticus presenting as a subacute progressive aphasia. *Seizure* 2002; **11**: 449–54.

DeToledo JC, Minagar A, Lowe MR. Persisting aphasia as the sole manifestation of partial status epilepticus. *Clin Neurol Neurosurg* 2000; **102**: 144–8.

Grimes DA, Guberman A. De novo aphasic status epilepticus. *Epilepsia* 1997; **38**: 945–9.

Kobayashi M, Takayama H, Mihara B, Sugishita M. Partial seizure with aphasic speech arrest caused by watching a popular animated TV program. *Epilepsia* 1999; **40**: 652–4.

Ozkaya G, Kurne A, Unal S, *et al*. Aphasic status epilepticus with periodic lateralized epileptiform discharges in a bilingual patient as a presenting sign of AIDS–toxoplasmosis complex. *Epilepsy Behav* 2006; **9**: 193–6.

Paquier PF, Van Dongen HR, Loonen CB. The Landau–Kleffner syndrome or 'acquired aphasia with convulsive disorder': long-term follow-up of six children and a review of the recent literature. *Arch Neurol* 1992; **49**: 354–9.

Rosenbaum DH, Siegel M, Barr WB, Rowan AJ. Epileptic aphasia. *Neurology* 1986; **36**: 822–5.

Trinka E, Unterberger I, Spiegel M, *et al*. De novo aphasic status epilepticus as presenting symptom of multiple sclerosis. *J Neurol* 2002; **249**: 782–3.

Wieshmann UC, Niehaus L, Meierkord H. Ictal speech arrest and parasagittal lesions. *Eur Neurol* 1997; **38**: 123–7.

4.4 Antiepileptic drug therapy causing cognitive impairment

Although reduction in seizure frequency as a consequence of prescribing antiepileptic drugs (AEDs) may unquestionably improve cognitive function, nonetheless AEDs feature in any list of medicines which may cause cognitive decline or even dementia (Farlow & Hake, 1998; Moore & O'Keefe, 1999). The cognitive side effects of chronic AED therapy, to which the elderly are more susceptible, have long been a topic of research interest (Devinsky, 1995; Vermeulen & Aldenkamp, 1995). The vexed questions of the effects of AEDs, particularly sodium valproate, on the IQ of children exposed in utero (Vinten *et al.*, 2005) and during development (Kasteleijn-Nolst Trinité & de Saint-Martin, 2004) remain highly topical but are not discussed here.

Sedation may be an important factor in adults receiving AEDs, as judged by increased reaction times and specific deficits in attention and working memory observed in some, but not all, patients taking drugs such as phenobarbitone, phenytoin, and benzodiazepines. Patients receiving monotherapy with phenytoin, sodium valproate, or carbamazepine who were tested before and after changes in drug dosage, either up or down, showed deficits in cognitive performance in the high serum level group, especially those receiving phenytoin or sodium valproate, whereas the carbamazepine group showed no change or even a trend towards improvement in the high serum level group (Thompson & Trimble, 1982, 1983). Volunteers receiving phenytoin, carbamazepine, sodium valproate, clonazepam, and clobazam have shown significant deficits, most marked with phenytoin and clonazepam. A large study in the USA comparing efficacy and toxicity of monotherapy with four antiepileptic drugs (phenobarbitone, primidone, phenytoin, and carbamazepine) found that, when controlling for age, education, and IQ, carbamazaepine had fewer cognitive effects than the other drugs (Mattson *et al.*, 1985), confirming previous smaller studies. However, other studies have not found a difference between carbamazepine and phenytoin when drug levels have been taken into account (Dodrill & Troupin, 1991). Polypharmacy is certainly associated with more severe adverse consequences for cognitive function (Trimble, 1987).

Newer antiepileptic drugs generally have improved side-effect profiles in comparison with previously used medications, but the increased scrutiny to which these medications have been subject has unfortunately shown that they are not exempt from cognitive side effects (Aldenkamp *et al.*, 2003). Lamotrigine, probably the most extensively studied from the cognitive perspective, seems well tolerated (Aldenkamp & Baker, 2001), and the same is probably true of gabapentin (Dodrill *et al.*, 1999) and oxcarbazepine. However, impaired attention, psychomotor slowing, and memory deficits have been recorded with topiramate, which seems more prone to cognitive side effects than lamotrigine or gabapentin (Martin *et al.*, 1999; Huppertz *et al.*, 2001), although this may be related to rapid drug titration in some studies. Pragmatic comparative drug trials have shown that memory disturbance is a common symptom and one of the most common adverse effects to result in treatment failure; this may be particularly the case with topiramate (Marson *et al.*, 2007a, b). Currently there are few studies evaluating cognitive side effects of vigabatrin, levetiracetam, tiagabine, and zonisamide (Aldenkamp *et al.*, 2003).

REFERENCES

Aldenkamp AP, Baker G. A systematic review of the effects of lamotrigine on cognitive function and quality of life. *Epilepsy Behav* 2001; **2**: 85–91.

Aldenkamp AP, De Krom M, Reijs R. Newer antiepileptic drugs and cognitive issues. *Epilepsia* 2003; **44** (suppl): 21–9.

Devinsky O. Cognitive and behavioral effects of antiepileptic drugs. *Epilepsia* 1995; **36** (suppl 2): 46–65.

Dodrill CB, Arnett JL, Hayes AG, *et al.* Cognitive abilities and adjustment with gabapentin: results of multi-site study. *Epilepsy Res* 1999; **35**: 109–21.

Dodrill CB, Troupin AS. Neuropsychological effects of carbamazepine and phenytoin: a reanalysis. *Neurology* 1991; **41**: 141–3.

Farlow MR, Hake AM. Drug-induced cognitive impairment. In: Biller J (ed.), *Iatrogenic Neurology*. Boston: Butterworth-Heinemann, 1998: 203–14.

Huppertz HJ, Quiske A, Schulze Bonhage A. Cognitive impairments due to add-on therapy with topiramate [in German]. *Nervenarzt* 2001; **72**: 275–80.

Kasteleijn-Nolst Trinité DGA, de Saint-Martin A. Cognitive aspects. In: Wallace SJ, Farrell K (eds.), *Epilepsy in Children* (2nd edition). London: Arnold, 2004: 433–46.

Marson AG, Al-Kharusi AM, Alwaidh M, *et al.* The SANAD study of effectiveness of carbamazepine, gabapentin, lamotrigine, oxcarbazepine, or topiramate for the treatment of partial epilepsy: an unblinded randomised controlled trial. *Lancet* 2007a; **369**: 1000–15.

Marson AG, Al-Kharusi AM, Alwaidh M, *et al.* The SANAD study of effectiveness of valproate, lamotrigine, or topiramate for generalised and unclassifiable epilepsy: an unblinded randomised controlled trial. *Lancet* 2007b; **369**: 1016–26.

Martin R, Kuzniecky R, Ho S, *et al.* Cognitive effects of topiramate, gabapentin, and lamotrigine in healthy young adults. *Neurology* 1999; **52**: 321–7.

Mattson RH, Cramer JA, Collins JF, *et al.* Comparison of carbamazepine, phenobarbital, phenytoin and primidone in partial and secondarily generalized tonic-clonic seizures. *N Engl J Med* 1985; **313**: 145–51.

Moore AR, O'Keefe ST. Drug-induced cognitive impairment in the elderly. *Drugs Aging* 1999; **15**: 15–28.

Thompson PJ, Trimble MR. Anticonvulsant drugs and cognitive functions. *Epilepsia* 1982; **23**: 531–44.

Thompson PJ, Trimble MR. Anticonvulsant serum levels: relationship to impairments of cognitive functioning. *J Neurol Neurosurg Psychiatry* 1983; **46**: 227–33.

Trimble MR. Anticonvulsant drugs and cognitive function: a review of the literature. *Epilepsia* 1987; **28** (suppl 3): 37–45.

Vermeulen J, Aldenkamp AP. Cognitive side-effects of chronic antiepileptic drug treatment: a review of 25 years of research. *Epilepsy Res* 1995; **22**: 65–95.

Vinten J, Adab N, Kini U, *et al.* Neuropsychological effects of exposure to anticonvulsant medication in utero. *Neurology* 2005; **64**: 949–54.

4.5 Treatment of cognitive problems in epilepsy

Treatment of cognitive complaints needs to be individualized to each patient with epilepsy, but some general guidelines may be enunciated. Optimizing seizure control with AEDs that have a good side-effect profile as far as cognitive function is concerned, and avoiding polypharmacy, is paramount. Treating confounding factors such as depression and sleep disorders is mandatory. However, it must be recognized that the underlying aetiology of seizures is often a major contributing factor, and one that may not be amenable to specific treatment. Whether cognitive enhancers such as cholinesterase inhibitors have anything to offer in this circumstance requires further study (Fisher *et al.*, 2001).

REFERENCES

Fisher RS, Bortz JJ, Blum DE, Duncan B, Burke H. A pilot study of donepezil for memory problems in epilepsy. *Epilepsy Behav* 2001; **2**: 330–4.

Neurogenetic disorders

Although great advances have been made in elucidating the genetic basis of neurological disorders in recent years, with profound implications not only for diagnosis but also for beginning to understand disease pathogenesis, nonetheless a clinical rather than a pathogenetic classification of disorders is used here, in part because the pathogenetic pathway from mutant gene to disease phenotype remains uncertain in many instances.

5.1   Hereditary dementias

Under this rubric, dementia syndromes with confirmed genetic basis, with or without additional neurological features, are included. Autosomal dominant Alzheimer's disease (see Section 2.1), frontotemporal dementia with parkinsonism linked to chromosome 17 (FTDP-17: Section 2.2.4) and hereditary forms of prion disease (Section 2.5.3) are discussed elsewhere, as are other genetic disorders which may result in dementia such as CADASIL (Section 3.6.2) and some of the hereditary cerebral amyloid angiopathies (Section 3.6.3).

5.1.1   Huntington's disease (HD)

The archetypal hereditary dementia is Huntington's disease (HD), although a number of the common neurodegenerative dementias may sometimes be inherited in an autosomal dominant manner (see Chapter 2). In his description of the disorder that now bears his name, George Huntington not only delineated the movement disorder, most usually chorea (cortical myoclonus and parkinsonism may also occur), the neuropsychiatric features, and the mode of inheritance, but also alluded to the gradually

progressive impairment of the mind (Huntington, 1872). Cognition is one of the four characteristics, along with motor function, behaviour, and functional abilities, assessed by the Unified Huntington's Disease Rating Scale (UHDRS), which has now become the universal scale for measuring HD function (Huntington's Study Group, 1996).

Collaborative studies have shown that HD results from a trinucleotide (CAG, polyglutamine, polyQ) repeat expansion on the *IT15* gene on chromosome 4 encoding the huntingtin protein (Huntington's Disease Collaborative Research Group, 1993). A significant inverse relationship exists between CAG repeat length and age at clinical onset. Clinical phenotype also varies with age of onset: juvenile disease (Westphal variant) has a prominent parkinsonian syndrome, whereas very late-onset disease may be associated with chorea and little intellectual impairment. Neuropathologically, there is a loss of medium spiny neurones and gliosis in the caudate nucleus and putamen, resulting in shrinkage of the caudate, which may be observed on structural brain imaging, as well as degenerative change in the cortex and hippocampus. Intranuclear inclusions immunopositive for huntingtin and ubiquitin are found (Vonsattel & Lianski, 2004). The availability of a diagnostic neurogenetic test has made possible the detection of presymptomatic cases in at-risk family members. HD phenocopies, without trinucleotide repeat in the huntingtin gene, do occur (Rosenblatt *et al.*, 1998). These cases may have insertions in the prion protein (*PRNP*) gene, or expansions in the genes encoding junctophilin-3 (*JPH3*) or TATA binding protein gene (*TBP*), the latter allelic with spinocerebellar ataxia type 17 (Stevanin *et al.*, 2003). As yet, no curative treatment is

Table 5.1. Neuropsychological deficits in Huntington's disease (HD).

Attention	↓ divided, sustained attention; working memory
Memory	'Subcortical pattern': impaired encoding and retrieval, recognition better than recall; impaired skill learning
Language	Letter fluency worse than category fluency
Perception	Visuoperceptual problems: defects in judging distance, spatial relationships
Praxis	Ideomotor apraxia
Executive function	Dysexecutive syndrome (impaired Stroop, Wisconsin Card Sorting); may contribute to many of the neuropsychological deficits observed

available for HD, and symptomatic treatments are limited in their effect. The natural history is one of relentless progression (Kosinski & Landwehrmeyer, 2005).

The cognitive disorder of HD has been extensively investigated (Craufurd & Snowden, 2003; Paulsen & Conybeare, 2005). Following the characterization of 'subcortical dementia' in progressive supranuclear palsy (Albert *et al.*, 1974; Section 2.4.2), the core deficits in HD have also been labelled as subcortical (McHugh & Folstein, 1975) and subsequent investigations have confirmed a pattern of deficits distinct from that in AD. Using the MMSE, HD patients perform more poorly than Alzheimer's disease patients on the attention item (serial sevens) but better on the orientation in time and memory items (Brandt *et al.*, 1988). Likewise, HD patients administered the Dementia Rating Scale show more impairment on the initiation/perseveration subtest and less impairment on the memory subtest than AD patients (Rosser & Hodges, 1994a). Reviewing a large number of studies of HD patients, Zakzanis (1998) reported deficits in memory acquisition and delayed recall, cognitive flexibility, abstraction, attention, and concentration. It may be that a dysexecutive syndrome accounts for the poor performance in many areas, reflective of pathological involvement of the basal ganglia and frontostriatal connections. The natural history of cognitive function is one of decline, but the rate is variable, as are the different domains affected. In one longitudinal study, over a 1-year period significant decline was detected in low-level psychomotor tasks, object recall, and verbal fluency, whereas executive function (WCST) remained stable (Snowden *et al.*, 2001).

Neuropsychological profile

The neuropsychological deficits typically seen in Huntington's disease are summarized in Table 5.1.

Attention

Impairments in attentional functions in HD are attested to by poor performance on WAIS subtests such as Digit Span and Digit Symbol which probe attention and working memory. Shifting of attention to new information may be particularly impaired, whereas attention to previously learned information is maintained with perseveration on previously correct responses (Lawrence *et al.*, 1996). This may be reflected in the clinical observation that HD patients perform worse when required to divide attention between tasks or stimuli. Selective and progressive attentional and executive dysfunctions are features of early HD (Ho *et al.*, 2003), and assessment of attentional tasks may be used to monitor progression of disease (Lemiere *et al.*, 2004).

Memory

Learning and memory difficulties are a common complaint of HD patients and their relatives. There is a problem with encoding and retrieval, since verbal recognition memory is preserved relative to recall

(Butters *et al.*, 1986). This may relate to inefficient encoding strategies, reflective of executive dysfunction. Retention of information over a delay period is relatively intact, hence there is no abnormal forgetting (Massman *et al.*, 1990), and on remote memory tests there is no temporal gradient. Compared to AD patients, HD patients matched for overall level of dementia had less impairment of delayed verbal and figural episodic memory but were worse on letter fluency, suggesting a double dissociation of semantic and episodic memory impairment (Hodges *et al.*, 1990). Semantic memory and delayed recall memory are relatively unaffected in early HD (Rohrer *et al.*, 1999; Ho *et al.*, 2003) but visuospatial memory may be impaired (Lawrence *et al.*, 1996).

Implicit memory as tested by skill learning is impaired, indicating a role for the basal ganglia in such learning processes, particularly 'open-loop' skills, a finding which may possibly be related to working memory deficits.

Language

Naming errors in HD seem to be largely visually based, reflecting disrupted perceptual analysis, whilst phonemic processes remain relatively intact (Hodges *et al.*, 1991). This contrasts with the semantic breakdown observed in AD, and is corroborated by verbal fluency tests showing greater impairment in letter fluency rather than semantic fluency in HD even early in the disease (Hodges *et al.*, 1990; Randolph *et al.*, 1993; Rosser & Hodges, 1994b), presumably related to frontostriatal dysfunction. Late deficits in confrontation naming are more likely due to visuoperceptual deficits and retrieval slowing rather than a disintegration of semantic knowledge (Rohrer *et al.*, 1999).

The motor disorder of HD may affect phonation, speech output becoming increasingly limited as the disease progresses. Apathy and psychomotor slowing may also contribute to this loss of speech. There may also be impaired comprehension of affective and propositional speech prosody (Speedie *et al.*, 1990).

Perception

Visuospatial disorder may be evident on object assembly and block design tasks and tests of pattern and spatial recognition memory, but again these deficits may reflect problems with other processes such as planning (Lawrence *et al.*, 2000). A defect in the perception of personal (egocentric) space has been consistently documented, with difficulty judging distances and spatial relationship to other objects (Brouwers *et al.*, 1984), the clinical correlate of which is a tendency to bump into things; it may also contribute to falls. Visuospatial memory may be impaired early in HD (Lawrence *et al.*, 1996).

Praxis

Although the assessment of praxis may be difficult in the context of the motor disorder of HD, nonetheless occasional studies have been undertaken. Shelton and Knopman (1991) found ideomotor apraxia to be common in a small cohort of patients with long-standing disease (mean duration > 10 years), particularly for imitation of non-symbolic movements, whereas recognition of gestures was preserved. These changes were thought to be primarily subcortical in origin. Hamilton *et al.* (2003), however, found apraxia to be more common in patients with greater neurological involvement and longer disease duration, suggesting that apraxia resulted from damage to corticostriate pathways rather than restricted basal ganglia involvement as in early disease, which fits better with the notion of apraxia as a feature of cortical dementias.

Executive function

Progressive impairment in executive function is found in early HD (Lawrence *et al.*, 1996; Ho *et al.*, 2003) and is associated with bilateral striatal (caudate) and extrastriatal (insular) atrophy (Peinemann *et al.*, 2005). Typical of patients with executive deficits, verbal fluency tests show poor category fluency but worse letter fluency, the reverse of the pattern seen in AD (Rosser & Hodges, 1994b), plus impairments on the Stroop Test and the WCST (Lemiere *et al.*, 2004). This dysexecutive syndrome may account for many of the cognitive impairments documented in HD, caused by striatal and corticostriatal involvement. Assessment of executive functions may be used to monitor progression of disease (Lemiere *et al.*, 2004).

Presymptomatic gene mutation carriers
Testing of presymptomatic carriers of the HD gene mutation has become possible with the characterization of the CAG trinucleotide repeat mutation on chromosome 4 (Huntington's Disease Collaborative Research Group, 1993), prior studies having relied on linkage. Campodonico *et al.* (1996) found stability in neuropsychological tests over a 2-year period in asymptomatic carriers, with a suggestion that patients nearing clinical onset showed deficits in sustained attention and mental processing speed. A larger study found that whereas some carriers were cognitively no different from controls, others had poorer performance on learning and memory tests, significantly associated with CAG repeat length, suggesting that cognitive deficits may be an early, subclinical, manifestation of disease (Hahn-Barma *et al.*, 1998). These preclinical deficits were suggested to be highly specific by Lawrence *et al.* (1998) for attentional set shifting and semantic verbal fluency, reflecting impaired striatofrontal mechanisms. In another study, carriers performed worse on digit symbol, picture arrangement and arithmetic tests and also showed mild impairment on reaction time tasks (Kirkwood *et al.*, 2000). A prospective study of genetically defined disease carriers found impairments in attentional, visuoperceptual, and executive functions compared to controls (Lemiere *et al.*, 2004). Clearly these observations of presymptomatic carriers have implications for preventative therapeutic strategies and monitoring of efficacy of therapeutic measures. Nonetheless, despite these findings, it remains the case that in clinical practice HD almost invariably presents as a consequence of movement disorder rather than because of cognitive decline (Larner, 2008).

REFERENCES

Albert ML, Feldman RG, Willis AL. The 'subcortical dementia' of progressive supranuclear palsy. *J Neurol Neurosurg Psychiatry* 1974; **37**: 121–30.

Brandt J, Folstein SE, Folstein MF. Differential cognitive impairment in Alzheimer's disease and Huntington's disease. *Ann Neurol* 1988; **23**: 555–61.

Brouwers P, Cox C, Martin A, Chase T, Fedio P. Differential perceptual–spatial impairment in Huntington's and Alzheimer's dementia. *Arch Neurol* 1984; **41**: 1073–6.

Butters N, Wolfe J, Granholm E, Martone M. An assessment of verbal recall, recognition, and fluency abilities in patients with Huntington's disease. *Cortex* 1986; **22**: 11–32.

Campodonico JR, Codori AM, Brandt J. Neuropsychological stability over two years in asymptomatic carriers of the Huntington's disease mutation. *J Neurol Neurosurg Psychiatry* 1996; **61**: 621–4.

Craufurd D, Snowden JS. Neuropsychological and neuropsychiatric aspects of Huntington's disease. In: Bates G, Harper PS, Jones L (eds.), *Huntington's Disease* (3rd edition). Oxford: Oxford University Press, 2003: 62–94.

Hahn-Barma V, Deweer B, Dürr A, *et al.* Are cognitive changes the first symptoms of Huntington's disease? A study of gene carriers. *J Neurol Neurosurg Psychiatry* 1998; **64**: 172–7.

Hamilton JM, Haaland KY, Adair JC, Brandt J. Ideomotor limb apraxia in Huntington's disease: implications for corticostriate involvement. *Neuropsychologia* 2003; **41**: 614–21.

Ho AK, Sahakian BJ, Brown RG, *et al.* Profile of cognitive progression in early Huntington's disease. *Neurology* 2003; **61**: 1702–6.

Hodges JR, Salmon DP, Butters N. Differential impairment of semantic and episodic memory in Alzheimer's and Huntington's diseases: a controlled prospective study. *J Neurol Neurosurg Psychiatry* 1990; **53**: 1089–95.

Hodges JR, Salmon DP, Butters N. The nature of the naming deficit in Alzheimer's and Huntington's disease. *Brain* 1991; **114**: 1547–58.

Huntington G. On chorea. *Med Surg Rep* 1872; **26**: 317–21.

Huntington's Disease Collaborative Research Group. A novel gene containing a trinucleotide repeat that is expanded and unstable on Huntington's disease chromosomes. *Cell* 1993; **72**: 971–83.

Huntington's Study Group. Unified Huntington's Disease Rating Scale: reliability and consistency. *Mov Disord* 1996; **11**: 136–42.

Kirkwood SC, Siemers E, Hodes ME, *et al.* Subtle changes among presymptomatic carriers of the Huntington's disease gene. *J Neurol Neurosurg Psychiatry* 2000; **69**: 773–9.

Kosinski CM, Landwehrmeyer B. Huntington's disease. In: Beal MF, Lang AE, Ludolph A (eds.), *Neurodegenerative Diseases: Neurobiology, Pathogenesis and Therapeutics*. Cambridge: Cambridge University Press, 2005: 847–60.

Larner AJ. Monogenic Mendelian disorders in general neurological practice. *Int J Clin Pract* 2008; **62**: in press.

Lawrence AD, Hodges JR, Rosser AE, *et al.* Evidence for specific cognitive deficits in preclinical Huntington's disease. *Brain* 1998; **121**: 1329–41.

Lawrence AD, Sahakian BJ, Hodges JR, *et al.* Executive and mnemonic functions in early Huntington's disease. *Brain* 1996; **119**: 1633–45.

Lawrence AD, Watkins LH, Sahakian BJ, *et al.* Visual object and visuospatial cognition in Huntington's disease: implications for information processing in corticostriatal circuits. *Brain* 2000; **123**: 1349–64.

Lemiere J, Decruyenaere M, Evers-Kiebooms G, Vandenbussche E, Dom R. Cognitive changes in patients with Huntington's disease (HD) and asymptomatic carriers of the HD mutation: a longitudinal follow-up study. *J Neurol* 2004; **251**: 935–42.

McHugh PR, Folstein MF. Psychiatric symptoms of Huntington's chorea: a clinical and phenomenological study. In: Benson DF, Blumer D (eds.), *Psychiatric Aspects of Neurological Disease*. New York: Raven Press, 1975: 267–85.

Massman PJ, Delis DC, Butters N, Levin BE, Salmon DP. Are all subcortical dementias alike? Verbal learning and memory in Parkinson's and Huntington's disease patients. *J Clin Exp Neuropsychol* 1990; **12**: 729–44.

Paulsen JS, Conybeare RA. Cognitive changes in Huntington's disease. *Adv Neurol* 2005; **96**: 209–25.

Peinemann A, Schuller S, Pohl C, *et al.* Executive dysfunction in early stages of Huntington's disease is associated with striatal and insular atrophy: a neuropsychological and voxel-based morphometric study. *J Neurol Sci* 2005; **239**: 11–19.

Randolph C, Braun AR, Goldberg TE, Chase T. Semantic fluency in Alzheimer's, Parkinson's, Huntington's disease: dissociation of storage and retrieval failures. *Neuropsychology* 1993; **7**: 82–8.

Rohrer D, Salmon DP, Wixted JT, Paulsen JS. The disparate effects of Alzheimer's disease and Huntington's disease on semantic memory. *Neuropsychology* 1999; **13**: 381–8.

Rosenblatt A, Ranen NG, Rubinsztein DG, *et al.* Patients with features similar to Huntington's disease, without CAG expansion in huntingtin. *Neurology* 1998; **51**: 215–20.

Rosser AE, Hodges JR. The Dementia Rating Scale in Alzheimer's disease, Huntington's disease and progressive supranuclear palsy. *J Neurol* 1994a; **241**: 531–6.

Rosser AE, Hodges JR. Initial letter and semantic category fluency in Alzheimer's disease, Huntington's disease and progressive supranuclear palsy. *J Neurol Neurosurg Psychiatry* 1994b; **57**: 1389–94.

Shelton PA, Knopman DS. Ideomotor apraxia in Huntington's disease. *Arch Neurol* 1991; **48**: 35–41.

Snowden J, Craufurd D, Griffiths H, Thompson J, Neary D. Longitudinal evaluation of cognitive disorder in Huntington's disease. *J Int Neuropsychol Soc* 2001; **7**: 33–44.

Speedie LJ, Brake N, Folstein SE, Bowers D, Heilman KM. Comprehension of prosody in Huntington's disease. *J Neurol Neurosurg Psychiatry* 1990; **53**: 607–10.

Stevanin G, Fujigasaki H, Lebre AS, *et al.* Huntington's disease like phenotype due to trinucleotide repeat expansions in the TBP and JPH3 genes. *Brain* 2003; **126**: 1599–603.

Vonsattel JPG, Lianski M. Huntington's disease. In: Esiri MM, Lee VMY, Trojanowski JQ (eds.), *The Neuropathology of Dementia* (2nd edition). Cambridge: Cambridge University Press, 2004: 376–401.

Zakzanis KK. The subcortical dementia of Huntington's disease. *J Clin Exp Neuropsychol* 1998; **20**: 565–78.

5.1.2 Dentatorubropallidoluysian atrophy (DRPLA)

This autosomal dominant trinucleotide repeat disorder due to a CAG (polyglutamine) expansion in the gene encoding atrophin-1 on chromosome 12p13.31 often has a clinical presentation identical to Huntington's disease, with movement disorders including chorea, dystonia, myoclonus, and parkinsonism, as well as cerebellar ataxia, psychosis, and epilepsy; the latter may be commoner than in HD. Likewise, cognitive dysfunction similar to that in HD is seen, including slowed thinking, difficulty retrieving information and in sequencing tasks, progressing to a more severe dementia (Ross *et al.*, 2005), in other words a subcortical pattern of deficits. Chiefly described in reports from Japan, DRPLA has also been seen in European and North American families, in which clinical features are noted to be diverse even within individual families (Warner *et al.*, 1995).

REFERENCES

Ross CA, Ellerby LM, Wood JD, Nucifora FC Jr. Dentatorubral-pallidoluysian atrophy (DRPLA): model for Huntington's disease and other polyglutamine diseases. In: Beal MF, Lang AE, Ludolph A (eds.), *Neurodegenerative Diseases: Neurobiology, Pathogenesis and Therapeutics.* Cambridge: Cambridge University Press, 2005: 861–70.

Warner TT, Williams LD, Walker RW, *et al.* A clinical and molecular genetic study of dentatorubropallidoluysian atrophy in four European families. *Ann Neurol* 1995; **37**: 452–9.

5.1.3 Familial British dementia (FBD)

Familial British dementia, previously known as Worster-Drought syndrome, is an autosomal dominant progressive dementia syndrome with associated cerebellar ataxia and spastic paraparesis with pathological evidence of deposition of cerebrovascular amyloid distinct from that observed in Alzheimer's disease (Worster-Drought *et al.*, 1933; Plant *et al.*, 2004). It results from a mutation in the *BRI* gene on the long arm of chromosome 13, in which substitution in a stop codon increases the open reading frame, resulting in the production of an amyloidogenic C-terminal peptide, A-Bri (Vidal *et al.*, 1999). This condition is sometimes classified with the cerebral amyloid angiopathies (see Section 3.6.3).

Memory impairment early in the course of the disease is marked, ultimately progressing to global dementia. Personality change, either irritability or depression, may also be an early manifestation (Plant *et al.*, 2004). In a study of patients at risk, cognitive problems were identified in some patients thought to be affected clinically (with limb/gait ataxia, mild spastic paraparesis). Impairment of delayed recognition and, particularly, recall memory was found, with additional impairments in delayed visual recall in some patients. General intelligence, naming, frontal lobe functions, and perception were preserved. These changes were associated with deep white matter hyperintensities and lacunar infarcts on MR brain imaging (Mead *et al.*, 2000).

REFERENCES

Mead S, James-Galton M, Revesz T, *et al.* Familial British dementia with amyloid angiopathy: early clinical, neuropsychological and imaging findings. *Brain* 2000; **123**: 975–91.

Plant GT, Ghiso J, Holton JL, Frangione B, Revesz T. Familial and sporadic cerebral amyloid angiopathies associated with dementia and the BRI dementias. In: Esiri MM, Lee VMY, Trojanowski JQ (eds.), *The Neuropathology of Dementia* (2nd edition). Cambridge: Cambridge University Press, 2004: 330–52.

Vidal R, Frangione B, Rostagno A, *et al.* A stop-codon mutation in the *BRI* gene associated with familial British dementia. *Nature* 1999; **399**: 776–81.

Worster-Drought C, Hill TR, McMenemey WH. Familial presenile dementia with spastic paralysis. *J Neurol Psychopathol* 1933; **14**: 27–34.

5.1.4 Familial Danish dementia (FDD)

Originally known as heredopathia ophthalmo-oto-encephalica, this autosomal dominant disorder is characterized by cataracts and ocular haemorrhages around the age of 30 years, impaired hearing and hearing loss in the 40s or 50s, cerebellar ataxia in the 40s, and paranoid psychosis and dementia in the 50s. Once the neurological disease is established, clinical manifestations are similar to those of familial British dementia (Plant *et al.*, 2004). It results from mutation of the *BRI* gene with a 10-nucleotide duplication resulting in an out-of-frame stop codon giving rise to an extended precursor protein with an amyloidogenic C-peptide,

A-Dan (Vidal *et al.*, 2000), which is found in the amyloid deposits in the brain (Holton *et al.*, 2002). Like FBD, it may be classified with the cerebral amyloid angiopathies (Section 3.6.3). Detailed accounts of the neuropsychological profile in this condition have not been identified.

REFERENCES

Holton JL, Lashley T, Ghiso J, *et al.* Familial Danish dementia: a novel form of cerebral amyloidosis associated with deposition of both amyloid-Dan and amyloid-*β*. *J Neuropathol Exp Neurol* 2002; **61**: 254–67.

Plant GT, Ghiso J, Holton JL, Frangione B, Revesz T. Familial and sporadic cerebral amyloid angiopathies associated with dementia and the BRI dementias. In: Esiri MM, Lee VMY, Trojanowski JQ (eds.), *The Neuropathology of Dementia* (2nd edition). Cambridge: Cambridge University Press, 2004: 330–52.

Vidal R, Revesz T, Rostagno A, *et al.* A decamer duplication in the 3′ region of the BRI gene originates an amyloid peptide that is associated with dementia in a Danish kindred. *Proc Natl Acad Sci USA* 2000; **97**: 4920–5.

5.1.5   Familial encephalopathy with neuroserpin inclusion bodies (FENIB)

This rare autosomal dominant disorder is one of the serpinopathies linked to a point mutation in the gene on chromosome 3 encoding neuroserpin, a serine proteinase inhibitor, the mutant protein undergoing polymerization. FENIB is characterized pathologically by cytoplasmic neuroserpin inclusions (Collins bodies) within the deep cortical layers, substantia nigra, and subcortical nuclei. Clinical phenotype is determined by genotype: neuroserpin mutations causing greater conformational change (G392E) cause early-onset progressive myoclonus epilepsy, whereas lesser degrees of conformational change (S49P) cause dementia in the fifth decade (Davis *et al.*, 1999, 2002).

Neuropsychological assessment of patients with the S49P mutation in the neuroserpin gene showed frontal or frontal-subcortical impairment in mildly to moderately affected individuals, with impaired attention, concentration, and response regulation functions, whilst recall memory was not as affected as other cognitive domains. A more global pattern of impairment was seen in more severely affected individuals. This pattern was corroborated by SPECT imaging studies which showed exclusively frontal anomalies in the less affected patients, with more global but patchy hypoperfusion in those more severely affected (Bradshaw *et al.*, 2001).

REFERENCES

Bradshaw CB, Davis RL, Shrimpton AE, *et al.* Cognitive deficits associated with a recently reported familial neurodegenerative disease: familial encephalopathy with neuroserpin inclusion bodies. *Arch Neurol* 2001; **58**: 1429–34.

Davis RL, Shrimpton AE, Carrell RW, *et al.* Association between conformational mutations in neuroserpin and onset and severity of dementia. *Lancet* 2002; **359**: 2242–7.

Davis RL, Shrimpton AE, Holohan PD, *et al.* Familial dementia caused by polymerization of mutant neuroserpin. *Nature* 1999; **401**: 376–9.

5.1.6   Polycystic lipomembranous osteodysplasia with sclerosing leukoencephalopathy (PLOSL), Nasu–Hakola disease, presenile dementia with bone cysts

This autosomal recessive disorder, described in both Japan and Finland, is characterized by large-scale destruction of cancellous bone resulting in bone cysts in the third decade of life, causing pain, swelling, and sometimes fracture of the wrists and ankles; and presenile dementia in the fourth decade, sometimes with epileptic seizures. MR brain imaging reveals frontal myelin loss and massive gliosis ('sclerosing leukoencephalopathy') as well as basal ganglia calcification. The condition is genetically heterogeneous, with mutations being identified in the *DAP12* gene on chromosome 19q13.1

(deletions, point mutations, and single-base deletions) in some families (Paloneva *et al.*, 2001; Kondo *et al.*, 2002), and in the *TREM2* gene (Klünemann *et al.*, 2005), both encoding different subunits of a multisubunit receptor complex, resulting in an identical phenotype (Bianchin *et al.*, 2004).

The cognitive impairment may be of frontal lobe type, sometimes without preceding osseous symptoms (Paloneva *et al.*, 2001). Healthy subjects heterozygous for a *TREM2* mutation have been reported with a deficit of visuospatial memory, with basal ganglia hypoperfusion on functional neuroimaging (SPECT), not seen in homozygotes for the wild-type allele (Montalbetti *et al.*, 2005).

REFERENCES

Bianchin MM, Capella HM, Chaves DL, *et al.* Nasu–Hakola disease (polycystic lipomembranous osteodysplasia with sclerosing leukoencephalopathy – PLOSL): a dementia associated with bone cystic lesions. From clinical to genetic and molecular aspects. *Cell Mol Neurobiol* 2004; **24**: 1–24.

Klünemann HH, Ridha BH, Magy L, *et al.* The genetic causes of basal ganglia calcification, dementia, and bone cysts: DAP12 and TREM2. *Neurology* 2005; **64**: 1502–7.

Kondo T, Takahashi K, Kohara N, *et al.* Heterogeneity of presenile dementia with bone cysts (Nasu–Hakola disease): three genetic forms. *Neurology* 2002; **59**: 1105–7.

Montalbetti L, Ratti MT, Greco B, *et al.* Neuropsychological tests and functional nuclear neuroimaging provide evidence of subclinical impairment in Nasu–Hakola disease heterozygotes. *Funct Neurol* 2005; **20**: 71–5.

Paloneva J, Autti T, Raininko R, *et al.* CNS manifestations of Nasu–Hakola disease: a frontal dementia with bone cysts. *Neurology* 2001; **56**: 1552–8.

5.1.7 Fahr's syndrome (striatopallidal calcification)

This rubric encompasses a heterogeneous group of conditions, both familial and sporadic, variably characterized by calcification of the basal ganglia, dentate nucleus, and deeper cortical layers, which may be asymptomatic or associated with any combination of dementia, seizures, movement disorder (parkinsonism, dystonia, tremor, ataxia), with or without endocrine parathyroid disorder of calcium metabolism. The familial idiopathic syndrome seems to be often associated with intellectual decline, with impairment of recent memory and memory retention, as well as parkinsonism and cerebellar ataxia (Kobari *et al.*, 1997). Cases of Fahr's syndrome presenting with subacute dementia and without a movement disorder have been reported (Benke *et al.*, 2004; Modrego *et al.*, 2005), characterized in one case by executive deficits, anterograde amnesia, attentional impairment, and neuropsychiatric features, with the functional imaging correlate of reduced glucose metabolism in the basal ganglia and frontal lobes (Benke *et al.*, 2004). One wonders if there might be overlap here with polycystic lipomembranous osteodysplasia with sclerosing leukoencephalopathy (Nasu–Hakola disease), a condition characterized by presenile dementia with basal ganglia calcification.

REFERENCES

Benke T, Karner S, Seppi K, *et al.* Subacute dementia and imaging correlates in a case of Fahr's disease. *J Neurol Neurosurg Psychiatry* 2004; **75**: 1163–5.

Kobari M, Nogawa S, Sugimoto Y, Fukuuchi Y. Familial idiopathic brain calcification with autosomal dominant inheritance. *Neurology* 1997; **48**: 645–9.

Modrego PJ, Mojonero J, Serrano M, Fayed N. Fahr's syndrome presenting with pure and progressive presenile dementia. *Neurol Sci* 2005; **26**: 367–9.

5.1.8 Inclusion body myopathy associated with Paget's disease of bone and frontotemporal dementia (IBMPFD)

This rare autosomal dominant disorder maps to chromosome 9p21.1–p12 and results from mutations in the gene encoding valosin-containing protein (VCP), a member of the AAA-ATPase superfamily, which has many roles in cellular metabolism including the ubiquitin–proteasome pathway (Watts *et al.*, 2004; Haubenberger *et al.*, 2005; Kimonis & Watts, 2005; Schröder *et al.*, 2005). The clinical findings are heterogeneous, with 90% of cases having myopathy, 40% Paget's disease of bone, and 30% dementia of frontotemporal type. Intrafamilial heterogeneity has been noted. The neuropathology of the dementia is character- ized by the presence of neuronal inclusions con- taining both ubiquitin and VCP (Schröder *et al.*, 2005).

REFERENCES

Haubenberger D, Bittner RE, Rauch SS, *et al.* Inclusion body myopathy and Paget disease is linked to a novel mutation in the VCP gene. *Neurology* 2005; **65**: 1304–5.

Kimonis VE, Watts GDJ. Autosomal dominant inclusion body myopathy, Paget disease of bone, and frontotem- poral dementia. *Alzheimer Dis Assoc Disord* 2005; **19** (suppl 1): S44–7.

Schröder R, Watts GDJ, Mehta SG, *et al.* Mutant valosin- containing protein causes a novel type of frontotem- poral dementia. *Ann Neurol* 2005; **57**: 457–61.

Watts GDJ, Wymer J, Kovach MJ, *et al.* Inclusion body myopathy associated with Paget disease of bone and frontotemporal dementia is caused by mutant valosin- containing protein. *Nat Genet* 2004; **36**: 377–81.

5.1.9   Kufor–Rakeb syndrome (PARK9)

Unlike the clinically similar pallido-pyramidal syndrome (Davidson, 1954), dementia may be a feature of this very rare autosomal recessive nigrostriatal-pallido-pyramidal degeneration syn- drome linked to chromosome 1p36 (Al-Din *et al.*, 1994). Detailed description of the dementia was not given, but considering the topography of disease a frontal-subcortical pattern might be anticipated. The condition has been described as PARK9, resulting from mutations in a neuronal P-type ATPase gene, *ATP13A2*, whose product may be located in lysosomes (Ramirez *et al.*, 2006).

REFERENCES

Al-Din NAS, Wriekat A, Mubaidin A, Dasouki M, Hiari M. Pallido-pyramidal degeneration, supranuclear upgaze paresis and dementia: Kufor–Rakeb syndrome. *Acta Neurol Scand* 1994; **89**: 347–52.

Davidson C. Pallido-pyramidal disease. *J Neuropathol Exp Neurol* 1954; **13**: 50–9.

Ramirez A, Heimbach A, Gründemann J, *et al.* Hereditary parkinsonism with dementia is caused by mutations in ATP13A2, encoding a lysosomal type 5 P-type ATPase. *Nat Genet* 2006; **38**: 1184–91.

5.1.10   Urbach–Wiethe disease (lipoid proteinosis)

This rare autosomal recessive condition is charac- terized by bilateral calcification of the anterior medial temporal lobe, especially the amygdala, but with sparing of the hippocampus. It has permitted an analysis of the contribution of the amygdala to cognitive function. Clinical studies suggest impaired learning and recall of odour–figure asso- ciations but no amnesia as such (Markowitsch *et al.*, 1994), and also impairments in emotional judgment and memory (Siebert *et al.*, 2003). Amygdala damage may also contribute to the cognitive sequelae of herpes simplex encephalitis (Caparros-Lefebvre *et al.*, 1996).

REFERENCES

Caparros-Lefebvre D, Girard-Buttoz I, Reboul S, *et al.* Cognitive and psychiatric impairment in herpes simplex virus encephalitis suggest involvement of the amygdalo-frontal pathways. *J Neurol* 1996; **243**: 248–56.

Markowitsch HJ, Calabrese P, Würker M, *et al.* The amygdala's contribution to memory: a study on two patients with Urbach–Wiethe disease. *Neuroreport* 1994; **5**: 1349–52.

Siebert M, Markowitsch HJ, Bartel P. Amygdala, affect and cognition: evidence from 10 patients with Urbach– Wiethe disease. *Brain* 2003; **126**: 2627–37.

5.1.11 Fragile X syndrome (FRAX), fragile X tremor/ataxia syndrome (FXTAS)

Fragile X syndrome (FRAX) is the commonest genetically determined cause of intellectual disability in males (Davies, 1989), resulting from a trinucleotide (CGG) repeat expansion in the 5' promoter region of the *Fragile Site Mental Retardation 1* (*FMR1*) gene located on the X chromosome (Verkerk *et al.*, 1991). The mechanism by which the mutation causes mental retardation, and the normal function of *FMR1*, remain unknown. Healthy male patients with FRAX showed poorer attention and short-term memory function than a comparison group of Down's syndrome patients (Schapiro *et al.*, 1995). Women with FRAX are worse than controls on tests of executive function (Bennetto *et al.*, 2001).

Smaller numbers of repeats, 50–200, are termed premutations, and are associated with the fragile X tremor/ataxia syndrome (FXTAS). Clinically this is characterized by progressive cerebellar ataxia and tremor (this may be postural, action, or resting), with or without parkinsonism, peripheral neuropathy, and autonomic features, features which do not occur in FRAX and which have caused frequent misdiagnosis of the condition, for example as other tremor or ataxia syndromes (Hall *et al.*, 2005). MR brain imaging typically shows high-signal-intensity lesions on T_2-weighted images in the cerebellar peduncles and in white matter inferior and lateral to the deep cerebellar nuclei, with additional cerebellar and cortical atrophy (Brunberg *et al.*, 2002; Jacquemont *et al.*, 2003).

Cognitive impairment and dementia may also be a feature of FXTAS, specifically in the domains of short-term memory and executive function, impairments which are included in suggested diagnostic criteria (Jacquemont *et al.*, 2003). FXTAS has on occasion been misdiagnosed as a dementia syndrome of Alzheimer's or vascular type (Hall *et al.*, 2005). FXTAS has also been described in women: they are not demented (Hagerman *et al.*, 2004), but it has been suggested that some perform poorly on certain tests of visual selective attention (Steyaert *et al.*, 2003).

REFERENCES

Bennetto L, Pennington BF, Porter D, Taylor AK, Hagerman RJ. Profile of cognitive functioning in women with the fragile X mutation. *Neuropsychology* 2001; **15**: 290–9.

Brunberg JA, Jacquemont S, Hagerman RJ, *et al*. Fragile X premutation carriers: characteristic MR imaging findings of adult male patients with progressive cerebellar and cognitive dysfunction. *AJNR Am J Neuroradiol* 2002; **23**: 1757–66.

Davies KE (ed.). *The Fragile X Syndrome*. Oxford: Oxford University Press, 1989.

Hagerman RJ, Leavitt BR, Farzin F, *et al*. Fragile X-associated tremor/ataxia syndrome (FXTAS) in females with the FMR1 premutation. *Am J Hum Genet* 2004; **74**: 1051–6.

Hall DA, Berry KE, Jacquemont S, *et al*. Initial diagnoses given to persons with the fragile X associated tremor/ataxia syndrome (FXTAS). *Neurology* 2005; **65**: 299–301.

Jacquemont S, Hagerman RJ, Leehey M, *et al*. Fragile X premutation tremor/ataxia syndrome: molecular, clinical and neuroimaging correlates. *Am J Hum Genet* 2003; **72**: 869–78.

Schapiro MB, Murphy DG, Hagerman RJ, *et al*. Adult fragile X syndrome: neuropsychology, brain anatomy, and metabolism. *Am J Med Genet* 1995; **60**: 480–93.

Steyaert J, Legius E, Borghgraef M, Fryns JP. A distinct neurocognitive phenotype in female fragile-X premutation carriers assessed with visual attention tasks. *Am J Med Genet A* 2003; **116**: 44–51.

Verkerk AJ, Pieretti M, Sutcliffe JS, *et al*. Identification of a gene (FMR1) containing a CGG repeat coincident with a breakpoint cluster region exhibiting length variation in fragile X syndrome. *Cell* 1991; **65**: 905–14.

5.2 Hereditary ataxias

Classically the cerebellum has been viewed as a component of the motor system, with damage resulting in motor signs, first clearly defined by Gordon Holmes (1922), of localizing value (ataxia, dysdiadochokinesia, nystagmus). More recently, a role for the cerebellum in cognition has been increasingly acknowledged, with the description of a 'cerebellar cognitive affective syndrome', particularly in association with posterior lobe and vermis lesions, characterized by executive dysfunction (set-shifting, planning, verbal fluency, abstract reasoning, working memory), and difficulties with spatial cognition, memory, and language, as well as personality change (Schmahmann & Sherman, 1998).

In this section, hereditary ataxias are considered according to their pattern of inheritance, although a pathogenetic classification of the hereditary ataxias has been proposed (De Michele *et al.*, 2004). So-called idiopathic late-onset cerebellar ataxias, possibly with added cognitive problems, may in fact be caused by multiple system atrophy (MSA-C: see Section 2.4.4), fragile X tremor/ataxia syndrome (FXTAS: Section 5.1.11), or gluten ataxia with or without coeliac disease (Bürk *et al.*, 2001; Section 8.2.2).

REFERENCES

Bürk K, Bösch S, Müller CA, *et al.* Sporadic cerebellar ataxia associated with gluten sensitivity. *Brain* 2001; **124**: 1013–19.

De Michele G, Coppola G, Cocozza S, Filla A. A pathogenetic classification of hereditary ataxias: is the time ripe? *J Neurol* 2004; **251**: 913–22.

Holmes G. The Croonian lectures on the clinical symptoms of cerebellar disease and their interpretation. *Lancet* 1922; **i**: 1177–82; 1231–7; **ii**: 59–65; 111–15.

Schmahmann JD, Sherman JC. The cerebellar cognitive affective syndrome. *Brain* 1998; **121**: 561–79.

5.2.1   Autosomal dominant hereditary ataxias, spinocerebellar ataxias (SCA)

The phenotypic classification of autosomal dominant cerebellar ataxias (ADCA) proposed by Harding acknowledged the concurrence of dementia in some patients with these conditions, specifically in type I, whereas type II was characterized by having pigmentary maculopathy and type III a pure ataxia (Harding, 1984). This nosology has been superseded by a genotypic classification of the spinocerebellar ataxias (SCA) based on the discovery of gene loci and specific genetic

mutations responsible for some of these syndromes (Paulson, 2005). At time of writing at least 28 loci have been defined. SCAs are characterized by ataxia of gait and limb, ataxic dysarthria, spasticity, and decreased vibration perception, with additional parkinsonism, tremor, neuropathy, ophthalmoparesis, and seizures, with cognitive impairment in some cases. Marked cerebellar atrophy, sometimes with cerebral cortical atrophy, is seen on structural brain imaging. Variability of phenotype despite identical genetic mutation may occur. Several SCAs may fall within the old clinical classification of ADCA type I (i.e. with cognitive impairment) including SCAs 1–4, 12, and 17. Clues to the particular SCA may be obtained from the clinical examination: the presence of early and/or prominent dementia suggests that SCA2 or SCA17 may be the cause. A frontal lobe-like syndrome may occur in SCA1; dementia may be present in elderly patients with SCA12; and cognitive difficulties have been described in SCAs 6, 8, and 19.

Classification of the dominant hereditary ataxias also includes the episodic ataxias, channelopathies, and the prion disease Gerstmann–Straussler–Scheinker disease (GSS: see Section 2.5.3).

SCA1

Generally intellect remains intact until the late stages of disease in SCA1, associated with a CAG/polyQ mutation in the ataxin-1 gene at 6p22.3, when behavioural changes and a frontal lobe-like syndrome may occur. One study found impairments of verbal memory and executive dysfunction with relative preservation of visuospatial memory and attention, a pattern labelled typical of frontal-subcortical dementia (Bürk *et al.*, 2001). As for other SCAs, cognitive impairments were not related to age of onset, disease duration, or trinucleotide repeat length.

SCA2

Cognitive changes are prominent in SCA2, associated with a CAG/polyQ mutation in the ataxin-2 gene at 12q24.12. In one series, 25% of patients were demented, and the cognitive defects were also apparent in non-demented individuals (Bürk *et al.*, 1999). Impairments have been noted in frontal executive function, as measured by the Stroop Test, verbal fluency, and the Wisconsin Card Sorting Test, with visuospatial memory and attention spared; these changes may be found despite a normal MMSE (Bürk *et al.*, 1999; Storey *et al.*, 1999; Boesch *et al.*, 2000). Verbal memory function has been reported to be impaired in some cases but not in others. Cognitive impairments are not related to motor disability (Bürk *et al.*, 1999) or trinucleotide repeat size (Storey *et al.*, 1999). A correlation of deficits with disease duration has been reported in one series (Boesch *et al.*, 2000) but not in another (Storey *et al.*, 1999).

SCA3, Machado–Joseph disease (MJD)

This is probably the commonest dominantly inherited ataxia in the world, due to a CAG/polyQ mutation in the ataxin-3 gene at 14q32.12. In addition to ataxia, there is levodopa-responsive parkinsonism, and variable peripheral involvement, ophthalmoparesis, lingual and facial fasciculations. Cognitive impairments have also been described on occasion. Deficits in visual attentional function with slowed processing of visual information were reported using a computerized test battery, along with inability to shift attention to previously irrelevant stimuli; learning and visual memory were normal. A frontal-subcortical pattern of impairments was claimed, apparently independent of motor dysfunction (Maruff *et al.*, 1996). Abnormal behaviour, uncooperativeness, crying, slow thought processes, hallucinations, and delusions were reported in four Japanese patients (Ishikawa *et al.*, 2002).

SCA6

SCA6 results from CAG/polyQ mutation in the alpha1A voltage-dependent calcium channel (*CACNL1A4*) gene at chromosome 19p13.2, and is allelic with some cases of familial hemiplegic migraine and episodic ataxia type 2. This common SCA is generally a 'pure' cerebellar ataxia (hence originally classified as ADCA type III), but a case has been reported with slowly progressive mental disorders labelled as schizophrenia and dementia (Tashiro *et al.*, 1999).

SCA7

SCA7 results from CAG/polyQ mutation in the ataxin-7 gene at chromosome 3p14.1. The clinical phenotype is marked by progressive visual loss due to retinal dystrophy, and hence the condition was originally classified as ADCA type II. Dementia has been mentioned as a symptom in some cases (Walker & Farrell, 2006).

SCA8

Executive, visuospatial, and affective problems, with normal MMSE, have been described in addition to ataxia in a mother and son with SCA8 due to a combined CTA/CTG expansion on chromosome 13q2; the neuropsychological features, rather than ataxia, were the major clinical symptom (Stone *et al.*, 2001). Two of seven patients with SCA8 reported from Portugal were said to have mild to moderate memory impairment (Silveira *et al.*, 2000).

SCA12

Dementia has been reported in some patients in the later stages of SCA12, due to a CAG mutation in the *PPP2R2B* gene at 5q32. Disorientation, memory loss, inability to calculate, and perseveration were the clinical features (O'Hearn *et al.*, 2001).

SCA17

Cognitive decline and dementia, as well as extra-pyramidal features, are common in SCA17 (Rolfs *et al.*, 2003), due to a CAG/polyQ mutation in the TATA binding protein gene (*TBP* or *TFIID*) at chromosome 6q27, and behavioural disorder and dementia may dominate the early stages of the disease. A frontal picture, with distractibility, poor judgment, and impaired verbal fluency, has been reported (Bruni *et al.*, 2004).

SCA19

Cognitive difficulties are an occasional feature of this disorder, linked to 1p21–q21 (Verbeek *et al.*, 2002).

REFERENCES

Boesch SM, Globas C, Bürk K, Poewe W, Dichgans J. Cognitive deficits in spinocerebellar ataxia type 2 (SCA2): a comparative study in two founder populations. *Mov Disord* 2000; **15** (suppl 3): 235 (abstract P1092).

Bruni AC, Takahashi-Fujigasaki J, Maltecca F, *et al.* Behavioral disorder, dementia, ataxia, and rigidity in a large family with TATA Box-binding protein mutation. *Arch Neurol* 2004; **61**: 1314–20.

Bürk K, Bosch S, Globas C, *et al.* Executive dysfunction in spinocerebellar ataxia type 1. *Eur Neurol* 2001; **46**: 43–8.

Bürk K, Globas C, Bösch S, *et al.* Cognitive deficits in spinocerebellar ataxia 2. *Brain* 1999; **122**: 769–77.

Harding AE. *The Hereditary Ataxias and Related Disorders.* Edinburgh: Churchill Livingstone, 1984.

Ishikawa A, Yamada M, Makino K, *et al.* Dementia and delirium in 4 patients with Machado-Joseph disease. *Arch Neurol* 2002; **59**: 1804–8.

Maruff P, Tyler P, Burt T, *et al.* Cognitive deficits in Machado–Joseph disease. *Ann Neurol* 1996; **40**: 421–7.

O'Hearn E, Holmes SE, Calvert PC, Ross CA, Margolis RL. SCA-12: tremor with cerebellar and cortical atrophy is associated with a CAG repeat expansion. *Neurology* 2001; **56**: 299–303.

Paulson HL. Autosomal dominant cerebellar ataxia. In: Beal MF, Lang AE, Ludolph A (eds.), *Neurodegenerative Diseases: Neurobiology, Pathogenesis and Therapeutics.* Cambridge: Cambridge University Press, 2005: 709–18.

Rolfs A, Koeppen AH, Bauer I, *et al.* Clinical features and neuropathology of autosomal dominant spinocerebellar ataxia (SCA17). *Ann Neurol* 2003; **54**: 367–75.

Silveira I, Alonso I, Guimaraes L, *et al.* High germinal instability of the (CTG)n at the SCA8 locus of both expanded and normal alleles. *Am J Hum Genet* 2000; **66**: 830–40.

Stone J, Smith L, Watt K, Barron L, Zeman A. Incoordinated thought and emotion in spinocerebellar ataxia type 8. *J Neurol* 2001; **248**: 229–32.

Storey E, Forrest SM, Shaw JH, Mitchell P, McKinley Gardner RJ. Spinocerebellar ataxia type 2: clinical features of a pedigree displaying prominent frontal-executive dysfunction. *Arch Neurol* 1999; **56**: 43–50.

Tashiro H, Suzuki SO, Hitotsumatsu T, Iwaki T. An autopsy case of spinocerebellar ataxia type 6 with mental symptoms of schizophrenia and dementia. *Clin Neuropathol* 1999; **18**: 198–204.

Verbeek DS, Schelhaas JH, Ippel EF, *et al.* Identification of a novel locus (SCA19) in a Dutch autosomal dominant cerebellar ataxia family on chromosome region 1p21–q21. *Hum Genet* 2002; **111**: 388–93.

Walker M, Farrell D. Spinocerebellar ataxia type 7 (SCA7). *Pract Neurol* 2006; **6**: 44–7.

5.2.2   Autosomal recessive hereditary ataxias

Friedreich's ataxia (FA)

The most common autosomal recessive cause of ataxia, Friedreich's ataxia (FA) is characterized by ataxia, dysarthria, axonal polyneuropathy and pyramidal weakness of the legs (absent ankle jerks and upgoing plantars), optic atrophy, scoliosis, and cardiac conduction abnormalities, usually with onset before the age of 20 years. Intronic trinucleotide repeat expansions in the frataxin gene on chromosome 9q13 resulting in disordered mitochondrial function are the cause of FA. The clinical phenotype has broadened as a result of the discovery of the causative genetic mutations (Dürr, 2002; Puccio & Koenig, 2005).

Any assessment of neuropsychological function in FA must take account of possible confounders such as dysarthria and fatigue, and any educational shortcomings engendered by physical disability. Nonetheless, studies suggest that FA is attended by cognitive impairments, such as lengthened mental reaction times and colour–word interference in the Stroop task. One group found no impairment in tests sensitive to neocortical (particularly prefrontal cortex) function, including verbal fluency, Wisconsin Card Sorting, Tower of Hanoi, and picture arrangement (White *et al.*, 2000), whereas another group found deficits in letter fluency, as well as impaired acquisition and consolidation of verbal information and alterations in visuoperceptual and visuoconstructive abilities (Wollmann *et al.*, 2002). All agree that cerebellar degeneration and interruption of cerebellar afferent and efferent connections is probably responsible for these findings.

Ataxia telangiectasia (AT)

This childhood-onset autosomal recessive syndrome is characterized by progressive ataxia, oculomotor apraxia requiring head thrusts to achieve ocular fixation, dysarthria, telangiectasia, and a tendency to develop recurrent infections (especially sinopulmonary) and malignancies. The molecular defect is in the *ATM* gene on chromosome 11, which encodes a protein required for DNA repair (Spacey *et al.*, 2000; Gatti *et al.*, 2005). Cognitive status is said to be normal in most cases, some patients completing university-level education, and significant neuropsychological impairments have been said to be uncommon. However, Colvin and Lennox (1997) reported frontal lobe dysfunction in a series of 18 AT patients as assessed with Wisconsin Card Sorting Test, Tower of London Test, verbal fluency, and similarities. Impairments of visual memory assessed with the Warrington Recognition Memory Test, and failure on some elements of the VOSP, were attributed to impaired oculomotor function.

Autosomal recessive spastic ataxia of Charlevoix–Saguenay (ARSACS)

This autosomal recessive disorder of childhood, initially reported from northeastern Quebec, Canada, is characterized by childhood onset of a slowly progressive pyramidal syndrome, dysarthria, ataxia, abnormal eye movements (nystagmus), retinal striation (= hypermyelinated retinal fibres), sphincter involvement, mitral incompetence, and motor neuropathy. It may be classified as a 'complicated' hereditary spastic paraparesis, or as an early-onset autosomal recessive cerebellar ataxia with retained reflexes. Pedigrees from Quebec and Tunisia showed linkage to chromosome 13q11–12 (Mrissa *et al.*, 2000), whence positional cloning techniques permitted characterization of the sacsin gene (Engert *et al.*, 2000). Many sacsin gene mutations have now been reported from pedigrees throughout the world, expanding the spectrum of sacsinopathies (Gomez, 2004). Two siblings reported from Japan had a unique phenotype of dementia, ophthalmoplegia, and absence of prominent retinal myelinated fibres (Hara *et al.*, 2005).

Ataxia with vitamin E deficiency (AVED)

This autosomal recessive disorder manifests as spinocerebellar ataxia and polyneuropathy without evidence of cognitive impairment, suggesting that vitamin E is not crucial to cognitive function.

REFERENCES

Colvin IB, Lennox GG. Cognitive function in ataxia telangiectasia. *J Neurol Neurosurg Psychiatry* 1997; **62**: 210 (abstract).

Dürr A. Friedreich's ataxia: treatment within reach. *Lancet Neurol* 2002; **1**: 370–4.

Engert JC, Berube P, Mercier J, *et al.* ARSACS, a spastic ataxia common in northeastern Quebec, is caused by mutations in a new gene encoding an 11.5-kb ORF. *Nat Genet* 2000; **24**: 120–5.

Gatti RA, Crawford TO, Mandir AS, Perlman S, Mount HTJ. Ataxia telangiectasia. In: Beal MF, Lang AE, Ludolph A (eds.), *Neurodegenerative Diseases: Neurobiology, Pathogenesis and Therapeutics*. Cambridge: Cambridge University Press, 2005: 738–48.

Gomez CM. ARSACS goes global. *Neurology* 2004; **62**: 10–11.

Hara K, Onodera O, Endo M, *et al.* Sacsin-related autosomal recessive ataxia without prominent retinal myelinated fibers in Japan. *Mov Disord* 2005; **20**: 380–2.

Mrissa N, Belal S, Ben Hamida M, *et al.* Linkage to chromosome 13q11-12 of an autosomal recessive cerebellar ataxia in a Tunisian family. *Neurology* 2000; **54**: 1408–14.

Puccio H, Koenig M. Friedreich's ataxia and other autosomal recessive ataxias. In: Beal MF, Lang AE, Ludolph A (eds.). *Neurodegenerative Diseases: Neurobiology, Pathogenesis and Therapeutics.* Cambridge: Cambridge University Press, 2005: 719–37.

Spacey SD, Gatti RA, Bebb G. The molecular basis and clinical management of ataxia telangiectasia. *Can J Neurol Sci* 2000; **27**: 184–91.

White M, Lalonde R, Botez-Marquard T. Neuropsychologic and neuropsychiatric characteristics of patients with Friedreich's ataxia. *Acta Neurol Scand* 2000; **102**: 222–6.

Wollmann T, Barroso J, Monton F, Nieto A. Neuropsychological test performance of patients with Friedreich's ataxia. *J Clin Exp Neuropsychol* 2002; **24**: 677–86.

5.3   Hereditary spastic paraplegia

The hereditary spastic paraplegias (HSP) are a heterogeneous group of inherited motor system disorders, typically presenting with lower limb spasticity and, to a lesser extent, weakness. Clinically, HSP may be divided into pure (uncomplicated) and complicated types, the latter manifesting other neurological features in addition to spasticity, such as seizures, amyotrophy, extrapyramidal signs, peripheral neuropathy, and cognitive impairment, sometimes amounting to dementia. Subtle cognitive deficits have also been detected in so-called 'pure' HSP types. To date around 20 genetic loci linked to HSP have been described, with dominant, recessive, and X-linked inheritance, and deterministic mutations have been described in at least 10 genes, encoding the proteins L1-CAM, proteolipid protein (PLP), atlastin, spastin, paraplegin, spartin, maspardin, hsp60, KIF5A, and NIPA1 (McDermott & Shaw, 2002; Fink, 2003). Cognitive impairment has been noted in both autosomal dominant (Webb & Hutchinson, 1998) and autosomal recessive HSP (Ferrer *et al.*, 1995).

Spastic paraparesis may be a feature of other monogenic Mendelian disorders which may also be associated with cognitive impairment, such as autosomal dominant Alzheimer's disease (see Section 2.1) associated with certain of the presenilin-1 mutations (Larner & Doran, 2006), some of the hereditary cerebral amyloid angiopathies (Section 3.6.3), and autosomal recessive spastic ataxia of Charlevoix–Saguenay (ARSACS: Section 5.2.2). Spastic paraparesis has also been reported in Krabbe disease (Section 5.5.2).

REFERENCES

Ferrer I, Olivé M, Rivera R, *et al.* Hereditary spastic paraparesis with dementia, amyotrophy and peripheral neuropathy: a neuropathological study. *Neuropathol Appl Neurobiol* 1995; **21**: 255–61.

Fink JK. The hereditary spastic paraplegias: nine genes and counting. *Arch Neurol* 2003; **60**: 1045–9.

Larner AJ, Doran M. Clinical phenotypic heterogeneity of Alzheimer's disease associated with mutations of the presenilin-1 gene. *J Neurol* 2006; **253**: 139–58.

McDermott CJ, Shaw PJ. Hereditary spastic paraplegia. *Int Rev Neurobiol* 2002; **53**: 191–204.

Webb S, Hutchinson M. Cognitive impairment in families with pure autosomal dominant hereditary spastic paraparesis. *Brain* 1998; **121**: 923–9.

5.3.1   SPG4

The commonest form of autosomal dominant HSP is that linked to the SPG4 locus on chromosome 2p where the gene that encodes spastin is found. Although classified as a pure form of HSP, cognitive deficits have been noted in patients, sometimes amounting to a global dementia with a profile similar to that in subcortical dementias (Webb *et al.*, 1998). Mild cognitive problems may be the first clinical manifestation in carriers of spastin gene mutations. Studies in Irish families reported cognitive decline affecting orientation, memory, and language that was age-dependent (Byrne *et al.*, 2000) and progressive over time (McMonagle *et al.*, 2004), whereas French studies found that cognitive decline was correlated with disease progression and not with age (Tallaksen *et al.*, 2003). These researchers found only mild, asymptomatic, cognitive loss, particularly affecting executive functions, more frequently observed in patients with missense rather than truncating spastin mutations. A report of a large series of patients with spastin mutations made no mention of any cognitive impairments (McDermott *et al.*, 2006).

REFERENCES

Byrne P, McMonagle P, Webb S, *et al.* Age-related cognitive decline in hereditary spastic paraparesis linked to chromosome 2p. *Neurology* 2000; **54**: 1510–17.

McDermott CJ, Burness CE, Kirby J, *et al.* Clinical features of hereditary spastic paraplegia due to spastin mutation. *Neurology* 2006; **67**: 45–51.

McMonagle P, Byrne P, Hutchinson M. Further evidence of dementia in SPG4-linked autosomal dominant hereditary spastic paraplegia. *Neurology* 2004; **62**: 407–10.

Tallaksen CME, Guichart-Gomez E, Verpillat P, *et al.* Subtle cognitive impairment but no dementia in patients with spastin mutations. *Arch Neurol* 2003; **60**: 1113–18.

Webb S, Coleman D, Byrne P, *et al.* Autosomal dominant hereditary spastic paraparesis with cognitive loss linked to chromosome 2p. *Brain* 1998; **121**: 601–9.

5.3.2 SPG21, mast syndrome

Mast syndrome is an autosomal recessive, complicated, form of HSP with a clinical phenotype of onset in the second decade with paraplegia, dysarthria, athetosis, and dementia. It was originally described in the Old Order Amish community (Cross & McKusick, 1967), but possible non-Amish cases have been reported with bradyphrenia and comprehension difficulties in their 40s, progressing to rare, inappropriate, single-syllable answers in the 50s (D'Hooge, 1992). It is slowly progressive, with cerebellar and extrapyramidal features emerging in advanced disease. It maps to chromosome 15q22.31 and frameshift mutations have been identified in a gene that encodes a protein product named maspardin (Simpson *et al.*, 2003).

REFERENCES

Cross HE, McKusick VA. The mast syndrome: a recessively inherited form of presenile dementia with motor disturbances. *Arch Neurol* 1967; **16**: 1–13.

D'Hooge M. Probable cases of mast syndrome in a non-Amish family. *J Neurol Neurosurg Psychiatry* 1992; **55**: 1210.

Simpson MA, Cross H, Proukakis C, *et al.* Maspardin is mutated in mast syndrome, a complicated form of hereditary spastic paraplegia associated with dementia. *Am J Hum Genet* 2003; **73**: 1147–56.

5.4 Hereditary movement disorders

5.4.1 Wilson's disease (hepatolenticular degeneration)

Wilson's disease is an autosomal recessive disorder of copper metabolism resulting from mutations in the gene *ATP7B*, encoding a copper-binding membrane-bound ATPase, resulting in elevated blood and urine copper and reduced blood caeruloplasmin levels. The condition usually presents in young adults with hepatic and/or neurological disease due to accumulation of copper in affected tissues. In the brain, although copper deposition occurs throughout, it is the basal ganglia which are particularly vulnerable, resulting in movement disorders (parkinsonism, dystonia, grimacing, excessive salivation); likewise the cerebellum (ataxia, wing-beating tremor, dysarthria). Copper deposition in Descemet's membrane may be observed as Kayser–Fleischer rings, a reliable sign of brain copper deposition (LeWitt & Brewer, 2005). Neuropsychiatric features are also common, such as personality change, depression, and occasionally psychosis (Brewer, 2005). Motor and neuropsychiatric features might possibly confound neuropsychological testing in Wilson's disease.

In his seminal paper on the disorder that now bears his name, Kinnier Wilson (1912) noted a distinct pattern of neurobehavioural disturbances without agnosia, apraxia, or severe memory loss in association with disease of the basal ganglia. The cognitive impairments in patients with neurological and/or hepatic symptoms may be mild (Rathbun, 1996), or involvement may be widespread, including impaired memory, visuo-spatial processing, and frontal-executive function (Medalia *et al.*, 1988; Seniów *et al.*, 2002). Rate of information processing may be spared, although response latencies are prolonged, probably as a consequence of the motor disorder (Littman *et al.*, 1995). Neuropsychological deficits may be present early in the course of the disease (Goldstein *et al.*, 1968), but patients with exclusive hepatic involvement do not differ from controls and adequate early treatment may prevent cognitive decline (Lang *et al.*, 1990). If untreated, dementia develops with disease progression, hence the need to screen all younger patients with movement disorders for abnormalities of copper metabolism. Once established, the dementia is generally held to be irreversible, although anecdotal reports of cognitive (as well as motor) improvement after chelation therapy (Rosselli *et al.*, 1987) and liver transplantation (Polson *et al.*, 1987, case 2) have appeared.

REFERENCES

Brewer GJ. Behavioral abnormalities in Wilson's disease. *Adv Neurol* 2005; **96**: 262–74.

Goldstein NP, Ewert JC, Randall RV, Gross JB. Psychiatric aspects of Wilson's disease (hepatolenticular degeneration): results of psychometric tests during long-term therapy. *Am J Psychiatry* 1968; **124**: 1555–61.

Lang C, Müller D, Claus D, Druschky KF. Neuropsychological findings in treated Wilson's disease. *Acta Neurol Scand* 1990; **81**: 75–81.

LeWitt PA, Brewer GJ. Neurological aspects of Wilson's disease. In: Beal MF, Lang AE, Ludolph A (eds.), *Neurodegenerative Diseases: Neurobiology, Pathogenesis and Therapeutics*. Cambridge: Cambridge University Press, 2005: 890–908.

Littman E, Medalia A, Senior G, Scheinberg IH. Rate of information processing in patients with Wilson's disease. *J Neuropsychiatry Clin Neurosci* 1995; **7**: 68–71.

Medalia A, Isaacs Glaberman K, Scheinberg IH. Neuropsychological impairment in Wilson's disease. *Arch Neurol* 1988; **45**: 502–4.

Polson RJ, Rolles K, Calne RY, Williams R, Marsden D. Reversal of severe neurological manifestations of Wilson's disease following orthotopic liver transplantation. *Q J Med* 1987; **64**: 685–91.

Rathbun JK. Neuropsychological aspects of Wilson's disease. *Int J Neurosci* 1996; **85**: 221–9.

Rosselli M, Lorenzana P, Rosselli A, Vergara I. Wilson's disease, a reversible dementia: case report. *J Clin Exp Neuropsychol* 1987; **9**: 399–406.

Seniów J, Bak T, Gajda J, Poniatowska R, Czlonkowska A. Cognitive functioning in neurologically symptomatic and asymptomatic forms of Wilson's disease. *Mov Disord* 2002; **17**: 1077–83.

Wilson SAK. Progressive lenticular degeneration: a familial nervous disease associated with cirrhosis of the liver. *Brain* 1912; **34**: 295–509.

5.4.2 Neurodegeneration with brain accumulation of iron-1 (NBAI-1), Hallervorden–Spatz disease

Hallervorden and Spatz were the first to describe a familial syndrome, now known to be of autosomal recessive inheritance, of dysarthria and progressive dementia with brown discoloration of the globus pallidus and substantia nigra at postmortem. The name Hallervorden–Spatz disease was used for this condition (Halliday, 1995) but has fallen from favour because of Hallervorden's association with unethical practices during the Nazi era, the term neurodegeneration with brain accumulation of iron-1 (NBAI-1) now being used (Pearce, 2006).

A distinction was drawn between Hallervorden–Spatz disease and Hallervorden–Spatz syndrome (Halliday, 1995), the former being childhood cases of either familial or sporadic origin with a fairly homogeneous phenotype of dystonia, dysarthria, rigidity, choreoathetosis, pigmentary retinopathy, and, in about a quarter of cases, cognitive decline. Hallervorden–Spatz syndrome was used for 'atypical' cases, usually of later onset (second to third decade), with speech difficulty, with or without extra-pyramidal and pyramidal signs, and in some cases with cognitive decline said to be reminiscent of frontotemporal dementia, with personality change, impulsivity, violent outbursts, and emotional lability

(Halliday, 1995). Typical pathological findings are pallidal iron deposition, axonal spheroids, and gliosis. T_2-weighted MR brain scans show decreased signal intensity in the pallidal nuclei with central hyperintensity, the 'eye-of-the-tiger' sign, which is highly suggestive although not specific. Such imaging findings have permitted diagnosis of more cases and broadened the phenotype (Hickman *et al.*, 2001). Mutations in the gene encoding pantothenate kinase (*PANK2*) on chromosome 20p13 have been identified in NBAI-1 (Zhou *et al.*, 2001), in both classic cases and in around one-third of atypical late-onset cases (Hayflick *et al.*, 2003).

The neuropsychological profile is, as might be expected, of frontal-subcortical type, with bradyphrenia, reduced verbal fluency, judgment difficulties, and attentional impairment, but with relative preservation of memory. Phenotype may be variable, even in siblings sharing the same mutation (Marelli *et al.*, 2005).

REFERENCES

Halliday W. The nosology of Hallervorden–Spatz disease. *J Neurol Sci* 1995; **134** (suppl): 84–91.

Hayflick SJ, Westaway SK, Levinson B, *et al.* Genetic, clinical, and radiographic delineation of Hallervorden–Spatz syndrome. *N Engl J Med* 2003; **348**: 33–40.

Hickman SJ, Ward NS, Surtees RA, Stevens JM, Farmer SF. How broad is the phenotype of Hallervorden–Spatz disease? *Acta Neurol Scand* 2001; **103**: 201–3.

Marelli C, Piacentini S, Garavaglia B, Girotti F, Albanese A. Clinical and neuropsychological correlates in two brothers with pantothenate kinase-associated neurodegeneration. *Mov Disord* 2005; **20**: 208–12.

Pearce JMS. Neurodegeneration with brain iron accumulation: a cautionary tale. *Eur Neurol* 2006; **56**: 66–8.

Zhou B, Westaway SK, Levinson B, *et al.* A novel pantothenate kinase gene is defective in Hallervorden–Spatz syndrome. *Nature Genet* 2001; **28**: 345–9.

5.4.3 Neuroacanthocytosis

There are various neuroacanthocytosis syndromes (Danek, 2004), of which chorea-acanthocytosis is a multisystem neurodegenerative disorder inherited as an autosomal recessive condition linked to chromosome 9q21 and associated with mutations in the *VPS13A* gene, encoding the protein chorein. The clinical phenotype includes movement disorders (orofaciolingual dystonia, chorea, parkinsonism), axonal polyneuropathy, epileptic seizures, and neuropsychiatric abnormalities, as well as cognitive impairments. Salient investigation findings are acanthocytes on fresh blood films (more than one film may need to be examined) and raised creatine phosphokinase, but there is no abnormality of lipid metabolism (Hardie *et al.*, 1991; Danek *et al.*, 2005; Storch *et al.*, 2005).

Personality change, such as impulsive and distractible behaviour or apathy and loss of insight, may be observed. We have encountered a patient who was served with an Anti-Social Behaviour Order because of personality problems due to undiagnosed neuroacanthocytosis (Doran *et al.*, 2006). Consistent with this suggestion of frontal lobe dysfunction, tests of executive function may be impaired sufficient to amount to a subcortical dementia (Kartsounis & Hardie, 1996). Hence in both its clinical and neuropsychological features, neuroacanthocytosis may resemble Huntington's disease.

REFERENCES

Danek A (ed.). *Neuroacanthocytosis Syndromes.* Dordrecht: Springer, 2004.

Danek A, Jung HH, Melone MAB, *et al.* Neuroacanthocytosis: new developments in a neglected group of dementing disorders. *J Neurol Sci* 2005; **229–30**: 171–86.

Doran M, Harvie AK, Larner AJ. Antisocial behaviour orders: the need to consider underlying neuropsychiatric disease. *Int J Clin Pract* 2006; **60**: 861–2.

Hardie RJ, Pullon HW, Harding AE, *et al.* Neuroacanthocytosis: a clinical, haematological and pathological study of 19 cases. *Brain* 1991; **114**: 13–49.

Kartsounis LD, Hardie RJ. The pattern of cognitive impairments in neuroacanthocytosis. *Arch Neurol* 1996; **53**: 77–80.

Storch A, Kornhass M, Schwarz J. Testing for acanthocytosis: a prospective reader-blinded study in movement disorder patients. *J Neurol* 2005; **252**: 84–90.

5.4.4   Neuroferritinopathy

Mutations in the gene encoding ferritin light polypeptide (FLP) or ferritin light chain (FTL) have been associated with a variety of autosomal dominant movement disorders, including dystonia, chorea, and akinetic-rigid syndrome. The extrapyramidal features may resemble Huntington's disease or parkinsonism. There is a low serum ferritin with brain aggregates of ferritin and iron (Curtis *et al.*, 2001; Vidal *et al.*, 2004).

Although few pedigrees have been reported thus far, cognitive decline does seem to be associated with neuroferritinopathy, at least in some cases. In one case, frontal lobe function was particularly affected (perseveration, poor cognitive estimates, impaired non-verbal abstract reasoning, and some word-retrieval difficulties), although the patient had been treated with high-dose anticholinergic agents for the movement disorder before cognitive decline occurred (Wills *et al.*, 2002). In a French family, two of the seven members had a frontal syndrome and another was demented (Chinnery *et al.*, 2003), and in another family the index case had a frontal syndrome and dementia (Vidal *et al.*, 2004). The index case in a Portuguese family had non-progressive mental retardation with IQ of 60 (Maciel *et al.*, 2005). Overall, cognitive impairment seems to be absent or subtle in the early stages, unlike the situation in Huntington's disease, with subcortical-frontal dysfunction developing later (Chinnery *et al.*, 2007).

REFERENCES

Chinnery PF, Crompton DE, Birchall D, *et al.* Clinical features and natural history of neuroferritinopathy caused by the FTL1 460InsA mutation. *Brain* 2007; **130**: 110–19.

Chinnery P, Curtis A, Fey C, *et al.* Neuroferritinopathy in a French family with late onset dominant dystonia. *J Med Genet* 2003; **40**: e69.

Curtis AR, Fey C, Morris CM, *et al.* Mutation in the gene encoding ferritin light polypeptide causes dominant adult-onset basal ganglia disease. *Nat Genet* 2001; **28**: 350–4.

Maciel P, Cruz VT, Constante M, *et al.* Neuroferritinopathy: missense mutation in FTL causing early-onset bilateral pallidal involvement. *Neurology* 2005; **65**: 603–5.

Vidal R, Ghetti B, Takao M, *et al.* Intracellular ferritin accumulation in neural and extraneural tissue characterizes a neurodegenerative disease associated with a mutation in the *Ferritin Light Polypeptide* gene. *J Neuropath Exp Neurol* 2004; **63**: 363–80.

Wills AJ, Sawle GV, Guilbert PR, Curtis ARJ. Palatal tremor and cognitive decline in neuroferritinopathy. *J Neurol Neurosurg Psychiatry* 2002; **73**: 91–2.

5.4.5   Acaeruloplasminaemia

This autosomal recessive condition results from the absence of caeruloplasmin ferroxidase activity due to mutations in the caeruloplasmin gene, with subsequent effects on iron metabolism. There is low serum iron, raised ferritin, absent caeruloplasmin, and increased liver iron on biopsy, and although serum copper is low this is in proportion to reduced caeruloplasmin, as normal urine and liver copper indicate that there is no copper overload. Unlike the situation with haemochromatosis, neurological presentations are common in acaeruloplasminaemia, usually with a movement disorder (dystonia, chorea, ataxia), with imaging evidence of iron deposition in the brain, particularly the basal ganglia. A role for caeruloplasmin in brain iron metabolism is therefore likely (Harris *et al.*, 1996).

Occasional cases of dementia have been reported in association with acaeruloplasminaemia (Morita *et al.*, 1992; Logan *et al.*, 1994; Harris *et al.*, 1996). The limited information available on the pattern of cognitive impairment indicates defects in immediate and delayed recall of verbal material, inability to learn new verbal material, with preservation of long-term memory, at least initially. The findings were said to be 'similar to subcortical dementia' (Logan *et al.*, 1994; Harris *et al.*, 1996).

REFERENCES

Harris ZL, Migas MC, Hughes AE, Logan JI, Gitlin JD. Familial dementia due to a frameshift mutation in the caeruloplasmin gene. *Q J Med* 1996; **89**: 355–9.

Logan JI, Harveyson KB, Wisdom GB, Hughes AE, Archbold GPR. Hereditary caeruloplasmin deficiency, dementia and diabetes mellitus. *Q J Med* 1994; **87**: 663–70.

Morita H, Inoue A, Yanagisawa N. A case of caeruloplasmin deficiency which showed dementia, ataxia and iron deposition in the brain [in Japanese]. *Rinsho Shinkeigaku* 1992; **32**: 483–7.

5.4.6 Essential tremor (ET)

Classic hereditary essential tremor (ET), in which similarly affected family members are found in at least three generations, is typified by early onset, complete penetrance by age 65 years, invariable onset of tremor in the hands, and absence of rigidity, rest tremor, persistent unilateral tremor, and isolated head, tongue, voice, jaw, or leg tremor (Bain *et al.*, 1994). The role of genetic factors has been confirmed by the demonstration of linkage of ET to loci on chromosomes 3q and 2p. However, many cases clinically labelled as ET either lack a family history (non-familial or sporadic ET), suggesting that environmental factors may contribute to aetiology, or vary from the classical clinical phenotype (Louis, 2005). Such cases are sometimes labelled as 'possible ET' although other diagnoses need to be borne in mind, such as enhanced physiological tremor, early Parkinson's disease, or dystonic tremor (Schrag *et al.*, 2000).

Although ET is generally considered a monosymptomatic tremor disorder, administration of neuropsychological tests has revealed subclinical impairments in tests sensitive to frontal lobe function. One study noted impaired verbal fluency, naming, mental set-shifting, verbal memory, and working memory. Deficits did not correlate with tremor severity. Prefrontal cortical involvement, perhaps encompassing frontocerebellar circuits, was surmised (Lombardi *et al.*, 2001). Impairments in attentional and conceptual thinking tasks were noted in another study, akin to those seen in idiopathic Parkinson's disease (PD), prompting the suggestion that this frontal lobe dysfunction may reflect dysregulation of frontal-subcortical dopamine pathways (Gasparini *et al.*, 2001). Although ET and PD are clinically and genetically unrelated (Plumb & Bain, 2007), the occasional concurrence of familial ET and restless legs syndrome (Larner & Allen, 1997) may support the idea of dopaminergic dysfunction. Lacritz *et al.* (2002) found mild cognitive impairment in about half of a small cohort of ET patients being evaluated for tremor surgery (hence a highly selected group), with deficits identified in cognitive flexibility, figural fluency, and selective attention. Attentional problems were also identified in another study (Duane & Vermilion, 2002).

Although these studies have some shortcomings in terms of selection bias and, in some, lack of appropriate control data, nonetheless they do suggest cognitive impairments in ET, albeit mild, affecting frontal-subcortical or cerebellar-frontal circuitry.

REFERENCES

Bain PG, Findley LJ, Thompson PD, *et al.* A study of hereditary essential tremor. *Brain* 1994; **117**: 805–24.

Duane DD, Vermilion KJ. Cognitive deficits in patients with essential tremor. *Neurology* 2002; **58**: 1706.

Gasparini M, Bonifati V, Fabrizio E, *et al.* Frontal lobe dysfunction in essential tremor: a preliminary study. *J Neurol* 2001; **248**: 399–402.

Lacritz LH, Dewey R Jr, Giller C, Cullum CM. Cognitive functioning in individuals with benign essential tremor. *J Int Neuropsychol Soc* 2002; **8**: 125–9.

Larner AJ, Allen CMC. Hereditary essential tremor and restless legs syndrome. *Postgrad Med J* 1997; **73**: 254.

Lombardi WJ, Woolston DJ, Roberts JW, Gross RE. Cognitive deficits in patients with essential tremor. *Neurology* 2001; **57**: 785–90.

Louis ED. Essential tremor. *Lancet Neurol* 2005; **4**: 100–10.

Plumb M, Bain P. *Essential Tremor: the Facts.* Oxford: Oxford University Press, 2007.

Schrag A, Münchau A, Bhatia KP, Quinn NP, Marsden CD. Essential tremor: an overdiagnosed condition? *J Neurol* 2000; **247**: 955–9.

5.4.7 Restless legs syndrome (RLS)

The negative impact of restless legs syndrome (RLS) on sleep may also affect cognitive functions, particularly those thought to be mediated by prefrontal cortex (Pearson *et al.*, 2006), producing deficits similar to those seen with sleep deprivation (Durmer & Dinges, 2005). Possible associations of RLS with Parkinson's disease, essential tremor (Larner & Allen, 1997), and migraine (Larner, 2007) might also contribute to observed cognitive deficits (see Sections 2.4, 5.4.6, and 3.7.2, respectively).

REFERENCES

Durmer JS, Dinges DF. Neurocognitive consequences of sleep deprivation. *Semin Neurol* 2005; **25**: 117–29.

Larner AJ. Migraine with aura and restless legs syndrome. *J Headache Pain* 2007; **8**: 141–2.

Larner AJ, Allen CMC. Hereditary essential tremor and restless legs syndrome. *Postgrad Med J* 1997; **73**: 254.

Pearson VE, Allen RP, Dean T, *et al.* Cognitive deficits associated with restless legs syndrome (RLS). *Sleep Med* 2006; **7**: 25–30.

5.4.8 Tourette syndrome (TS), obsessive-compulsive disorder (OCD)

There is a high concordance of Tourette syndrome (TS) and the related obsessive-compulsive disorder (OCD) in monozygotic twins, although the genetic basis remains to be determined. The psychopathology of Tourette syndrome includes both anxiety and depression (Robertson, 2000; Jankovic, 2001). A correlation between obsessive-compulsive symptoms and performance on the Wisconsin Card Sorting Test has been noted in children with TS (Bornstein, 1991). A Tourette-like syndrome of vocal motor tics has been reported in fronto-temporal dementia (see Section 2.2), responding to clonidine (Stewart & Williams, 2003).

Neuropsychological testing has been undertaken in patients with OCD. When corrected for comorbidity with anxiety and depression, these suggest selective impairments on tests of spatial working and recognition memory, speed of motor initiation and execution during problem solving, but with preserved verbal memory and language tasks. The deficits may perhaps be related to difficulties in inhibitory functions (Chamberlain *et al.*, 2005), or in sustaining attention and forming internal representations of stimuli, reflecting abnormal frontal-basal ganglia connections (Maruff *et al.*, 2002).

REFERENCES

Bornstein RA. Neuropsychological correlates of obsessive characteristics in Tourette syndrome. *J Neuropsychiatry Clin Neurosci* 1991; **3**: 157–62.

Chamberlain SR, Blackwell AD, Fineberg NA, Robbins TW, Sahakian BJ. The neuropsychology of obsessive compulsive disorder: the importance of failures in cognitive and behavioural inhibition as candidate endophenotypic markers. *Neurosci Biobehav Rev* 2005; **29**: 399–419.

Jankovic J. Tourette's syndrome. *N Engl J Med* 2001; **345**: 1184–92.

Maruff P, Purcell R, Pantelis C. Obsessive-compulsive disorder. In: Harrison JE, Owen AM (eds.), *Cognitive Deficits in Brain Disorders*. London: Martin Dunitz, 2002: 249–72.

Robertson MM. Tourette syndrome, associated conditions and the complexities of treatment. *Brain* 2000; **123**: 425–62.

Stewart JT, Williams LS. Tourette's-like syndrome and dementia. *Am J Psychiatry* 2003; **160**: 1356–7.

5.5 Hereditary metabolic disorders

This section encompasses those disorders once styled as 'inborn errors of metabolism'.

5.5.1 Mitochondrial disorders

Mitochondrial disorders are a heterogeneous group, with respect to both phenotype and genotype. Both peripheral and central nervous systems may be affected, the former including myopathy and peripheral neuropathy, the CNS features including epilepsy, migraine, stroke-like episodes, ophthalmoplegia, ataxia, and spasticity, as well as cognitive impairment. There may also be involvement of other systems, such as cardiomyopathy, diabetes mellitus, pigmentary retinal degeneration, and sensorineural hearing loss. Various more or less characteristic phenotypes may be identified, including Kearns–Sayre syndrome, chronic progressive external ophthalmoplegia (CPEO), the syndrome of mitochondrial encephalomyopathy, lactic acidosis, and stroke-like episodes (MELAS), and the syndrome of myoclonic epilepsy and ragged red fibres (MERRF). At the level of genotype, mitochondrial disorders may result from mutations (deletions, point mutations) within the small mitochondrial genome or within nuclear genes (autosomal, X-linked) which encode mitochondrial respiratory chain proteins (Schapira & DiMauro, 2002; Finsterer, 2006).

The possibility that neuropsychological deficits might be common in mitochondrial disorders was suggested by Kartsounis et al. (1992), who noted in a series of 36 patients with myopathies and encephalomyopathies that 14 patients were thought to be cognitively impaired on clinical grounds, but 21 were found to have general intellectual decline on testing and a further 5 of the remaining 15 had focal cognitive deficits, in the domains of language, memory, or perception (frontal lobe tests were not administered in this series). Turconi et al. (1999) found no global cognitive decline in 16 patients with mitochondrial encephalomyopathies but selective impairments of visuospatial skills and short-term memory, unrelated to clinical phenotype and genetic mutations. Kornblum et al. (2000) studied 18 patients with progressive external ophthalmoplegia and Kearns–Sayre syndrome. None had general intellectual deterioration, but disturbances were identified in visual construction, vigilance and concentration, abstraction/flexibility, and verbal/visual memory, suggesting the presence of frontal and parieto-occipital deficits.

In MELAS, repeated cerebral infarctions may ultimately lead to dementia (Montagna et al., 1988).

A subcortical dementia resembling Binswanger's disease (see Section 3.2), but without lipohyalinosis, in association with mitochondrial DNA variants has been described under the rubric of disseminated neocortical and subcortical encephalopathy (DNSE: Haferkamp et al., 1998).

REFERENCES

Finsterer J. Central nervous system manifestations of mitochondrial disorders. *Acta Neurol Scand* 2006; **114**: 217–38.

Haferkamp O, Rosenau W, Scheuerle A, *et al.* Disseminated neocortical and subcortical encephalopathy (DNSE) with widespread activation of macrophages: a new dementia disorder? Autopsy report of two postmenopausal women from families with mitochondrial DNA mutations. *Clin Neuropathol* 1998; **17**: 85–94.

Kartsounis LD, Truong DD, Morgan Hughes JA, Harding AE. The neuropsychological features of mitochondrial myopathies and encephalomyopathies. *Arch Neurol* 1992; **49**: 158–60.

Kornblum C, Bosbach S, Wagner M, *et al.* Neuropsychological testing of patients with PEO and Kearns–Sayre syndrome reveals distinct frontal and parieto-occipital deficits. *J Neurol* 2000; **247** (suppl 3): III/73 (abstract P266).

Montagna P, Gallassi R, Medori R, *et al.* MELAS syndrome: characteristic migrainous and epileptic features and maternal transmission. *Neurology* 1988; **38**: 751–4.

Schapira AHV, DiMauro S (eds.). *Mitochondrial Disorders in Neurology* (2nd edition). Boston: Butterworth-Heinemann, 2002.

Turconi AC, Benti R, Castelli E, *et al.* Focal cognitive impairment in mitochondrial encephalomyopathies: a neuropsychological and neuroimaging study. *J Neurol Sci* 1999; **170**: 57–63.

5.5.2 Leukodystrophies

Leukodystrophies are genetic metabolic diseases which generally present in early childhood, often at the time of myelination. Occasionally, however, these disorders may present in adulthood (Baumann & Turpin, 2000), and dementia may be one feature of the clinical phenotype. These conditions may be recessive (e.g. metachromatic leukodystrophy) or sex-linked (e.g. X-linked adrenoleukodystrophy). This is a heterogeneous group, including lysosomal and peroxisomal disorders.

Metachromatic leukodystrophy (MLD)

Reduced enzymatic activity of arylsulphatase A (ARSA) due to mutations in the *ARSA* gene result in accumulation of sulphatide in Schwann cells and oligodendroglia with peripheral and central demyelination, causing peripheral neuropathy and leukodystrophy. Depending on the degree of residual enzyme activity, disease may range from severe, late infantile, to mild, adult-onset. Cases of MLD with adult-onset dementia have been reported. These may vary in the pattern of cognitive impairment: cases with amnesia, visuospatial dysfunction, and attentional difficulties, with medial temporal and frontal cortical hypometabolism on functional imaging, are reported (Johannsen *et al.*, 2001), as are cases with more typical frontal features of behavioural change, apathy, and psychosis akin to schizophrenia, with frontal hypoperfusion on functional imaging (Fukutani *et al.*, 1999; Salmon *et al.*, 1999). Concurrent peripheral neuropathy may be a clue to diagnosis, although cases with adult-onset dementia without neuropathy have been reported (Marcão *et al.*, 2005).

X-linked adrenoleukodystrophy (X-ALD)

X-linked adrenoleukodystrophy (X-ALD) is a peroxisomal disorder associated with mutations in the ATP-binding cassette (*ABCD1*) gene, which encodes a peroxisomal membrane protein. The clinical phenotype varies, dependent on the age of presentation: children most often have rapidly progressive cerebral disease, whereas adults most often present with adrenomyeloneuropathy (AMN), these two phenotypes accounting for more than 75% of all cases. Adult cerebral disease is the least frequently observed phenotype (Moser *et al.*, 2005).

X-ALD cases presenting with adult-onset dementia have only rarely been reported. Features suggestive of frontal lobe dysfunction have been prominent in many of these cases (Powers *et al.*, 1980; Esiri *et al.*, 1984; Sereni *et al.*, 1987; Panegyres *et al.*, 1989; Larner, 2003). Patients presenting with marked personality change and labelled as having manic-depressive psychosis (Angus *et al.*, 1994) or mania with disinhibition, impulsivity, hypersexuality, and perseveration (Garside *et al.*, 1999) may possibly represent the same phenotype. Presentation with Balint syndrome and dementia has also been described (Uyama *et al.*, 1993). The pathogenesis of these features is presumably the functional disconnection of cortical regions by an advancing wave of inflammatory demyelination, either anterior or posterior, which is the typical pathological substrate of X-ALD. A correlation between frontal type dementia and an anterior pattern of white matter change on MR imaging has been noted in one case (Larner, 2003).

With developments in diagnostic techniques, particularly neuroimaging and neurogenetic testing, X-ALD may now be diagnosed in asymptomatic but at-risk individuals. Study of neurologically and radiologically asymptomatic boys has shown overall normal cognitive function, with the emergence of subtle visual perceptual and visuomotor deficits with age in a few (Cox *et al.*, 2005). Early therapeutic intervention might be predicted to preserve cognitive function, and there is some evidence to support the view that bone marrow transplantation may preserve neuropsychological outcome (Shapiro *et al.*, 1995).

Alexander's disease and Rosenthal fibre encephalopathy (RFE)

Alexander's disease is typically a disease of childhood characterized by megalencephaly and relentless neurological deterioration, with a leukodystrophy and the neuropathological finding of Rosenthal fibres, eosinophilic cytoplasmic inclusions within astrocyte processes adjacent to areas of demyelination. These are immunopositive for glial fibrillary acidic protein (GFAP), ubiquitin, and heat shock proteins such as hsp27 and $\alpha\beta$-crystallin. Mutations in the gene encoding GFAP on chromosome 17 have been associated with the condition (Brenner *et al.*, 2001), including occasional adult-onset cases (Namekawa *et al.*, 2002).

Rosenthal fibre encephalopathy (RFE) is the name used for a condition in which the pathological finding of Rosenthal fibres occurs without clinical features of demyelinating lesions typical of Alexander's disease. Rosenthal fibres are typically found in subependymal, subpial, and perivascular regions, often confined to the brainstem, and often in the context of systemic illness (Wilson *et al.*, 1996).

Occasional adult-onset cases of Alexander's disease and RFE have been described (Jacob *et al.*, 2003), some with dementia, for example in a patient with learning disability who developed further cognitive decline, ataxia, and dysarthria (Walls *et al.*, 1984). A review of adult-onset cases (Jacob *et al.*, 2003) suggested that dementia was more common in RFE (4/11) than in Alexander's disease (2/15).

Pelizaeus–Merzbacher disease (PMD)

Pelizaeus–Merzbacher disease (PMD) is an X-linked recessive disorder of myelin due to deficiency of proteolipid protein (PLP) which usually presents in the first months of life with a combination of a movement disorder (head tremor, laryngeal stridor, choreoathetosis, spastic paraparesis) and intellectual decline. Various forms have been described, including a late-onset form known as Löwenberg–Hill syndrome (Bruyn *et al.*, 1985). Point mutations, duplications, and deletions of the *PLP* gene have been identified, as have cases with the clinical phenotype of PMD but normal *PLP* gene, suggesting that other regulatory genes may also be involved in disease pathogenesis (Garbern *et al.*, 1999).

Adult cases with dementia and movement disorder are unusual. Cases with or without *PLP* gene mutation have been described, as has a case of dementia, gait disorder, and MR evidence of leukodystrophy in the mother of a man with PMD, presumably a manifesting carrier (Saito *et al.*, 1993; Nance *et al.*, 1996; Sasaki *et al.*, 2000).

Krabbe disease (globoid cell leukodystrophy)

This autosomal recessive leukodystrophy results from deficiency of the lysosomal enzyme galactocerebroside β-galactosidase (GALC) due to mutations in the encoding gene located on chromosome 14q24.3–q32.1. In addition to the infantile and late-infantile/juvenile forms that account for most cases, an adult form is also described, manifesting with spastic paraparesis. Dementia, optic atrophy, and peripheral neuropathy also develop, although a protracted course with apparently preserved intellect has been reported (Jardim *et al.*, 1999). Bone marrow transplantation may be effective in preventing dementia if performed early enough (Shapiro *et al.*, 1995).

18q deletion (18q–) syndrome

Deletion of the long arm of chromosome 18, also known as de Grouchy syndrome (OMIM #601808), produces a variable phenotype encompassing learning disability, short stature, variable dysmorphism, and neurological symptoms and signs (de Grouchy *et al.*, 1964). Magnetic resonance brain imaging shows white matter abnormalities with incomplete myelination and poor differentiation of grey and white matter, features ascribed to loss of the myelin basic protein gene (*MBP*) which lies on chromosome 18q. Rare deletions in which the *MBP* gene is retained have normal-appearing white matter. For this reason, the condition has been classified with the leukodystrophies. Occasional cases presenting in adult life have been reported, but these are due to seizure disorder rather than cognitive decline (Adab & Larner, 2006). Lower cognitive ability predicts larger 18q deletion size (Semrud Clikeman *et al.*, 2005)

REFERENCES

Adab N, Larner AJ. Adult-onset seizure disorder in 18q deletion syndrome. *J Neurol* 2006; **253**: 527–8.

Angus B, de Silva R, Davidson R, Bone I. A family with adult-onset cerebral adrenoleucodystrophy. *J Neurol* 1994; **241**: 497–9.

Baumann N, Turpin JC. Adult-onset leukodystrophies. *J Neurol* 2000; **247**: 751–9.

Brenner M, Johnson AB, Boespflug-Tanguy O, *et al.* Mutations in GFAP, encoding glial fibrillary acidic protein, are associated with Alexander disease. *Nat Genet* 2001; **27**: 117–20.

Bruyn GW, Weenink HR, Bots GT, Teepen JL, van Wolferen WJ. Pelizaeus–Merzbacher disease: the Löwenberg–Hill type. *Acta Neuropathol (Berl)* 1985; **67**: 177–89.

Cox CS, Dubey P, Raymond GV, *et al.* Cognitive evaluation of neurologically asymptomatic boys with X-linked adrenoleukodystrophy. *Arch Neurol* 2005; **63**: 69–73.

de Grouchy J, Royer P, Salmon C, Lamy M. Délétion partielle des bras longs du chromosome 18. *Pathol Biol* 1964; **12**: 579–82.

Esiri MM, Hyman NM, Horton WL, Lindenbaum RH. Adrenoleukodystrophy: clinical, pathological and biochemical findings in two brothers with the onset of cerebral disease in adult life. *Neuropath Appl Neurobiol* 1984; **10**: 429–45.

Fukutani Y, Noriki Y, Sasaki K, *et al.* Adult-type metachromatic leukodystrophy with a compound heterozygote mutation showing character change and dementia. *Psychiatry Clin Neurosci* 1999; **53**: 425–8.

Garbern J, Cambi F, Shy M, Kamholz J. The molecular pathogenesis of Pelizaeus–Merzbacher disease. *Arch Neurol* 1999; **56**: 1210–14.

Garside S, Rosebush PI, Levinson AJ, Mazurek MF. Late-onset adrenoleukodystrophy associated with long-standing psychiatric symptoms. *J Clin Psychiatry* 1999; **60**: 460–8.

Jacob J, Robertson NJ, Hilton DA. The clinicopathological spectrum of Rosenthal fibre encephalopathy and Alexander's disease: a case report and review of the literature. *J Neurol Neurosurg Psychiatry* 2003; **74**: 807–10.

Jardim LB, Giugliani R, Pires RF, *et al.* Protracted course of Krabbe disease in an adult patient bearing a novel mutation. *Arch Neurol* 1999; **56**: 1014–17.

Johannsen P, Ehlers L, Hansen HJ. Dementia with impaired temporal glucose metabolism in late-onset metachromatic leukodystrophy. *Dement Geriatr Cogn Disord* 2001; **12**: 85–8.

Larner AJ. Adult-onset dementia with prominent frontal lobe dysfunction in X-linked adrenoleukodystrophy with R152C mutation in ABCD1 gene. *J Neurol* 2003; **250**: 1253–4.

Marcão AM, Wiest R, Schindler K, *et al.* Adult onset metachromatic leukodystrophy without electroclinical peripheral nervous system involvement: a new mutation in the ARSA gene. *Arch Neurol* 2005; **62**: 309–13.

Moser HW, Raymond GV, Dubey P. Adrenoleukodystrophy: new approaches to a neurodegenerative disease. *JAMA* 2005; **294**: 3131–4.

Namekawa M, Takiyama Y, Aoki Y, *et al.* Identification of GFAP gene mutation in hereditary adult-onset Alexander's disease. *Ann Neurol* 2002; **52**: 779–85.

Nance MA, Boyadjiev S, Pratt VM, *et al.* Adult-onset neurodegenerative disorder due to proteolipid protein gene mutation in the mother of a man with Pelizaeus–Merzbacher disease. *Neurology* 1996; **47**: 1333–5.

Panegyres PK, Goldswain P, Kakulas BA. Adult-onset adrenoleukodystrophy manifesting as dementia. *Am J Med* 1989; **87**: 481–3.

Powers JM, Schaumburg HH, Gaffney CL. Kluver–Bucy syndrome caused by adreno-leukodystrophy. *Neurology* 1980; **30**: 1231–2.

Saito Y, Ando T, Doyu M, Takahashi A, Hashizume Y. An adult case of classical Pelizaeus–Merzbacher disease: magnetic resonance images and neuropathological findings [in Japanese]. *Rinsho Shinkeigaku* 1993; **33**: 187–93.

Salmon E, van der Linden M, Maerfens-Noordhout A, *et al.* Early thalamic and cortical hypometabolism in adult-onset dementia due to metachromatic leukodystrophy. *Acta Neurol Belg* 1999; **99**: 185–8.

Sasaki A, Miyanaga K, Ototsuji M, *et al.* Two autopsy cases with Pelizaeus–Merzbacher disease phenotype of adult onset, without mutation of proteolipid protein gene. *Acta Neuropathol (Berl)* 2000; **99**: 7–13.

Semrud Clikeman M, Thompson NM, Schaub BL, *et al.* Cognitive ability predicts degree of genetic abnormality in participants with 18q deletions. *J Int Neuropsychol Soc* 2005; **11**: 584–90.

Sereni C, Ruel M, Iba-Zizen T, *et al.* Adult adrenoleukodystrophy: a sporadic case? *J Neurol Sci* 1987; **80**: 121–8.

Shapiro EG, Lockman LA, Balthazor M, Krivit W. Neuropsychological outcomes of several storage diseases with and without bone marrow transplantation. *J Inherit Metab Dis* 1995; **18**: 413–29.

Uyama E, Iwagoe H, Maeda J, *et al.* Presenile onset cerebral adrenoleukodystrophy presenting as Balint's syndrome and dementia. *Neurology* 1993; **43**: 1249–51.

Walls TJ, Jones RA, Cartlidge NEF, Saunders M. Alexander's disease with Rosenthal fibre formation in an adult. *J Neurol Neurosurg Psychiatry* 1984; **47**: 399–403.

Wilson SP, Al-Sarraj S, Bridges LR. Rosenthal fiber encephalopathy presenting with demyelination and Rosenthal fibers in a solvent abuser: adult Alexander's disease? *Clin Neuropathol* 1996; **15**: 13–16.

5.5.3 Lysosomal storage disorders

Around 40 lysosomal storage disorders affecting the brain are described (Platt & Walkley, 2004). Learning disability/mental retardation is a feature in many of these disorders, but some may present in adulthood with cognitive impairment as a feature (Coker, 1991). Some of these are mentioned elsewhere: e.g. metachromatic leukodystrophy Krabbe disease (see Section 5.5.2).

Acid maltase deficiency (glycogenosis type IIb)

This autosomal recessive lysosomal disorder of glycogen storage results from deficiency of the lysosomal enzyme acid α-glucosidase, or acid maltase, due to mutation of the gene located on chromosome 17 which encodes this protein. The clinical phenotype is variable, with age of onset ranging from infancy to adulthood, with myopathy, cardiomyopathy, and organomegaly. Adult-onset disease (Engel's disease) may present with respiratory failure due to diaphragmatic involvement (Trend *et al.*, 1985). One case of adult-onset acid maltase deficiency (AMD) associated with low IQ and impairments of frontal lobe function has been reported; other family members with AMD did not have dementia. As the authors point out, this may be a fortuitous association, but equally acid maltase is expressed in brain as well as in muscle, and brain levels may be low (Prevett *et al.*, 1992).

Anderson–Fabry disease (Fabry's disease, angiokeratoma corporis diffusum, hereditary dystonic lipidosis)

This autosomal recessive lysosomal storage disorder is due to mutations in the gene encoding α-galactosidase A, with resultant enzyme deficiency leading to accumulation of glycosphingolipids such as ceramide trihexoside in the vascular endothelium and smooth muscle cells of visceral tissues including brain, and in body fluids. The resultant multisystem disease has a broad phenotype, with neurological (peripheral and central nervous system), dermatological, renal, ocular, gastro-enterological, cardiac, and respiratory features (Mehta, 2002), with variable age at diagnosis.

A slowly progressive vascular dementia has been described (Mendez *et al.*, 1997) with multiple cognitive deficits including memory impairment, anomia, perseveration, and visuospatial difficulties, with additional behavioural changes. This is due to multiple subcortical strokes and diffuse ischaemic white matter disease due to pathological involvement of small penetrating arteries, hypertension (secondary to renal disease), and cardiogenic emboli. Although this is an extremely rare presentation of Anderson–Fabry disease, a case-registry series reported dementia in 18% of patients, in all cases associated with recurrent strokes or transient ischaemic attacks (MacDermott *et al.*, 2001). Prevention may be feasible with enzyme replacement therapy.

Gangliosidosis

Late-onset GM2 gangliosidosis, also known as late-onset Tay–Sachs disease, resulting from autosomal recessive hexosaminidase A deficiency, may result in cognitive dysfunction in about half of patients, with impaired executive and memory function. Studies disagree as to whether dementia occurs at all (Zaroff *et al.*, 2004), or is common (Frey *et al.*, 2005).

Gaucher's disease

A rare adult neuronopathic form of this autosomal recessive disease, due to deficiency of β-glucocerebrosidase, is recognized (Guimarães *et al.*, 2003), causing akinetic-rigid syndrome, supranuclear gaze palsy, myoclonus, seizures, and cognitive decline. There is elevated serum acid phosphatase and bone marrow infiltration with lipid-laden fibroblasts known as Gaucher's cells. A possible link between Gaucher's disease and the synucleinopathies (see Section 2.4) has been postulated, based on the finding of synuclein-positive Lewy bodies in Gaucher's patients with parkinsonism and an increased incidence of Lewy body disorders in the relatives of Gaucher's probands. Carriers of glucocerebrosidase mutations have a wide spectrum of parkinsonian disorders including dementia with Lewy bodies (Hruska *et al.*, 2006).

Neuronal ceroid lipofuscinosis (NCL), Kuf's disease

The neuronal ceroid lipofuscinoses (NCL) are a large group of neurodegenerative disorders with onset between infancy and adulthood, characterized by accumulation of autofluorescent inclusion bodies in neurones and other tissues (Wisniewski *et al.*, 2001a,b). Kuf's disease is the name often applied to adult-onset variants, which may be sporadic or inherited, and manifest with a progressive myoclonus epilepsy and cognitive decline and dementia or with movement disorders such as facial dyskinesia (Berkovic *et al.*, 1988). Families with disease onset in the fourth decade, heralded by seizures and with subsequent dementia, have been reported (Josephson *et al.*, 2001). In addition to the various pathological inclusions (fingerprint, curvilinear, rectilinear, granular osmiophilic), neuritic plaques and possibly neurofibrillary tangles may also be seen in Kuf's disease (Wisniewski *et al.*, 1979), leading to the suggestion of an overlapping pathogenesis with Alzheimer's disease (Larner, 1996). Various genetic loci have been identified in the neuronal ceroid lipofuscinoses, with both autosomal recessive and dominant patterns of inheritance (Wisniewski *et al.*, 2001a; Mole *et al.*, 2005).

Niemann-Pick disease type C

This autosomal recessive disorder is a lipidosis, resulting from a defect in cellular trafficking of cholesterol, leading to the accumulation of cholesterol and sphingolipids in late endosomes/lysosomes. It results from mutations in the genes *NPC1* and *NPC2*. The clinical phenotype of the former is broad, including dystonia, supranuclear gaze palsy, ataxia, dysarthria, seizures, and progressive cognitive decline with onset from the first to the fifth decade (Uc *et al.*, 2000; Battisti *et al.*, 2003). Mutations in the gene encoding the cholesterol binding protein HE1 (*NPC2*) have been reported to cause dementia in the 30s with focal frontal involvement. Tau-positive neurofibrillary tangles as well as lysosomal inclusions were seen at postmortem (Klünemann *et al.*, 2002).

Sanfilippo syndrome (mucopolysaccharidosis III)

This autosomal recessive disorder, associated with excessive urinary excretion of heparan sulphate, comes in four biochemical and genetic variants, all due to deficiencies of different enzymes, usually causing childhood-onset dementia and neurobehavioural problems. The clinical phenotype is variable, and type B cases with dementia onset in the third or fourth decade have been reported (van Schrojenstein-de Valk & van de Kamp, 1987). Bone marrow transplantation provides no benefit and is therefore not recommended (Shapiro *et al.*, 1995).

REFERENCES

Battisti C, Tarugi P, Dotti MT, *et al.* Adult onset Niemann–Pick type C disease: a clinical, neuroimaging and molecular genetic study. *Mov Disord* 2003; **18**: 1405–9.

Berkovic SF, Carpenter S, Andermann F, *et al.* Kufs' disease: a critical reappraisal. *Brain* 1988; **111**: 27–62.

Coker SB. The diagnosis of childhood neurodegenerative disorders presenting as dementia in adults. *Neurology* 1991; **41**: 794–8.

Frey LC, Ringel SP, Filley CM. The natural history of cognitive dysfunction in late-onset GM2 gangliosidosis. *Arch Neurol* 2005; **62**: 989–94.

Guimarães J, Amaral O, Sá Miranda MC. Adult-onset neuronopathic form of Gaucher's disease: a case report. *Parkinsonism Relat Disord* 2003; **9**: 261–4.

Hruska KS, Goker-Alpan O, Sidransky E. Gaucher disease and the synucleinopathies. *J Biomed Biotechnol* 2006; **2006**: 78549 [*sic*].

Josephson SA, Schmidt RE, Millsap P, McManus DQ, Morris JC. Autosomal dominant Kufs' disease: a cause of early onset dementia. *J Neurol Sci* 2001; **188**: 51–60.

Klünemann HH, Elleder M, Kaminski WE, *et al.* Frontal lobe atrophy due to a mutation in the cholesterol binding protein HE1/NPC2. *Ann Neurol* 2002; **52**: 743–9.

Larner AJ. Alzheimer's disease, Kuf's disease, tellurium, and selenium. *Med Hypotheses* 1996; **47**: 73–5.

MacDermott KD, Holmes A, Miners AH. Anderson–Fabry disease: clinical manifestations and impact of disease in a cohort of 98 hemizygous males. *J Med Genet* 2001; **38**: 750–60.

Mehta A. New developments in the management of Anderson–Fabry disease. *Q J Med* 2002; **95**: 647–53.

Mendez MF, Stanley TM, Medel NM, Li Z, Tedesco DT. The vascular dementia of Fabry's disease. *Dement Geriatr Cogn Disord* 1997; **8**: 252–7.

Mole SE, Williams RE, Goebel HH. Correlations between genotype, ultrastructural morphology and clinical phenotype in the neuronal ceroid lipofuscinoses. *Neurogenetics* 2005; **6**: 107–26.

Platt FM, Walkley SU (eds.). *Lysosomal Disorders of the Brain: Recent Advances in Molecular and Cellular Pathogenesis and Treatment.* Oxford: Oxford University Press, 2004.

Prevett M, Enevoldson TP, Duncan JS. Adult onset acid maltase deficiency associated with epilepsy and dementia: a case report. *J Neurol Neurosurg Psychiatry* 1992; **55**: 509.

Shapiro EG, Lockman LA, Balthazor M, Krivit W. Neuropsychological outcomes of several storage diseases with and without bone marrow transplantation. *J Inherit Metab Dis* 1995; **18**: 413–29.

Trend PStJ, Wiles CM, Spencer GT, *et al.* Acid maltase deficiency in adults. *Brain* 1985; **108**: 845–60.

Uc EY, Wenger DA, Jankovic J. Niemann–Pick disease type C: two cases and an update. *Mov Disord* 2000; **15**: 1199–203.

van Schrojenstein-de Valk HMJ, van de Kamp JJP. Follow-up on seven adult patients with mild Sanfilippo B disease. *Am J Med Genet* 1987; **28**: 125–30.

Wisniewski K, Jervis GA, Moretz RC, Wisniewski HM. Alzheimer neurofibrillary tangles in diseases other than senile and presenile dementia. *Ann Neurol* 1979; **5**: 288–94.

Wisniewski KE, Kida E, Golabek AA, *et al.* Neuronal ceroid lipofuscinoses: classification and diagnosis. *Adv Genet* 2001a; **45**: 1–34.

Wisniewski KE, Zhong N, Philippart M. Pheno/genotypic correlations in neuronal ceroid lipofuscinoses. *Neurology* 2001b; **57**: 576–81.

Zaroff CM, Neudorfer O, Morrison C, *et al.* Neuropsychological assessment of patients with late onset GM2 gangliosidosis. *Neurology* 2004; **62**: 2283–6.

5.5.4 Cerebrotendinous xanthomatosis (CTX)

This autosomal recessive lipid storage disorder results from mutations in the mitochondrial enzyme 27-sterol hydroxylase on chromosome 2p, causing impaired bile acid synthesis. Brain imaging shows global atrophy and demyelination, such that some authorities classify CTX with the leukodystrophies. Spasticity, ataxia, and peripheral neuropathy are included amongst the neurological features as well as dementia, with onset in the third decade. A survey of 32 patients found low IQ in 66%, and in 81% of 181 patients reported in the literature (Verrips *et al.*, 2000a,b). No detailed neuropsychological profile has been identified, although a subcortical pattern might be expected.

REFERENCES

Verrips A, Hoefsloot LH, Steenbergen GCH, *et al.* Clinical and molecular genetic characteristics of patients with cerebrotendinous xanthomatosis. *Brain* 2000a; **123**: 908–19.

Verrips A, van Engelen BGM, Wevers RA, *et al.* Presence of diarrhea and absence of tendon xanthomas in patients with cerebrotendinous xanthomatosis. *Arch Neurol* 2000b; **57**: 520–4.

5.5.5 Haemochromatosis

Genetic, primary, or hereditary haemochromatosis is an autosomal recessive disorder characterized by iron overload with pathological deposition in liver and pancreas, with resulting liver impairment and diabetes mellitus respectively. Iron does not normally cross the blood–brain barrier, and elevated brain iron content is rarely if ever a feature of haemochromatosis, the clinical correlate being that neurological symptoms are also rare, despite systemic iron overload equivalent to that seen in acaeruloplasminaemia (see Section 5.4.5). Cognitive features may be seen in hereditary movement disorders associated with abnormal iron metabolism (e.g. neuroferritinopathy, acaeruloplasminaemia), and iron content is reported to be increased in the striatum in Huntington's disease and in the posterior putamen in parkinsonian-type multiple system atrophy.

Cases of haemochromatosis presenting with dementia and ataxia have been reported in the context of advanced liver disease, progressing to death within 2 years of the onset of neurological features (Jones & Hedley-Whyte, 1983). Two cases with mild systemic features and concurrent dementia of frontotemporal type (one semantic dementia, one frontal variant) have been reported, with the suggestion that this may reflect linkage of genetic diseases, rather than a toxic consequence of abnormal iron metabolism, although in the absence of brain pathology the matter remains unresolved (Harvey et al., 1997). One patient had sensorineural hearing loss, which may be significant (see superficial siderosis of the nervous system, Section 3.4.3).

The association of these cases might reflect chance concurrence. It has been argued that movement disorders occurring in the context of hereditary haemochromatosis should prompt a search for another cause (Russo et al., 2004), and the same is probably true of cognitive impairment, although this might be anticipated as a consequence of complications such as hepatic failure and/or diabetes mellitus.

REFERENCES

Harvey RJ, Summerfield JA, Fox NC, Warrington EK, Rossor MN. Dementia associated with haemochromatosis: a report of two cases. *Eur J Neurol* 1997; **4**: 318–22.

Jones HR, Hedley-Whyte ET. Idiopathic hemochromatosis (IHC): dementia and ataxia as presenting signs. *Neurology* 1983; **33**: 1479–83.

Russo N, Edwards M, Andrews T, O'Brien M, Bhatia KP. Hereditary haemochromatosis is unlikely to cause movement disorders. A critical review. *J Neurol* 2004; **251**: 849–52.

5.5.6   Lafora body disease

This autosomal recessive progressive myoclonic epilepsy syndrome typically presents in the 10- to 18-year-old age group, with epileptic seizures, myoclonus, and neurological deterioration with cognitive impairment and eventually dementia, with typical Lafora body inclusions in brain, liver, skin, and muscle. Deterministic mutations have been demonstrated in two genes, *EPM2A* and *EPM2B*, encoding the proteins laforin and malin respectively (Minassian et al., 1998; Chan et al., 2003), which colocalize to the endoplasmic reticulum. Delayed onset up to about the age of 25 years has been infrequently reported (Messouak et al., 2002; Baykan et al., 2005). Mutations in certain exons of the laforin gene may be associated with an earlier onset (Ganesh et al., 2002).

REFERENCES

Baykan B, Striano P, Gianotti S, et al. Late-onset and slow-progressing Lafora disease in four siblings with EPM2B mutation. *Epilepsia* 2005; **46**: 1695–7.

Chan EM, Young EJ, Ianzano L, et al. Mutations in NHLRC1 cause progressive myoclonus epilepsy. *Nat Genet* 2003; **35**: 125–7.

Ganesh S, Delgado-Escueta AV, Suzuki T, et al. Genotype–phenotype correlations for EPM2A mutations in Lafora's progressive myoclonus epilepsy: exon 1 mutations associate with an early-onset cognitive deficit subphenotype. *Hum Mol Genet* 2002; **11**: 1263–71.

Messouak O, Yahyaoui M, Benabdeljalil M, et al. La maladie de Lafora à révélation tardive. *Rev Neurol Paris* 2002; **158**: 74–6.

Minassian BA, Lee JR, Herbrick JA, et al. Mutations in a gene encoding a novel protein tyrosine phosphatase cause progressive myoclonus epilepsy. *Nat Genet* 1998; **20**: 171–4.

5.5.7   Polyglucosan body disease

Glycogen storage disease type IV, also known as amylopectinosis or Andersen's disease, is an autosomal recessive disorder associated with deficiency of the glycogen branching enzyme (GBE) encoded on chromosome 3p14. The clinical phenotype is extremely heterogeneous (Moses & Parvari, 2002), ranging from progressive liver cirrhosis and death in childhood, through cardiomyopathic and benign myopathic variants, to an adult-onset neurodegenerative disorder, polyglucosan body disease (PGBD). This latter is a rare disorder, often characterized by a combination of upper and lower motor neurone signs, the latter due to an axonal sensorimotor peripheral neuropathy, along with urinary incontinence and other motor disorders. Nerve biopsy may be diagnostic, showing the typical polyglucosan bodies, which may also be seen in dermal sweat glands or brain tissue. Dementia has been reported on occasion in PGBD (Robertson *et al.*, 1998), apparently of frontal type (Boulan Predseil *et al.*, 1995), sometimes associated with white matter changes on MR imaging (Berkhoff *et al.*, 2001). Familial cases are reported (Bigio *et al.*, 1997). Mild cognitive impairment has been documented in an individual heterozygous for a point mutation in the GBE gene and with other clinical features suggesting manifesting heterozygote status (Ubogu *et al.*, 2005).

REFERENCES

Berkhoff M, Weis J, Schroth G, Sturzenegger M. Extensive white-matter changes in case of adult polyglucosan body disease. *Neuroradiology* 2001; **43**: 234–6.

Bigio EH, Weiner MF, Bonte FJ, White CL. Familial dementia due to adult polyglucosan body disease. *Clin Neuropathol* 1997; **16**: 227–34.

Boulan Predseil P, Vital A, Brochet B, *et al.* Dementia of frontal lobe type due to adult polyglucosan body disease. *J Neurol* 1995; **242**: 512–16.

Moses SW, Parvari R. The variable presentations of glycogen storage disease type IV: a review of clinical, enzymatic and molecular studies. *Curr Mol Med* 2002; **2**: 177–88.

Robertson NP, Wharton S, Anderson J, Scolding NJ. Adult polyglucosan body disease associated with extrapyramidal syndrome. *J Neurol Neurosurg Psychiatry* 1998; **65**: 788–90.

Ubogu EE, Hong STK, Akman HO, *et al.* Adult polyglucosan body disease: a case report of a manifesting heterozygote. *Muscle Nerve* 2005; **32**: 675–81.

5.5.8 Porphyria

Although a recognized cause of various neurological and neuropsychiatric syndromes, including delirium in response to precipitating factors such as infection or drugs (Crimlisk, 1997; Peters & Sarkany, 2005), it is not clear that any one of the porphyrias causes or leads to dementia, although there may be complaints of poor memory. This is mentioned because of the popular association of porphyria with the madness of King George III, but the evidence for him having had this condition is not compelling.

REFERENCES

Crimlisk HL. The little imitator – porphyria: a neuropsychiatric disorder. *J Neurol Neurosurg Psychiatry* 1997; **62**: 319–28.

Peters TJ, Sarkany R. Porphyria for the general physician. *Clin Med* 2005; **5**: 275–81.

5.5.9 Unverricht–Lundborg disease (Baltic myoclonus)

This condition, due to mutations in the cystatin B gene, enters the differential diagnosis of progressive myoclonic epilepsy along with Lafora body disease, neuronal ceroid lipofuscinosis, and mitochondrial disorders, amongst others. In addition to the polymyoclonus and cerebellar ataxia, the phenotype may include a mild and slowly progressive dementia (Mazarib *et al.*, 2001).

REFERENCES

Mazarib A, Xiong L, Neufeld MY, *et al.* Unverricht–Lundborg disease in a five-generation Arab family: instability of dodecamer repeats. *Neurology* 2001; **57**: 1050–4.

5.6 Hereditary neurocutaneous syndromes (phakomatoses)

This category of hereditary disorders is characterized by involvement of ectodermal structures (nervous system, skin, eyes) with slow evolution during childhood and adolescence with a tendency to formation of benign tumours or hamartomas. The terminology may also sometimes be taken to include conditions with cutaneous angiomatosis and CNS abnormalities, such as ataxia telangiectasia (see Section 5.2.2) and Anderson–Fabry disease (Section 5.5.3).

5.6.1 Neurofibromatosis

Neurofibromatosis type 1 (NF1) is one of the commonest monogenic Mendelian disorders seen in general neurology outpatient practice, but reasons for consultation may often be incidental to the diagnosis of NF1 (Larner, 2008). However, many possible neurological problems may be encountered in both NF1 and NF2 (Huson & Hughes, 1994; Korf & Rubenstein, 2005). In a series of 103 NF1 patients aged between 6 and 75 years, IQ was lower than in control patients, although the impairment was generally mild. NF1 patients had poorer reading and impaired short-term memory, and on computerized tests had slower reaction times, higher error rates, and impaired attention. However, no particular profile emerged (Ferner *et al.*, 1996). Intellectual problems in NF1 are not thought to be progressive. Severe impairments are unusual and should mandate a search for another cause, either related to NF1 (such as tumour or hydrocephalus) or unrelated.

Deficits of spatial memory and navigation associated with bilateral hippocampal atrophy have been reported in bilateral vestibulopathy associated with neurofibromatosis type 2 (see Section 6.15).

REFERENCES

Ferner RE, Hughes RAC, Weinman J. Intellectual impairment in neurofibromatosis 1. *J Neurol Sci* 1996; **138**: 125–33.

Huson SM, Hughes RAC (eds.). *The Neurofibromatoses: a Pathogenetic and Clinical Overview*. London: Chapman & Hall, 1994.

Korf BR, Rubenstein AE. *Neurofibromatosis: a Handbook for Patients, Families, and Health Care Professionals* (2nd edition). New York: Thieme, 2005.

Larner AJ. Monogenic Mendelian disorders in general neurological practice. *Int J Clin Pract* 2008; **62**: in press.

5.6.2 Tuberous sclerosis

Tuberous sclerosis was initially identified as a syndrome of mental retardation, epilepsy, and facial angiofibroma, with the neuropathological finding of tubers. The phenotype has extended to less severe cases with the identification of linkage to genes (*TSC1*, *TSC2*) which may act as tumour suppressors, and the appreciation that subependymal nodules reflecting abnormal neuronal migration occur in the majority of cases. The different localization of these lesions might be predicted to cause differing deficits in individual patients. Neuropsychological studies in this heterogeneous disorder have confirmed this, with a possible emphasis on executive tasks related to prefrontal pathology (Harrison & Bolton, 2002). Many patients have normal cognition. Refractory seizures and presence of the *TSC2* mutation have been associated with adverse cognitive outcome (Winterkorn *et al.*, 2007).

REFERENCES

Harrison JE, Bolton PF. Cognitive dysfunction in tuberous sclerosis and other neuronal migration disorders. In: Harrison JE, Owen AM (eds.), *Cognitive Deficits in Brain Disorders*. London: Martin Dunitz, 2002: 325–39.

Winterkorn EB, Pulsifer MB, Thiele EA. Cognitive prognosis of patients with tuberous sclerosis complex. *Neurology* 2007; **68**: 62–4.

Inflammatory, immune-mediated, and systemic disorders

6.1 Multiple sclerosis (MS)

Multiple sclerosis (MS) is a common inflammatory demyelinating disorder of CNS white matter, the most common cause of neurological disability in young adults. Ultimately, it results from immune-mediated attack on the myelin–oligodendrocyte complex, although many features of pathogenesis remain unclear (Compston & Coles, 2002; Compston *et al.*, 2006). Viral infections may be a sufficient but not necessary triggering or exacerbating factor (Larner, 1986; Kennedy & Steiner, 1994; Dalgleish, 1997). Natural history studies indicate that the disease may follow a variable course, permitting classification into a number of groups, which are helpful in defining cohorts for study: relapsing–remitting disease (RRMS), when acute exacerbations resolve over time with no permanent disability, is common at disease onset, but this may evolve into secondary progressive disease (SPMS) when disability accrues between or in the absence of acute exacerbations; rarely, disease is relentlessly progressive from the onset, the primary progressive pattern (PPMS). Benign variants are also recognized. Diagnostic criteria for MS encompass the clinical, neuroradiological, and laboratory findings (McDonald *et al.*, 2001; Polman *et al.*, 2005).

Although MS is most commonly recognized as a cause of physical disability, cognitive impairment is also common. This was described by Charcot, and a large literature has subsequently developed, most particularly in the last two decades (Rao, 1986; Langdon, 1997; Thornton & Raz, 1997; Wishart & Sharpe, 1997; Feinstein, 1999; Foong & Ron, 2000; Kesselring & Klement, 2001; Bobholz & Gleason, 2006; Calabrese, 2006; Fischer & Rao, 2007). Cross-sectional community-based studies have shown that around 40–60% of patients with MS have cognitive deficits, even in the early stages of disease (McIntosh-Michaelis et al., 1991; Rao et al., 1991). Literature reviews suggest an even higher percentage (Peyser et al., 1990). Clearly all series are subject to some degree of selection bias, and obviously may mask individual variability, but nonetheless cognitive dysfunction appears to be common in MS.

Concomitant neurological and psychiatric features might contribute to this morbidity, including depression, fatigue, primary sensory abnormalities of vision or hearing, dominant hand dysfunction, or concurrent medications, factors which need to be considered when assessing subjective memory complaints in MS patients (Maor et al., 2001). Nonetheless, in many instances impairments occur independent of these factors, i.e. the disease per se is responsible. The neuropsychological domains most commonly affected are verbal and non-verbal memory, with impaired attention, reduced speed of information processing, and abstract reasoning and verbal fluency deficits, with or without mild visuospatial impairments. Since deficits typical of cortical dementia, such as aphasia, agnosia, and apraxia, seldom occur, the cognitive impairment in MS has been classified as a subcortical dementia.

Such is the frequency of cognitive deficits in MS, with their effects on quality of life and vocational status, that a systematic search has been recommended, using instruments sensitive to the most commonly affected domains. Since, typically for a white matter dementia, these deficits may be regarded as subcortical (Rao, 1996),

commonly used bedside neuropsychological tests such as the MMSE may be insensitive, particularly to early changes (Swirsky-Sacchetti et al., 1992). Recommended screening instruments include the Brief Repeatable Battery of Neuropsychological Tests (BRB-N: Rao, 1990; Rao et al., 1991) and the MS Inventory of Cognition (MUSIC: Calabrese, 2006). The Paced Auditory Serial Addition Test (PASAT) and its visual equivalent (PVSAT), Digit Symbol substitution, backward Digit Span, and the learning stage of the California Verbal Learning Test (CVLT) are suggested as elements to be included in meaningful batteries for neuropsychological screening (Lensch et al., 2006; Sartori & Edan, 2006). PASAT is also included in the Multiple Sclerosis Functional Composite (MSFC) scale. Impairments in these screening tests may be followed up with more comprehensive batteries such as the Minimal Assessment of Cognitive Function in MS (MACFIMS: Benedict et al., 2002) and WMS-R.

The relationship of cognitive impairment to the natural history, neurological signs, and neuroimaging correlates of MS has been extensively investigated. As regards natural history, cognitive impairment may be an early feature of disease. IQ decline and auditory attention deficits were found in one study of patients with clinically isolated syndromes of the kind which often evolve to MS (optic neuritis, brainstem and partial spinal cord syndromes), with a mean duration of symptoms of over 2 years (Callanan et al., 1989). Even in patients with symptoms of only a few days' duration, impaired auditory (PASAT) and visual (PVSAT) attention has been recorded, particularly in patients with radiological evidence of brain lesions (Feinstein et al., 1992b). Attention and non-verbal memory may be impaired in early disease (Schulz et al., 2006).

Cognitive impairments in newly diagnosed patients were also observed by Jønsson et al. (2006) in a group consisting mostly of patients with relapsing–remitting disease (RRMS), in which situation Zivadinov et al. (2001) showed a correlation of cognitive deterioration with brain parenchymal volume atrophy, suggesting that axonal loss was the key substrate for early development and progression. In acute relapses or disease exacerbations, attention and memory test performance may be compromised, but may improve with remission, with a decrease in gadolinium-enhanced MR lesion load (Foong *et al.*, 1998). Hence cognitive decline may be reversible in the early stages of disease.

A study of patients with primary progressive disease (PPMS) showed no change in mean cognitive scores over a 2-year follow-up period. One-third showed absolute cognitive decline on individual test scores, but only a weak relation between cognitive and MR imaging measures was found (Camp *et al.*, 2005). Comparing different MS types, cognitive deficits are reported to be more marked in secondary progressive as compared to RRMS (Heaton *et al.*, 1985). Comparing primary and secondary progressive disease (PPMS versus SPMS), Wacowius *et al.* (2005) reported PPMS patients to be more frequently and more severely affected than SPMS patients, with poorer performance in verbal learning and verbal fluency. However, a review of cross-sectional and longitudinal studies came to the conclusion that cognitive dysfunction was more frequent in SPMS than in PPMS or RRMS (Amato *et al.*, 2006).

Longitudinal studies suggest that cognitive deterioration occurs in a minority of MS patients, with considerable individual variation over time. Following up a cohort of patients with clinically isolated syndromes (Callanan *et al.*, 1989), Feinstein *et al.* (1992a) found that at the group level only visual memory had deteriorated significantly, whilst patients who had developed a chronic progressive course were more impaired on tests of verbal memory and auditory attention. Follow-up studies of patients with established MS have shown considerable individual variation, many patients not progressing, although some new deficits may become apparent in others (Jennekens-Schinkel *et al.*, 1990; Amato *et al.*, 1995; Hohol *et al.*, 1997). Those with cognitive impairment at baseline seem more likely to develop progressive cognitive decline, whereas those who are cognitively normal may remain so (Kujala *et al.*, 1997).

With respect to neurological dysfunction, the correlations with cognitive impairments are generally poor. For example, cognitive dysfunction far greater than neurological disability has been described in association with frontal release signs (Franklin *et al.*, 1989), or even in the absence of physical disability (Tinnefeld *et al.*, 2005). A rare 'cortical variant' of MS has also been reported, presenting with a progressive dementia with prominent amnesia, with or without aphasia, alexia, and agraphia, often with prominent mood disturbance (Zarei *et al.*, 2003). Presumably this syndrome correlates with small cortical lesions in MS, under-represented by MR imaging (Kidd *et al.*, 1999; Kutzelnigg & Lassmann, 2006).

With respect to neuroimaging correlates, total lesion score in terms of area or volume on MR imaging shows significant correlation with cognitive dysfunction (Rao *et al.*, 1989a; Feinstein *et al.*, 1992b) and it is this overall burden rather than regional brain disease which is most important in determining cognitive deficits (Rovaris *et al.*, 1998). Longitudinal studies indicate that progression of brain pathology correlates with cognitive decline (Feinstein *et al.*, 1992a; Hohol *et al.*, 1997). Stable MR lesion scores seem to be associated with no cognitive decline. Brain atrophy may also be relevant: Rao *et al.* (1989a) showed an association between corpus callosum atrophy and reduced speed of information processing, and Zivadinov *et al.* (2001) showed a correlation between cognitive deterioration and brain parenchymal volume atrophy in RRMS. In a 5-year prospective cohort study of RRMS, T_1 lesion volumes were predictive of future cognitive impairment, and IQ decline and memory impairment were more severe in those with higher atrophy scores (Summers *et al.*, 2006). Hence both inflammatory and degenerative processes may contribute to cognitive dysfunction.

Neuropsychological profile

The cognitive profile in MS is heterogeneous, as for the neurological findings, so only a general picture can be given (Table 6.1).

Table 6.1. Neuropsychological deficits in multiple sclerosis (MS).

Attention	Impaired processing speed, working memory (backward Digit Span, PASAT)
General intelligence, IQ	↓ FSIQ vs. premorbid IQ; PIQ typically more impaired than VIQ
Memory	Impaired verbal and spatial learning, acquisition +/− encoding; semantic and implicit memory relatively preserved
Language	Aphasia rare
Perception	Visuospatial and visuoperceptual deficits may occur
Praxis	Praxis difficult to assess with concurrent motor deficits
Executive function	Dysexecutive syndrome common: impaired abstract reasoning, concept formation, and problem solving

Attention

Although simple tests of attention such as Digit Span may be normal in MS, analysis of the more demanding backwards component of this task demonstrates more impairment in MS patients than in controls (Rao *et al.*, 1991; Feinstein *et al.*, 1997). The capacity to store and access information held in working memory seems intact, although it may become impaired in disease exacerbations (Grant *et al.*, 1984) or if disease course becomes progressive (Beatty *et al.*, 1988). More stringent tests of attention may be abnormal even in early disease; for example, the PASAT is generally performed worse by MS patients than by controls (Feinstein *et al.*, 1992b; D'Esposito *et al.*, 1996), and likewise the visual version, PVSAT (Feinstein *et al.*, 1992b). Subclinical working memory dysfunction may be evident on neurophysiological studies measuring event-related potentials (Pelosi *et al.*, 1997).

These results may reflect an inability to devote sufficient attentional resources to process simultaneously the multiple components of these tasks. These are also tests of speed of information processing (as well as of arithmetical ability and short-term memory), such that fatigue is a potential confounder. In support of a defect in cognitive speed, slowed scanning of working memory (Reed–Sternberg paradigm) has been demonstrated (Rao *et al.*, 1989c), as has slowed information processing in both auditory and visual tasks when controlling for accuracy of task performance. On the basis of

these findings it has been suggested that impaired speed of information processing may be a key deficit in MS, with implications for rehabilitation strategies (Demaree *et al.*, 1999). Attentional deficits may be present even in the early stages of disease (Callanan *et al.*, 1989; Schulz *et al.*, 2006).

General intelligence, IQ

Measures of general intelligence in MS, virtually all using the NART to predict premorbid IQ, have consistently found a fall in IQ, but this is mainly related to measures on the performance scales, impairments in which may be related to sensorimotor dysfunction. Verbal IQ scores generally remain stable.

Memory

Although impairments in 'short-term memory' are present (considered under attention, above), deficits specifically of long-term (secondary) memory are probably the commonest memory impairment in MS (Rao *et al.*, 1989b; Feinstein, 1999; Calabrese, 2006). This refers to both verbal and non-verbal memory (Grant *et al.*, 1984; Rao *et al.*, 1991). Since deficits are more apparent on tests of recall than recognition, a defect of retrieval rather than encoding has been postulated, although there is also evidence of impaired acquisition or encoding of new information (DeLuca *et al.*, 1994; Thornton & Raz, 1997). As regards remote (retrograde) memory deficits, deficits in famous faces recognition tests have been reported by some authors (Beatty *et al.*, 1988) but not others (Rao *et al.*, 1991), although the patients in these two studies were not comparable. Impairments in verbal fluency also suggest a retrograde memory loss (Rao *et al.*, 1991). Implicit (procedural) memory seems relatively intact in MS (Beatty *et al.*, 1990; Grafman *et al.*, 1991).

Language

Although disorders of speech, dysarthria, are common in MS, disorders of language, aphasia, have been considered rare (Murdoch & Theodoros, 2000). However, careful assessment of language function may reveal abnormalities in patients with onset of cognitive decline (Kujala *et al.*, 1996). Aphasia, alexia, and agraphia may be present in the 'cortical variant' of MS, which presents with progressive dementia with prominent amnesia (Zarei *et al.*, 2003). A study of 2700 patients from three centres in France found 22 cases (0.81%) of acute aphasia in MS (Lacour *et al.*, 2004). This may rarely occur as a monosymptomatic presentation of MS (Erdem *et al.*, 2001; Di Majo *et al.*, 2002; Lacour *et al.*, 2004), or as a feature of acute exacerbation in association with new left hemisphere white matter lesions on MR imaging in established MS (Achiron *et al.*, 1992; Devere *et al.*, 2000). However, aetiologies other than acute inflammation need to be considered in MS patients with acute aphasia, including non-convulsive 'aphasic' status epilepticus (Primavera *et al.*, 1996; Trinka *et al.*, 2001), which has also been reported as the initial presenting symptom of MS (Trinka *et al.*, 2002) and of MS relapse (Spatt *et al.*, 1994). Second pathologies, as well as alternative aetiologies, may need to be ruled out (Larner & Lecky, 2007). It has also been suggested that aphasic presentations of MS may in fact be cases of acute disseminated encephalomyelitis (ADEM: Section 6.2; Brinar *et al.*, 2004).

Perception

Assessment of visuospatial and visuoconstructive functions is problematic in MS because of concurrent peripheral visual impairments; motor deficits may also contribute to testing difficulties. Impairments in tests reliant on complex spatial stimuli, such as Raven's Progressive Matrices, have been detected by some authors (Rao *et al.*, 1991) but not others (Jennekens-Schinkel *et al.*, 1990). Visual form agnosia has been reported on occasion (Okuda *et al.*, 1996).

Praxis

Motor deficits (weakness, spasticity) may confound assessment of praxis in MS. Apraxia has occasionally been mentioned as a symptom (Herscovitch *et al.*, 1984; Okuda *et al.*, 1996). Callosal disconnection syndromes seem to be rare in MS (Schnider *et al.*, 1993), notwithstanding the predilection for corpus callosum involvement so evident on MR brain imaging.

Executive function

Tests of planning, problem solving, concept formation, utilization of feedback, and abstract reasoning, all of which may be subsumed under the heading of 'executive function' or cognitive flexibility (even though different skills and neuroanatomical substrates may be implicated), have been found to be impaired in some MS patients. On the Wisconsin Card Sorting Test, MS patients may show poor performance (Heaton *et al.*, 1985; Rao *et al.*, 1987, 1991), sufficient to differentiate them from healthy controls, perhaps more so in chronic progressive disease. Problem solving with Raven's Progressive Matrices is also impaired (Rao *et al.*, 1991), although this also tests visuospatial skills. Tests of verbal fluency, such as the COWAT, are affected (Rao *et al.*, 1991).

Whether it may be inferred that these deficits reflect 'frontal lobe' dysfunction in MS has been harder to answer. Poor performance on executive tasks could not be attributed solely to frontal lobe MR changes in one study, suggesting that there is a general effect of cerebral dysfunction on tasks such as WCST (Foong *et al.*, 1997). Moreover, because of the links of frontal cortex to subcortical structures (thalamus, basal ganglia), remote lesions might produce these symptoms, e.g. white matter lesions undercutting frontal-subcortical circuits.

Treatment of neuropsychological deficits

Little is currently known about the optimal treatment of cognitive disorders in MS. Options include disease-modifying agents, symptomatic treatments, and cognitive rehabilitation techniques including cognitive behavioural therapy (Amato & Zipoli, 2003). Increasingly cognitive measures are being included as endpoints in therapeutic trials. Occasionally, acute focal deficits may resolve following administration of steroids (Rozewicz *et al.*, 1996; Devere *et al.*, 2000), but generally deficits are more likely to accrue. Trials of 'disease-modifying drugs' have sometimes suggested benefits in particular cognitive domains, for example with the interferons (e.g. Pliskin *et al.*, 1996; Fischer *et al.*, 2000; Barak & Achiron, 2002), or stability of cognitive function over time, for example with glatiramer (Weinstein *et al.*, 1999).

Cholinesterase inhibitors (ChEIs), established agents in the treatment of Alzheimer's disease, have been suggested for use in MS (Porcel & Montalban, 2006). Small trials suggest that ChEIs may be helpful in MS patients with mild cognitive impairments (Krupp *et al.*, 2004). Functional imaging studies suggesting that ChEIs may modulate functional adaptive neuroplasticity in the MS brain (Parry *et al.*, 2003) may lend some support to the rationale for ChEI use in MS. However, changes in brain activation patterns observed on fMRI during cognitive testing in MS patients compared with controls may be interpreted as compensatory, adaptive responses, reflecting inherent brain neuroplasticity (Staffen *et al.*, 2002). Such changes may need to be taken into account when assessing whether MS disease-modifying drugs or ChEIs have any effect on cognitive function.

REFERENCES

Achiron A, Ziv I, Djaldetti R, *et. al.* Aphasia in multiple sclerosis: clinical and radiologic correlations. *Neurology* 1992; **42**: 2195–7.

Amato MP, Ponziani G, Pracucci G, *et al.* Cognitive impairment in early-onset multiple sclerosis. *Arch Neurol* 1995; **52**: 168–72

Amato MP, Zipoli V. Clinical management of cognitive impairment in multiple sclerosis: a review of current evidence. *Int MS J* 2003; **10** (3): 72–83.

Amato MP, Zipoli V, Portaccio E. Multiple sclerosis-related cognitive changes: a review of cross-sectional and longitudinal studies. *J Neurol Sci* 2006; **245**: 41–6.

Barak Y, Achiron A. Effect of interferon-beta-1b on cognitive functions in multiple sclerosis. *Eur Neurol* 2002; **47**: 11–14.

Beatty WW, Goodkin DE, Monson N, Beatty PA. Implicit learning in patients with chronic-progressive multiple sclerosis. *Int J Clin Neuropsychol* 1990; **12**: 153–62.

Beatty WW, Goodkin DE, Monson N, Beatty PA, Hertsgaard D. Anterograde and retrograde amnesia in patients with chronic progressive multiple sclerosis. *Arch Neurol* 1988; **42**: 611–19.

Benedict RHB, Fischer JS, Archibald CJ, *et al.* Minimal neuropsychological assessment of MS patients: a consensus approach. *Clin Neuropsychol* 2002; **16**: 381–97.

Bobholz JA, Gleason A. Cognitive dysfunction in multiple sclerosis. In: Gauthier S, Scheltens P, Cummings JL (eds.), *Alzheimer's Disease and Related Disorders Annual 5*. London: Taylor & Francis, 2006: 165–80.

Brinar VV, Poser CM, Basic S, Petelin Z. Sudden onset aphasic hemiplegia: an unusual manifestation of disseminated encephalomyelitis. *Clin Neurol Neurosurg* 2004; **106**: 187–96.

Calabrese P. Neuropsychology of multiple sclerosis: an overview. *J Neurol* 2006; **253** (Suppl 1): I/10–15.

Callanan M, Logsdail SJ, Ron MA, Warrington EK. Cognitive impairment in patients with clinically isolated lesions of the type seen in multiple sclerosis: a psychometric and MRI study. *Brain* 1989; **112**: 361–74.

Camp SJ, Stevenson VL, Thompson AJ, *et al.* A longitudinal study of cognition in primary progressive multiple sclerosis. *Brain* 2005; **128**: 2891–8.

Compston A, Coles A. Multiple sclerosis. *Lancet* 2002; **359**: 1221–31.

Compston A, Confavreux C, Lassmann H, *et al. McAlpine's Multiple Sclerosis* (4th edition). London: Churchill Livingstone, 2006.

Dalgleish AG. Viruses and multiple sclerosis. *Acta Neurol Scand* 1997; **169** (suppl): 8–15.

DeLuca J, Barbieri-Berger S, Johnson SK. The nature of memory impairments in multiple sclerosis: acquisition versus retrieval. *J Clin Exp Neuropsychol* 1994; **16**: 183–9.

Demaree HA, DeLuca J, Gaudino EA, Diamond BJ. Speed of information processing as a key deficit in multiple sclerosis: implications for rehabilitation. *J Neurol Neurosurg Psychiatry* 1999; **67**: 661–3.

D'Esposito M, Onishi K, Thompson H, *et al.* Working memory impairments in multiple sclerosis: evidence from a dual-task paradigm. *Neuropsychology* 1996; **10**: 51–6.

Devere TR, Trotter JL, Cross AH. Acute aphasia in multiple sclerosis. *Arch Neurol* 2000; **57**: 1207–9.

Di Majo L, Bisceglia M, Lanzillo R, *et al.* Aphasia as a rare presentation of monosymptomatic demyelinating disease: case report and review of the literature. *Neurol Sci* 2002; **23**: 79–82.

Erdem H, Stålberg E, Caglar I. Aphasia in multiple sclerosis. *Ups J Med Sci* 2001; **106**: 205–10.

Feinstein A. *The Clinical Neuropsychiatry of Multiple Sclerosis.* Cambridge: Cambridge University Press, 1999: 96–196.

Feinstein A, Feinstein KJ, Gray T, O'Connor P. Neurobehavioral correlates of pathological crying and laughing in multiple sclerosis. *Arch Neurol* 1997; **54**: 1116–21.

Feinstein A, Kartsounis L, Miller D, Youl B, Ron M. Clinically isolated lesions of the type seen in multiple sclerosis: a cognitive, psychiatric and MRI follow-up study. *J Neurol Neurosurg Psychiatry* 1992a; **55**: 869–76.

Feinstein A, Youl B, Ron M. Acute optic neuritis: a cognitive and magnetic resonance imaging study. *Brain* 1992b; **115**: 1403–15.

Fischer JS, Priore RL, Jacobs LD, *et al.* Neuropsychological effects of interferon beta-1a in relapsing multiple sclerosis. Multiple Sclerosis Collaborative Research Group. *Ann Neurol* 2000; **48**: 885–92.

Fischer JS, Rao SM. Assessment of neuropsychological function in multiple sclerosis. In: Cohen JA, Rudick RA (eds.), *Multiple Sclerosis Therapeutics* (3rd edition). Abingdon: Informa Healthcare, 2007: 79–99.

Foong J, Ron M. Cognitive impairment and neuropsychological assessment in multiple sclerosis. *Int MS J* 2000; **7** (1): 31–4.

Foong J, Rozewicz L, Quaghebeur G, *et al.* Executive function in multiple sclerosis. The role of frontal lobe pathology. *Brain* 1997; **120**: 15–26.

Foong J, Rozewicz L, Quaghebeur G, *et al.* Neuropsychological deficits in multiple sclerosis after acute relapse. *J Neurol Neurosurg Psychiatry* 1998; **64**: 529–32.

Franklin GM, Nelson LM, Filley CM, Heaton RK. Cognitive loss in multiple sclerosis: case reports and review of the literature. *Arch Neurol* 1989; **46**: 162–7.

Grafman J, Rao S, Bernardin L, Leo GJ. Automatic memory processes in patients with multiple sclerosis. *Arch Neurol* 1991; **48**: 1072–5.

Grant I, McDonald WI, Trimble MR, Smith E, Reed R. Deficient learning and memory in early and middle phases of multiple sclerosis. *J Neurol Neurosurg Psychiatry* 1984; **47**: 250–5.

Heaton RK, Nelson LM, Thompson DS, Burks JS, Franklin GM. Neuropsychological findings in relapsing–remitting and chronic–progressive multiple sclerosis. *J Consult Clin Psychol* 1985; **53**: 103–10.

Herscovitch P, Trotter JL, Lemann W, Raichle ME. Positron emission tomography (PET) in active MS: demonstration of demyelination and diaschisis. *Neurology* 1984; **34** (suppl 1): 78.

Hohol MJ, Guttmann CRG, Orav J, *et al.* Serial neuropsychological assessment and magnetic resonance imaging analysis in multiple sclerosis. *Arch Neurol* 1997; **54**: 1018–25.

Jennekens-Schinkel A, Laboyrie PM, Lanser JB, van der Velde EA. Cognition in patients with multiple sclerosis: after four years. *J Neurol Sci* 1990; **99**: 229–47.

Jønsson A, Andresen J, Storr L, *et al.* Cognitive impairment in newly diagnosed multiple sclerosis patients: a 4-year follow-up study. *J Neurol Sci* 2006; **245**: 77–85.

Kennedy PGE, Steiner I. On the possible viral aetiology of multiple sclerosis. *Q J Med* 1994; **87**: 523–8.

Kesselring J, Klement U. Cognitive and affective disturbances in multiple sclerosis. *J Neurol* 2001; **248**: 180–3.

Kidd D, Barkhof F, McConnell R, *et al.* Cortical lesions in multiple sclerosis. *Brain* 1999; **122**: 17–26.

Krupp LB, Christodoulou C, Melville P, *et al.* Donepezil improved memory in multiple sclerosis in a randomized clinical trial. *Neurology* 2004; **63**: 1579–85.

Kujala P, Portin R, Ruutiainen J. Language functions in incipient cognitive decline in multiple sclerosis. *J Neurol Sci* 1996; **141**: 79–86.

Kujala P, Portin R, Ruutiainen J. The progress of cognitive decline in multiple sclerosis: a controlled 3-year follow-up. *Brain* 1997; **120**: 289–97.

Kutzelnigg A, Lassmann H. Cortical demyelination in multiple sclerosis: a substrate for cognitive deficits? *J Neurol Sci* 2006; **245**: 123–6.

Lacour A, De Seze J, Revenco E, *et al.* Acute aphasia in multiple sclerosis: a multicenter study of 22 patients. *Neurology* 2004; **62**: 974–7.

Langdon DW. Cognitive dysfunction in multiple sclerosis: what are we measuring and why does it matter? In: Thompson AJ, Polman C, Hohlfeld R (eds.), *Multiple*

Sclerosis: Clinical Challenges and Controversies. London: Martin Dunitz, 1997: 253–63.

Larner AJ. Aetiological role of viruses in multiple sclerosis: a review. *J R Soc Med* 1986; **79**: 412–17.

Larner AJ, Lecky BRF. Acute aphasia in MS revisited. *Int MS J* 2007; **14**: 76–7.

Lensch E, Matzke M, Peteriet HF, *et al.* Identification and management of cognitive disorders in multiple sclerosis: a consensus approach. *J Neurol* 2006; **253** (suppl 1): I/29–31.

McDonald WI, Compston A, Edan G, *et al.* Recommended diagnostic criteria for multiple sclerosis: guidelines from the International Panel on the Diagnosis of Multiple Sclerosis. *Ann Neurol* 2001; **50**: 121–7.

McIntosh-Michaelis SA, Wilkinson SM, Diamond ID, *et al.* The prevalence of cognitive impairment in a community survey of multiple sclerosis. *Br J Clin Psychol* 1991; **30**: 333–48.

Maor Y, Olmer L, Mozes B. The relation between objective and subjective impairment in cognitive function among MS patients: the role of depression. *Multiple Sclerosis* 2001; **7**: 131–5.

Murdoch B, Theodoros D (eds.). *Speech and Language Disorders in Multiple Sclerosis*. London: Whurr, 2000.

Okuda B, Tanaka H, Tachibana H, *et al.* Visual form agnosia in multiple sclerosis. *Acta Neurol Scand* 1996; **94**: 38–44.

Parry AMM, Scott RB, Palace J, Smith S, Matthews PM. Potentially adaptive functional changes in cognitive processing for patients with multiple sclerosis and their acute modulation by rivastigmine. *Brain* 2003; **126**: 2750–60.

Pelosi L, Geesken JM, Holly M, Hayward M, Blumhardt LD. Working memory impairment in early multiple sclerosis: evidence from an event-related potential study of patients with clinically isolated myelopathy. *Brain* 1997; **120**: 2039–58.

Peyser JM, Rao SM, LaRocca NG, Kaplan E. Guidelines for neuropsychological research in multiple sclerosis. *Arch Neurol* 1990; **47**: 94–7.

Pliskin NH, Hamer DP, Goldstein DS, *et al.* Improved delayed visual reproduction test performance in multiple sclerosis patients receiving interferon beta-1b. *Neurology* 1996; **47**: 1463–8.

Polman CH, Reingold SC, Edan G, *et al.* Diagnostic criteria for multiple sclerosis: 2005 revisions to the McDonald criteria. *Ann Neurol* 2005; **58**: 840–6.

Porcel J, Montalban X. Anticholinesterasics [*sic*] in the treatment of cognitive impairment in multiple sclerosis. *J Neurol Sci* 2006; **245**: 177–81.

Primavera A, Gianelli MV, Bandini F. Aphasic status epilepticus in multiple sclerosis. *Eur Neurol* 1996; **36**: 374–7.

Rao SM. Neuropsychology of multiple sclerosis: a critical review. *J Clin Exp Neuropsychol* 1986; **8**: 503–42.

Rao SM. *A Manual for the Brief Repeatable Battery of Neuropsychological Tests in Multiple Sclerosis*. New York: National Multiple Sclerosis Society, 1990.

Rao SM. White matter disease and dementia. *Brain Cogn* 1996; **31**: 250–68.

Rao SM, Hammeke TA, Speech TJ. Wisconsin Card Sorting Test performance in relapsing–remitting and chronic–progressive multiple sclerosis. *J Consult Clin Psychol* 1987; **55**: 263–5.

Rao SM, Leo GJ, Bernadin L, Unversagt F. Cognitive dysfunction in multiple sclerosis. I. Frequency, patterns and predictions. *Neurology* 1991; **41**: 685–91.

Rao SM, Leo GJ, Haughton VM, St Aubin-Faubert P, Bernadin L. Correlation of magnetic resonance imaging with neuropsychological testing in multiple sclerosis. *Neurology* 1989a; **39**: 161–6.

Rao SM, Leo GJ, St Aubin-Faubert P. On the nature of memory disturbance in multiple sclerosis. *J Clin Exp Neuropsychol* 1989b; **11**: 699–712.

Rao SM, St Aubin-Faubert P, Leo GJ. Information processing speed in patients with multiple sclerosis. *J Clin Exp Neuropsychol* 1989c; **11**: 471–7.

Rovaris M, Filippi M, Falautano M, *et al.* Relation between MR abnormalities and patterns of cognitive impairment in multiple sclerosis. *Neurology* 1998; **50**: 1601–8.

Rozewicz L, Langdon DW, Davie CA, Thompson AJ, Ron MA. Resolution of left hemisphere cognitive dysfunction in multiple sclerosis with magnetic resonance correlates: a case report. *Cognit Neuropsychiatry* 1996; **1**: 17–25.

Sartori E, Edan G. Assessment of cognitive dysfunction in multiple sclerosis. *J Neurol Sci* 2006; **245**: 169–75.

Schnider A, Benson F, Rosner LJ. Callosal disconnection in multiple sclerosis. *Neurology* 1993; **43**: 1243–5.

Schulz D, Kopp B, Kunkel A, Faiss JH. Cognition in the early stage of multiple sclerosis. *J Neurol* 2006; **253**: 1002–10.

Spatt J, Goldenberg G, Mamoli B. Simple dysphasic seizures as the sole manifestation of relapse in multiple sclerosis. *Epilepsia* 1994; **35**: 1342–5.

Staffen W, Mair A, Zauner H, *et al.* Cognitive function and fMRI in patients with multiple sclerosis: evidence for compensatory cortical activation during an attention task. *Brain* 2002; **125**: 1275–82.

Summers M, Anderson VM, Fisniku L, *et al.* Predicting cognitive impairment in relapsing–remitting multiple sclerosis. *J Neurol* 2006; **253** (suppl 2): II/7 (abstract O35).

Swirsky-Sacchetti T, Field HL, Mitchell DR, *et al.* The sensitivity of the Mini-Mental State Examination in the white matter dementia of multiple sclerosis. *J Clin Psychol* 1992; **48**: 779–86.

Thornton AE, Raz N. Memory impairment in multiple sclerosis: a quantitative review. *Neuropsychology* 1997; **11**: 357–66.

Tinnefeld M, Treitz FH, Haase CG, *et al.* Attention and memory dysfunctions in mild multiple sclerosis. *Eur Arch Psychiatry Clin Neurosci* 2005; **255**: 319–26.

Trinka E, Unterberger I, Luef G, *et al.* Acute aphasia in multiple sclerosis. *Arch Neurol* 2001; **58**: 133–4.

Trinka E, Unterberger I, Spiegel M, *et al.* De novo aphasic status epilepticus as presenting symptom of multiple sclerosis. *J Neurol* 2002; **249**: 782–3.

Wacowius U, Talley M, Silver N, Heinze HJ, Sailer M. Cognitive impairment in primary and secondary progressive multiple sclerosis. *J Clin Exp Neuropsychol* 2005; **27**: 65–77.

Weinstein A, Schwid SI, Schiffer RB, *et al.* Neuropsychologic status in multiple sclerosis after treatment with glatiramer. *Arch Neurol* 1999; **56**: 319–24.

Wishart H, Sharpe D. Neuropsychological aspects of multiple sclerosis: a quantitative review. *J Clin Exp Neuropsychol* 1997; **19**: 810–24.

Zarei M, Chandran S, Compston A, Hodges J. Cognitive presentation of multiple sclerosis: evidence for a cortical variant. *J Neurol Neurosurg Psychiatry* 2003; **74**: 872–7.

Zivadinov R, Sepcic J, Nasuelli D, *et al.* A longitudinal study of brain atrophy and cognitive disturbances in the early phase of relapsing–remitting multiple sclerosis. *J Neurol Neurosurg Psychiatry* 2001; **70**: 773–80.

6.2 Acute disseminated encephalomyelitis (ADEM)

Acute disseminated encephalomyelitis (ADEM) is an inflammatory CNS disorder of presumed autoimmune aetiology. Although affecting mainly children, sometimes following infection or immunization, ADEM is also well recognized in adults (Wang *et al.*, 1996; Schwarz *et al.*, 2001; Höllinger *et al.*, 2002). Although usually a monophasic illness, multiphasic and recurrent variants have occasionally been described, making it difficult to differentiate ADEM from a first episode of multiple sclerosis (MS). Suggested operational criteria (Schwarz *et al.*, 2001) may be confounded in clinical practice (John *et al.*, 2003). The clinical picture is heterogeneous, with encephalopathy, focal neurological signs, and even psychosis being the presenting features. Aphasia has been reported as a presenting feature with hemiplegia, hemisensory deficit, and facial palsy (Brinar *et al.*, 2004), prompting the suggestion that acute aphasic presentations of MS may in fact be cases of ADEM.

REFERENCES

Brinar VV, Poser CM, Basic S, Petelin Z. Sudden onset aphasic hemiplegia: an unusual manifestation of disseminated encephalomyelitis. *Clin Neurol Neurosurg* 2004; **106**: 187–96.

Höllinger P, Sturzenegger M, Mathis J, Schroth G, Hess CW. Acute disseminated encephalomyelitis in adults: a reappraisal of clinical, CSF, EEG, and MRI findings. *J Neurol* 2002; **249**: 320–9.

John L, Khaleeli AA, Larner AJ. Acute disseminated encephalomyelitis: a riddle wrapped in a mystery inside an enigma. *Int J Clin Pract* 2003; **57**: 235–7.

Schwarz S, Mohr A, Knauth M, Wildemann B, Storch-Hagenlocher B. Acute disseminated encephalomyelitis: a follow-up study of 40 adult patients. *Neurology* 2001; **56**: 1313–18.

Wang PN, Fuh JL, Liu HC, Wang SJ. Acute disseminated encephalomyelitis in middle-aged or elderly patients. *Eur Neurol* 1996; **36**: 219–23.

6.3 Sarcoidosis

Sarcoidosis is a systemic immunologically mediated disorder of uncertain aetiology characterized pathologically by non-caseating epithelioid cell granulomata. The organs most commonly affected are the lymph nodes, lungs, liver, spleen, skin, and eyes. Neurosarcoidosis as one feature of systemic sarcoidosis is relatively rare (5–15% of cases), isolated intracranial disease even more so, the commonest neurological features being hypothalamic involvement and cranial nerve palsy (Nowak & Widenka, 2001).

Dementia as a presenting manifestation of sarcoidosis has been reported to be rare. Schielke *et al.* (2001) identified only 10 cases in addition to their own report, in which frontal-subcortical deficits were evident: apathy, bradyphrenia, verbal perseveration, impaired speech fluency, as well as memory difficulties, with associated paratonia, grasp reflex, and motor perseveration. All had abnormal CSF indices (raised protein, white cell count) where these were tested. The importance of obtaining tissue confirmation of diagnosis prior to commencement of steroid therapy and exclusion of CNS tuberculosis was emphasized. These patients were noted to be older at age of onset (> 50 years) than expected for sarcoidosis (median 35 years). In this context, it should be remembered that chance concurrence of dementia and sarcoidosis may occur: a patient with relatively indolent pulmonary sarcoidosis who developed Alzheimer's disease has been seen in the author's clinic.

Against this apparent rarity, in a series of 68 patients with or without systemic sarcoidosis, cognitive decline was reported to be the clinical presentation of neurosarcoidosis in seven (10%) patients (Zajicek *et al.*, 1999). The alleged rarity of dementia as the presentation of neurosarcoidosis has also been questioned by Flowers *et al.* (2006), who reported five biopsy-confirmed patients. The index case presented at age 29 years with short-term and spatial memory difficulties. Neuropsychological assessment showed impaired mental tracking, concentration, cognitive speed, and memory retrieval, as well as subtle expressive language difficulties. Improvement was reported with immunosuppression, the authors suggesting that sarcoidosis is a treatable cause of cognitive impairment.

Neurosarcoidosis causing an isolated amnesic syndrome has been reported (Willigers & Kohler, 1993), but without neuropsychological assessment and with diagnosis based on histological appearances of a skin lesion. Focal cognitive deficits related to the rare presentation of sarcoidosis as a cerebral mass lesion ('sarcoid tumour': Larner *et al.*, 1999) or as cerebral haemorrhage related to thrombocytopenia (Larner, 1990) might also be anticipated.

REFERENCES

Flowers JM, Omer SM, Wren DW, Al-Memar AY. Neurosarcoidosis presenting with cognitive impairment: a series of five cases. *J Neurol Neurosurg Psychiatry* 2006; **77**: 128 (abstract 010).

Larner AJ. Life-threatening thrombocytopenia in sarcoidosis. *BMJ* 1990; **300**: 317–19.

Larner AJ, Ball JA, Howard RS. Sarcoid tumour: continuing diagnostic problems in the MRI era. *J Neurol Neurosurg Psychiatry* 1999; **66**: 510–12.

Nowak DA, Widenka DC. Neurosarcoidosis: a review of its intracranial manifestation. *J Neurol* 2001; **248**: 363–72.

Schielke E, Nolte C, Muller W, Bruck W. Sarcoidosis presenting as a rapidly progressive dementia: clinical and neuropathological evaluation. *J Neurol* 2001; **248**: 522–4.

Willigers P, Kohler P. Amnesic syndrome caused by neurosarcoidosis. *Clin Neurol Neurosurg* 1993; **95**: 131–5.

Zajicek JP, Scolding NJ, Foster O, *et al.* Central nervous system sarcoidosis: diagnosis and management. *Q J Med* 1999; **92**: 103–17.

6.4 Systemic lupus erythematosus (SLE)

Systemic lupus erythematosus (SLE) is a multisystem autoimmune disorder of the collagen vascular disease group, seldom associated with true vasculitis, with systemic, dermatological, rheumatological, renal, pulmonary, cardiac, and haematological, as well as neurological, complications (Scolding & Joseph, 2002). Diagnostic criteria for SLE have been formulated (Tan *et al.*, 1982) and revised (Hochberg, 1997).

Neurological features may affect both the CNS (delirium, psychosis, headache, cerebrovascular disease, myelopathy, movement disorder, demyelination, seizures, aseptic meningitis) and the PNS (cranial neuropathy, polyneuropathy, plexopathy, mononeuropathy/multiplex, Guillain–Barré syndrome, autonomic neuropathy, myasthenia gravis) (ACR Ad Hoc Committee on Neuropsychiatric Lupus Nomenclature, 1999; West, 2002). Because of the frequency of neuropsychiatric complications, nervous system involvement is sometimes referred to as 'NP-SLE'. What contribution antiphospholipid antibodies, which are found in 30% of SLE cases, make to these clinical features is uncertain (see Hughes' syndrome (primary antiphospholipid antibody syndrome), Section 3.6.8).

Cognitive dysfunction is said to be common in SLE: up to 66% of adult SLE patients without a history of NP-SLE have 'mild cognitive impairment', usually subclinical and conforming to no specific pattern, and many patients with a previous history of NP-SLE have significant cognitive dysfunction which may progress to dementia, possibly due to active CNS disease, 'burned-out' NP-SLE, and/or multiple infarcts (Carbotte *et al.*, 1986; Kozora *et al.*, 1996; Denburg *et al.*, 1997). One longitudinal study found cognitive impairment in around one-third of SLE patients in 'stable neurological condition' with or without neuropsychiatric symptoms, deficits which persisted at retest (mean interval between assessments 21.5 months), suggesting that cognitive impairment is a consistent finding of CNS involvement in SLE. No relationship with neuropsychiatric disorder, neuroradiological findings, disease activity, or use of immunosuppressive therapy was found. The most sensitive tests were those examining visuospatial reasoning and visuoconstructive function (Carlomagno *et al.*, 2000). Another study found that cognitive impairments in SLE patients included attentional skills, psychomotor speed, and abstract problem solving, in other words executive function. This was felt to be largely due to cerebral infarction, and hence potentially amenable to prevention with anticoagulation (Waterloo *et al.*, 2001). Focal, cortical-type, deficits may also occur: a case of Gerstmann syndrome (finger agnosia, right–left confusion,

agraphia, acalculia) with an appropriately placed white matter lesion (left parieto-occipital, underlying the angular gyrus) due to SLE has been reported (Jung *et al.*, 2001). An amnesic syndrome mimicking limbic encephalitis has also been reported (Stubgen, 1998). Relatively isolated autobiographical amnesia in a patient with SLE and temporal lobe epilepsy is reported (Kapur, 2001), but the cognitive syndrome may have been incidental to the SLE, since the limited clinical details were not suggestive of NP-SLE.

The possible role of inflammatory and hormonal factors in the cognitive impairments of SLE has been suggested by a study of patients without neuropsychiatric symptoms ('non-CNS SLE') who nonetheless had lower learning and attention scores, which were related to these biochemical measures (Kozora *et al.*, 2001). If inflammatory factors are involved in the pathogenesis of cognitive impairment, this may have implications for reversibility (Hanly *et al.*, 1997), other than in multi-infarct disease (Briley *et al.*, 1989).

REFERENCES

ACR Ad Hoc Committee on Neuropsychiatric Lupus Nomenclature. The American College of Rheumatology nomenclature and case definitions for neuropsychiatric lupus syndromes. *Arthritis Rheum* 1999; **42**: 599–608.

Briley DP, Coull BM, Goodnight SHJ. Neurological disease associated with antiphospholipid antibodies. *Ann Neurol* 1989; **25**: 221–7.

Carbotte RM, Denburg SD, Denburg JA. Prevalence of cognitive impairment in systemic lupus erythematosus. *J Nerv Ment Dis* 1986; **174**: 357–64.

Carlomagno S, Migliaresi S, Ambrosone L, *et al.* Cognitive impairment in systemic lupus erythematosus: a follow-up study. *J Neurol* 2000; **247**: 273–9.

Denburg SD, Carbotte RM, Denburg JA. Psychological aspects of systemic lupus erythematosus: cognitive function, mood, and self-report. *J Rheumatol* 1997; **24**: 998–1003.

Hanly JG, Cassell K, Fisk JD. Cognitive function in systemic lupus erythematosus: results of a 5-year prospective study. *Arthritis Rheum* 1997; **40**: 1542–3.

Hochberg MC. Updating the American College of Rheumatology revised criteria for the classification of systemic lupus erythematosus. *Arthritis Rheum* 1997; **40**: 1725.

Jung RE, Yeo RA, Sibbitt WL Jr, *et al.* Gerstmann syndrome in systemic lupus erythematosus: neuropsychological, neuroimaging and spectroscopic findings. *Neurocase* 2001; **7**: 515–21.

Kapur N. Autobiographical amnesia and temporal lobe pathology. In: Parkin AJ (ed.), *Case Studies in the Neuropsychology of Memory*. Hove: Psychology Press, 1997: 37–62 [at 43–7].

Kozora E, Laudenslager M, Lemieux A, West SG. Inflammatory and hormonal measures predict neuropsychological functioning in systemic lupus erythematosus and rheumatoid arthritis patients. *J Int Neuropsychol Soc* 2001; **7**: 745–54.

Kozora E, Thompson L, West S, *et al.* Analysis of cognitive and psychological deficits in systemic lupus erythematosus patients without overt central nervous system disease. *Arthritis Rheum* 1996; **39**: 2035–45.

Scolding NJ, Joseph FG. The neuropathology and pathogenesis of systemic lupus erythematosus. *Neuropathol Appl Neurobiol* 2002; **28**: 173–89.

Stubgen JP. Nervous system lupus mimics limbic encephalitis. *Lupus* 1998; **7**: 557–60.

Tan EM, Cohen AS, Fries JF, *et al.* The 1982 revised criteria for the classification of systemic lupus erythematosus. *Arthritis Rheum* 1982; **25**: 1271–7.

Waterloo K, Omdal R, Sjoholm H, *et al.* Neuropsychological dysfunction in systemic lupus erythematosus is not associated with changes in cerebral blood flow. *J Neurol* 2001; **248**: 595–602.

West SG. Systemic lupus erythematosus and the nervous system. In: Wallace DJ, Hahn BH (eds.), *Dubois' Lupus Erythematosus* (6th edition). Philadelphia: Lippincott Williams & Wilkins, 2002: 693–738 [esp. 702–3].

6.5   Sjögren's syndrome

Sjögren's syndrome is a chronic autoimmune disorder of the exocrine glands associated with lymphocytic infiltrates, occurring either alone (primary Sjögren's syndrome) or in the presence of another autoimmune disorder such as rheumatoid arthritis, SLE, or progressive systemic sclerosis (secondary Sjögren's syndrome). Extraglandular manifestations may occur in skin, lung, heart, kidneys, and nervous system, both central and peripheral (Fox, 2005). Diagnostic criteria (Vitali, 2003) include ocular and oral symptoms, objective evidence of dry eyes and salivary gland involvement, and laboratory abnormalities (at least one of anti SS-A (anti-Ro) or SS-B (anti-La), ANA, IgM RhF).

Neurological manifestations occur in about 20% of patients and include CNS involvement, cranial nerve palsies, myelopathy, peripheral neuropathy (especially sensory, including a ganglionopathy), and a multiple-sclerosis-like syndrome (Delalande *et al.*, 2004). Abnormalities may be found on neuropsychological tests, particularly of frontal lobe function and memory, which correlate with defects on functional imaging with SPECT when MR imaging is normal; hence it has been argued that neuropsychological testing is the most sensitive test for CNS involvement in Sjögren's (Belin *et al.*, 1999). However, similar deficits on functional imaging have been reported in patients with or without 'psychoneurological' symptoms (Lass *et al.*, 2000).

Isolated cognitive impairment has been described in Sjögren's syndrome. The pattern of neuropsychological impairment in one series of patients was fairly homogeneous, with either subcorticofrontal or corticosubcortical dysfunction. In the former group there was normal intellectual quotient, normal memory and visuoconstructional skills but impaired attention control, abstraction, response inhibition, and set-shifting abilities (i.e. dysexecutive frontal-type pattern); in the latter there was additional intellectual decline and poor visuoconstructional abilities, associated with overt signs of CNS involvement (spastic tetraparesis, pseudobulbar syndrome, cerebellar syndrome). MR brain imaging was normal or showed only non-specific punctate periventricular white matter high signal intensities on T_2-weighted scans, with normal findings in CSF or only mild protein elevation (Lafitte *et al.*, 2001). Cases mimicking Alzheimer's disease have also been reported, but retrospectively certain features were identified that argued against AD, including no disproportionate loss of memory or anomia, and presence of cognitive fluctuation, psychotic features, and somatic symptoms and signs such as tremor, hyperreflexia, and gait ataxia (Caselli *et al.*, 1993).

REFERENCES

Belin C, Moroni C, Caillat-Vigneron N, *et al.* Central nervous system involvement in Sjögren's syndrome: evidence from neuropsychological testing and HMPAO-SPECT. *Ann Med Interne Paris* 1999; **150**: 598–604.

Caselli RJ, Scheithauer BW, O'Duffy JD, *et al.* Chronic inflammatory meningoencephalitis should not be mistaken for Alzheimer's disease. *Mayo Clin Proc* 1993; **68**: 846–53.

Delalande S, de Seze J, Fauchais AL, *et al.* Neurologic manifestations in primary Sjögren's syndrome: a study of 82 patients. *Medicine (Baltimore)* 2004; **83**: 280–91.

Fox RI. Sjögren's syndrome. *Lancet* 2005; **366**: 321–31.

Lafitte C, Amoura Z, Cacoub P, *et al.* Neurological complications of primary Sjögren's syndrome. *J Neurol* 2001; **248**: 577–84.

Lass P, Krajka-Lauer J, Homziak M, *et al.* Cerebral blood flow in Sjögren's syndrome using 99Tcm-HMPAO brain SPET. *Nucl Med Commun* 2000; **21**: 31–5.

Vitali C. Classification criteria for Sjögren's syndrome. *Ann Rheum Dis* 2003; **62**: 94–5.

6.6 Behçet's disease

Behçet's disease is a recurrent systemic inflammatory disorder of unknown aetiology, diagnostic criteria for which include recurrent aphthous ulceration plus any two of genital ulceration, skin lesions (such as erythema nodosum), eye involvement (anterior or posterior uveitis or retinal vasculitis), and positive pathergy test (skin hypersensitivity to pin prick) (International Study Group for Behçet's Disease, 1990). Neuro-Behçet's disease, confined almost entirely to the central rather than the peripheral nervous system, occurs in about 5% of cases. Involvement may be defined as either parenchymal or non-parenchymal, the former affecting particularly the brainstem with ataxia, dysarthria, hemi-

paresis, and pyramidal signs, with accompanying or preceding cognitive and neuropsychiatric changes. Non-parenchymal involvement usually takes the form of intracranial hypertension due to dural sinus thrombosis, wherein cognitive evaluation is usually normal (Akman-Demir & Serdaroglu, 2002; Kidd *et al.*, 1999).

If sought, cognitive impairments may be common in neuro-Behçet's disease. For example, of 74 patients tested in a cohort of 200, 65 were abnormal, the most common impairments being in memory (verbal and visual), attention, and frontal lobe functions, with relative sparing of orientation, language, arithmetic, and visuospatial function (Akman-Demir *et al.*, 1999). In a more detailed analysis of 12 patients with neuro-Behçet's disease, memory deficit was the commonest finding, particularly delayed recall of both verbal and visual material, suggesting a retrieval deficit, although acquisition and storage were also affected. Attention and executive function deficits also occurred, whilst language and visuospatial function were largely spared. Neuropsychological deficits were evident before detectable changes on structural brain imaging, and insidious deterioration was observed independent of neurological relapses (Oktem-Tanör *et al.*, 1999). Another series noted cognitive and/or behavioural features in 16% of patients, a frequency less common than headache, upper motor neurone type weakness, and brainstem and cerebellar signs (Siva *et al.*, 2001). A case of Behçet's disease resembling herpes simplex encephalitis has been reported (Hasegawa *et al.*, 2005).

Cognitive deficits may also be common in Behçet's patients without overt neurological involvement: Monastero *et al.* (2004) found deficits in almost half of a cohort of 26 patients, memory being the domain most affected, although visuospatial skills were also impaired relative to controls. High disease activity and high prednisolone dosage were independently associated with cognitive impairment after adjustment for demographic variables.

Reports of dementia in neuro-Behçet's disease are rare (Wakayama, 2004), possibly because of the predilection for brainstem disease (although lesions isolated to the brainstem have been associated with cognitive impairment in cerebrovascular disease and central pontine myelinolysis). However, severe neurological prognosis, including dementia, has been reported to be the norm by some authors (Wechsler *et al.*, 1999).

REFERENCES

Akman-Demir G, Serdaroglu P. Neuro-Behçet's disease: a practical approach to diagnosis and treatment. *Pract Neurol* 2002; **2**: 340–7.

Akman-Demir G, Serdaroglu P, Taşçi B, and the Neuro-Behçet Study Group. Clinical patterns of neurological involvement in Behçet's disease: evaluation of 200 patients. *Brain* 1999; **122**: 2171–81.

Hasegawa T, Kanno S, Kato M, *et al.* Neuro-Behçet's disease presenting initially as mesiotemporal lesions mimicking herpes simplex encephalitis. *Eur J Neurol* 2005; **12**: 661–2.

International Study Group for Behçet's Disease. Criteria for the diagnosis of Behçet's disease. *Lancet* 1990; **335**: 1078–80.

Kidd D, Steuer A, Denman AM, Rudge P. Neurological complications in Behçet's syndrome. *Brain* 1999; **122**: 2183–94.

Monastero R, Camarda C, Pipia C, *et al.* Cognitive impairment in Behçet's disease patients without overt neurological involvement. *J Neurol Sci* 2004; **220**: 99–104.

Oktem-Tanör O, Baykan-Kurt B, Gurvit IH, Akman-Demir G, Serdaroglu P. Neuropsychological follow-up of 12 patients with neuro-Behçet disease. *J Neurol* 1999; **246**: 113–19.

Siva A, Kantarci OH, Saip S, *et al.* Behçet's disease: diagnostic and prognostic aspects of neurological involvement. *J Neurol* 2001; **248**: 95–103.

Wakayama Y. Dementia due to Behçet's disease [in Japanese]. *Nippon Rinsho* 2004; **62** (suppl): 445–8.

Wechsler B, Gerber S, Vidailhet M, Dormont D. Neurologic manifestations of Behçet's disease [in French]. *Ann Med Interne Paris* 1999; **150**: 555–61.

6.7   Rheumatoid arthritis (RhA)

CNS involvement is rare in rheumatoid arthritis (RhA), but not unheard of, as exemplified by meningeal or parenchymal nodules, vasculitis. Rheumatoid arthritis with cerebral vasculitis causing Gerstmann syndrome and dementia has been reported (Ramos & Mandybur, 1975). An inverse relation between RhA and Alzheimer's disease has been suggested, admittedly in a highly selected inpatient geriatric population (Jenkinson *et al.*, 1989).

Because of the rarity of CNS involvement, RhA patients are sometimes used in studies of cognitive deficits in other disorders in order to control for chronic, inflammatory, but non-CNS disease (e.g. Kozora *et al.*, 2001). However, in a study of the prevalence of cognitive impairment in multiple sclerosis, in a control group of RhA patients included to control for any possible effects of depression related to chronic illness, 12% of the RhA group were found to be impaired (McIntosh-Michaelis *et al.*, 1991). Whether inflammatory mediators may contribute to these deficits remains uncertain (Kozora *et al.*, 2001).

REFERENCES

Jenkinson ML, Bliss MR, Brain AT, Scott DL. Rheumatoid arthritis and senile dementia of the Alzheimer's type. *Br J Rheumatol* 1989; **28**: 86–8.

Kozora E, Laudenslager M, Lemieux A, West SG. Inflammatory and hormonal measures predict neuropsychological functioning in systemic lupus erythematosus and rheumatoid arthritis patients. *J Int Neuropsychol Soc* 2001; **7**: 745–54.

McIntosh-Michaelis SA, Wilkinson SM, Diamond ID, *et al.* The prevalence of cognitive impairment in a community survey of multiple sclerosis. *Br J Clin Psychol* 1991; **30**: 333–48.

Ramos M, Mandybur TI. Cerebral vasculitis and rheumatoid arthritis. *Arch Neurol* 1975; **32**: 271–5.

6.8   Scleroderma, systemic sclerosis

CNS involvement is rare in this disorder, which is characterized by excess collagen deposition in blood vessels. Occasional cases associated with dementia and cerebrovascular calcification have been reported (Héron *et al.*, 1998). A vasospastic mechanism was suggested in a patient with scleroderma and Raynaud's phenomenon who suffered two episodes of transient global amnesia (Nishida *et al.*, 1990).

REFERENCES

Héron E, Fornes P, Rance A, *et al*. Brain involvement in scleroderma: two autopsy cases. *Stroke* 1998; **29**: 719–21.

Nishida A, Kaiya H, Uematsu M, *et al*. Transient global amnesia and Raynaud's phenomenon in scleroderma. *Acta Neurol Scand* 1990; **81**: 550–2.

6.9 Relapsing polychondritis

This rare disorder, characterized by recurrent episodes of inflammation of the cartilage of ear, nose, trachea, and larynx, as enshrined in proposed clinical diagnostic criteria (McAdam *et al.*, 1976), may be complicated by systemic and cerebral vasculitis, with clinical presentations including aseptic meningitis, encephalopathy, seizures, stroke, and transient ischaemic attacks. Cases with cognitive impairment due to a non-paraneoplastic limbic encephalitis have been reported (Fujiki *et al.*, 2004; Ohta *et al.*, 2004; Irani *et al.*, 2006).

REFERENCES

Fujiki F, Tsuboi Y, Hashimoto K, *et al*. Non-herpetic limbic encephalitis associated with relapsing polychondritis. *J Neurol Neurosurg Psychiatry* 2004; **75**: 1646–7.

Irani SR, Soni A, Beynon H, Athwal BS. Relapsing 'encephalo' polychondritis. *Pract Neurol* 2006; **6**: 372–5.

McAdam LP, O'Hanlan MA, Bluestone R, Pearson CM. Relapsing polychondritis: prospective study of 23 patients and a review of the literature. *Medicine (Baltimore)* 1976; **55**: 193–215.

Ohta Y, Nagano I, Niiya D, *et al*. Nonparaneoplastic limbic encephalitis with relapsing polychondritis. *J Neurol Sci* 2004; **220**: 85–8.

6.10 Cerebral vasculitides

The vasculitides are inflammatory disorders of blood vessels, probably of autoimmune origin. Vasculitis may be exclusive to the CNS, as in primary or isolated angiitis of the CNS (PACNS), also known as intracranial vasculitis or, in older texts, granulomatous angiitis (Schmidley, 2000), but more commonly CNS involvement is part of a systemic disorder (Younger, 2004). Primary vasculitides include polyarteritis nodosa, Churg–Strauss syndrome, Wegener's granulomatosis, giant cell (temporal) arteritis, and Takayasu's arteritis. Connective tissue disorders may also be complicated by vasculitis, such as rheumatoid arthritis, systemic lupus erythematosus, Sjögren's syndrome, progressive systemic sclerosis, and dermatomyositis/polymyositis. Vasculitis is also recognized secondary to certain infections, neoplasias, and toxins/drugs (Moore & Richardson, 1998).

REFERENCES

Moore PM, Richardson B. Neurology of the vasculitides and connective tissue diseases. *J Neurol Neurosurg Psychiatry* 1998; **65**: 10–22.

Schmidley JW. *Central Nervous System Angiitis*. Boston: Butterworth-Heinemann, 2000.

Younger DS. Vasculitis of the nervous system. *Curr Opin Neurol* 2004; **17**: 317–36.

6.10.1 Primary angiitis of the CNS (PACNS)

Dementia may be a feature of pathologically confirmed PACNS (Koo & Massey, 1988; Chu *et al.*, 1998), and this disorder is occasionally the neuropathological substrate for dementia of unknown cause submitted to brain biopsy (Warren *et al.*, 2005). 'Rapidly progressive dementia' as the presentation of primary (isolated) angiitis of the CNS has been reported (Castelnovo *et al.*, 2001), although one wonders whether this was a disease-related encephalopathy, since intermittent confusion, and behavioural and psychiatric symptoms are not uncommon in PACNS. Dementia evolving in a patient with biopsy-proven but quiescent angiitis may reflect a second pathology such as Alzheimer's disease (Brotman *et al.*, 2000).

Cognitive problems are reported to be prominent in the rare syndrome of Aβ-related angiitis (ABRA), a granulomatous angiitis resembling PACNS with additional sporadic amyloid-β-peptide-related cerebral amyloid angiopathy. Alterations in mental status were common in ABRA and, although not systematically examined, were said to include confusion, and poor memory and concentration, sometimes progressing to frank dementia that was sometimes diagnosed premortem as Alzheimer's disease (Scolding *et al.*, 2005).

REFERENCES

Brotman DJ, Eberhart CG, Burger PC, McArthur JC, Hellmann DB. Primary angiitis of the central nervous system and Alzheimer's disease: clinically and pathologically evident in a single patient. *J Rheumatol* 2000; **27**: 2935–7.

Castelnovo G, Bouldy S, Vladut M, Marty-Double C, Labauge P. Rapidly progressive dementia disclosing primary angiitis of the central nervous system [in French]. *Ann Med Interne Paris* 2001; **152**: 273–5.

Chu CT, Gray L, Goldstein LB, Hulette CM. Diagnosis of intracranial vasculitis: a multi-disciplinary approach. *J Neuropathol Exp Neurol* 1998; **57**: 30–8.

Koo EH, Massey EW. Granulomatous angiitis of the central nervous system: protean manifestations and response to treatment. *J Neurol Neurosurg Psychiatry* 1988; **51**: 1126–33.

Scolding NJ, Joseph F, Kirby PA, *et al.* Aβ-related angiitis: primary angiitis of the central nervous system associated with cerebral amyloid angiopathy. *Brain* 2005; **128**: 500–15.

Warren JD, Schott JM, Fox NC, *et al.* Brain biopsy in dementia. *Brain* 2005; **128**: 2016–25.

6.10.2 Systemic vasculitides

The systemic vasculitides may be classified according to the size of the affected blood vessels (Scolding, 1999; Siva, 2001):

- large arteries: giant cell arteritis; Takayasu's arteritis
- medium arteries: Kawasaki disease; classical polyarteritis nodosa
- small vessels and medium arteries: Wegener's granulomatosis; Churg–Strauss syndrome; microscopic polyangiitis
- small vessels: Henoch–Schonlein purpura; essential cryoglobulinaemia; cutaneous leukocytoclastic vasculitis

Some of these systemic vasculitides may be accompanied by autoantibodies directed against constituents of the neutrophil azurophil granules (ANCA): cytoplasmic ANCA (c-ANCA) is associated with Wegener's granulomatosis with approximately 95% specificity; perinuclear ANCA (p-ANCA) directed at myeloperoxidase is found in microscopic polyangiitis and Churg–Strauss syndrome with lesser specificity. A distinction may be drawn between primary disorders and vasculitides occurring secondary to infection (e.g. hepatitis B, syphilis, HIV), drugs (e.g. sulphonamides, cocaine), or other connective tissue disorder (e.g. rheumatoid arthritis, SLE, Sjögren's syndrome). ANCA assays are sometimes positive in SLE (Joseph & Scolding, 2002).

Neurological presentations of systemic vasculitis are very diverse, but those affecting the CNS generally manifest as an acute or subacute encephalopathy, or as an 'MS-like' relapsing–remitting disorder with features atypical for multiple sclerosis such as seizures and headache, or as a rapidly progressive space-occupying lesion (Scolding *et al.*, 1997). Cognitive disorders are unusual, but occasionally described.

Occasional reports of dementia as a symptom, sometimes the presentation, of giant cell arteritis (GCA) have appeared, the dementia presumed to reflect multiple infarctions, sometimes in association with bilateral carotid artery occlusion, but without brain pathology to confirm the supposition (Howard *et al.*, 1984; Gamboa *et al.*, 1991; Mouritsen & Junker, 1991; Pascual *et al.*, 1992; Morris & Lockie, 2005). If this occurs it must be rare: GCA typically affects the extracranial carotid artery, and stroke is an uncommon vasculitic complication which usually involves the posterior intracranial circulation. Moreover, most patients with GCA are over 50 years of age so there may be other, confounding, factors which might contribute to cognitive decline. CNS involvement in Takayasu's arteritis is due to carotid stenosis, cerebral hypoperfusion, and subclavian steal syndrome.

Diffuse encephalopathy with cognitive decline and seizures or stroke-like episodes may occur in polyarteritis nodosa. Dementia in the context of lymphocytic meningitis and encephalitis has been reported in polyarteritis nodosa, reversing after immunosuppressive treatment (Harlé *et al.*, 1991). Encephalopathy and stroke-like episodes may occur in Churg–Strauss syndrome, although peripheral nervous system involvement is more common. Rapid-onset dementia with microscopic polyangiitis, ascribed to CNS small vessel disease but without pathological proof, and also causing peripheral neuropathy, has been described, with some patients improving cognitively following institution of immunosuppressive therapy (Capra *et al.*, 1998).

Cerebral vasculitis as a cause of Gerstmann syndrome and dementia in a patient with rheumatoid arthritis has been reported (Ramos & Mandybur, 1975). Cerebral vasculitis causing severe autobiographical amnesia but with preserved semantic memory has also been documented (Evans *et al.*, 1996).

In a group of non-demented patients with ANCA-associated small vessel vasculitides (Wegener's granulomatosis, Churg–Strauss syndrome, microscopic polyangiitis), neuropsychological testing revealed subclinical deficits in abstract reasoning, speed of information processing, and visual memory in just under a third of patients, the suggestion being that small vessel vasculitis may mediate subcortical brain damage (Mattioli *et al.*, 2002).

REFERENCES

Capra R, Gregorini G, Mattioli F, Santostefano M, Galluzzi S. Rapid onset dementia in patients with microscopic polyangiitis. *J Neurol* 1998; **245**: 397 (abstract P64).

Evans JJ, Breen EK, Antoun N, Hodges JR. Focal retrograde amnesia for autobiographical events following cerebral vasculitis: a connectionist account. *Neurocase* 1996; **2**: 1–12.

Gamboa F., Iriarte LM, Garcia-Bragado F, *et al.* Multiinfarct dementia in giant cell arteritis (temporal arteritis) [in Spanish]. *Med Clin Barc* 1991; **97**: 617–19.

Harlé JR, Disdier P, Ali Cherif A, *et al.* Curable dementia and panarteritis nodosa [in French]. *Rev Neurol Paris* 1991; **147**: 148–50.

Howard GF, Ho SU, Kim KS, Wallach J. Bilateral carotid artery occlusion resulting from giant cell arteritis. *Ann Neurol* 1984; **15**: 204–7.

Joseph FG, Scolding NJ. Cerebral vasculitis: a practical approach. *Pract Neurol* 2002; **2**: 80–93.

Mattioli F, Capra R, Rovaris M, *et al.* Frequency and patterns of subclinical cognitive impairment in patients with ANCA-associated small vessel vasculitides. *J Neurol Sci* 2002; **195**: 161–6.

Morris OC, Lockie P. Giant cell arteritis: presenting as stroke, transient ischaemic attack and dementia. *Aust Fam Physician* 2005; **34**: 653–5.

Mouritsen M, Junker P. Reversible dementia caused by giant cell arteritis [in Danish]. *Ugeskr Laeg* 1991; **153**: 2572.

Pascual JM, Cantero J, Boils P, Solanas JV, Redón J. Dementia as a presentation symptom of giant cell arteritis [in Spanish]. *An Med Interna* 1992; **9**: 39–40.

Ramos M, Mandybur TI. Cerebral vasculitis and rheumatoid arthritis. *Arch Neurol* 1975; **32**: 271–5.

Scolding N. Cerebral vasculitis. In: Scolding N (ed.), *Immunological and Inflammatory Disorders of the Central Nervous System*. Oxford: Butterworth-Heinemann, 1999: 210–57.

Scolding NJ, Jayne DRW, Zajicek JP, *et al.* Cerebral vasculitis: recognition, diagnosis and management. *Q J Med* 1997; **90**: 61–73.

Siva A. Vasculitis of the nervous system. *J Neurol* 2001; **248**: 451–68.

6.11 Sydenham's chorea, paediatric autoimmune neuropsychiatric disorders associated with streptococcal infections (PANDAS)

Postinfectious (post-streptococcal) movement and neuropsychiatric disorders of autoimmune origin have been increasingly recognized in recent times. The neuropsychiatric features usually reported have been those of obsessive-compulsive disorder, but the spectrum of psychiatric symptoms is widening (Martino & Giovannoni, 2005). Basal ganglia (striatal) involvement may be observed on structural and functional imaging (hyperperfusion and hypermetabolism). Neuropsychological deficits do not seem to be a clinical feature of these conditions, although dementia associated with striatal hypermetabolism and the detection of antistriatal antibodies which reversed with steroids has been reported (Léger et al., 2004). Cases clinically resembling Sydenham's chorea, with additional dementia associated with antiphospholipid antibodies, have also been described (Van Horn et al., 1996).

REFERENCES

Léger GC, Johnson N, Horowitz SW, et al. Dementia-like presentation of striatal hypermetabolic state with antistriatal antibodies responsive to steroids. Arch Neurol 2004; **61**: 754–7.

Martino D, Giovannoni G. Autoaggressive immune-mediated movement disorders. Adv Neurol 2005; **96**: 320–35.

Van Horn G, Arnett FC, Dimachkie MM. Reversible dementia and chorea in a young woman with the lupus anticoagulant. Neurology 1996; **46**: 1599–603.

6.12   Limbic encephalitis

Limbic encephalitis is a syndrome of subacute onset characterized by cognitive decline, particularly memory impairment, due to limbic system involvement, with or without additional epileptic seizures of temporal lobe origin and MR imaging evidence of signal change in the limbic system, particularly the hippocampus. Initially described as a remote effect of occult neoplasia (paraneoplasia), a similar picture may also result from infective and autoimmune pathologies (Schott, 2006).

REFERENCES

Schott JM. Limbic encephalitis: a clinician's guide. Pract Neurol 2006; **6**: 143–53.

6.12.1   Paraneoplastic limbic encephalitis (PNLE)

Paraneoplastic limbic encephalitis (PNLE) was first described as such in the 1960s (Corsellis et al., 1968). The syndrome is most often associated with lung tumours but also with breast and testicular neoplasms, and a variety of onconeural antibodies may be found, including anti-Hu, anti-Ma2, and ANNA-3, although their absence does not exclude the diagnosis (Gultekin et al., 2000; Lawn et al., 2003). Whole-body PET scanning may identify an occult tumour when other imaging modalities have been negative (Rees et al., 2001). Detailed reports of neuropsychological assessment in PNLE are relatively few, perhaps because of concurrent confusion, altered consciousness, and psychiatric features precluding assessment. Martin et al. (1996) found severe anterograde amnesia for both verbal and visual information but preserved visual perception and construction, language, speed of information processing, and verbal abstract reasoning, all consistent with pathology confined to the mesial temporal lobes. A case with topographical disorientation as well as amnesia in association with anti-Hu antibodies has been reported, with MR signal change not only in the anteromedial temporal lobes bilaterally but also in the right retrosplenial region and inferior precuneus (Hirayama et al., 2003). More widespread deficits and imaging changes may have prognostic implications: Bak et al. (2001) reported two patients with PNLE, one with pure anterograde amnesia and normal MRI who recovered completely with tumour remission, the other with dense anterograde and extensive retrograde amnesia with anomia and executive impairments, with atrophy of hippocampus and amygdala on MR imaging and frontotemporal hypoperfusion on SPECT, who showed no cognitive recovery following tumour regression.

REFERENCES

Bak TH, Antoun N, Balan KK, Hodges JR. Memory lost, memory regained: neuropsychological findings and neuroimaging in two cases of paraneoplastic limbic encephalitis with radically different outcomes. *J Neurol Neurosurg Psychiatry* 2001; **71**: 40–7.

Corsellis JA, Goldberg GJ, Norton AR. 'Limbic encephalitis' and its association with carcinoma. *Brain* 1968; **91**: 481–96.

Gultekin SH, Rosenfeld MR, Voltz R, *et al.* Paraneoplastic limbic encephalitis: neurological symptoms, immunological findings and tumour association in 50 patients. *Brain* 2000; **123**: 1481–94.

Hirayama K, Taguchi Y, Sato M, Tsukamoto T. Limbic encephalitis presenting with topographical disorientation and amnesia. *J Neurol Neurosurg Psychiatry* 2003; **74**: 110–12.

Lawn ND, Westmoreland BF, Kiely MJ, *et al.* Clinical, magnetic resonance imaging, and electroencephalographic findings in paraneoplastic limbic encephalitis. *Mayo Clin Proc* 2003; **78**: 1363–8.

Martin RC, Haut MW, Goeta Kreisler K, Blumenthal D. Neuropsychological functioning in a patient with paraneoplastic limbic encephalitis. *J Int Neuropsychol Soc* 1996; **2**: 460–6.

Rees JH, Hain SF, Johnson MR, *et al.* The role of [18F] fluoro-2-deoxyglucose-PET scanning in the diagnosis of paraneoplastic neurological disorders. *Brain* 2001; **124**: 2223–31.

6.12.2   Non-paraneoplastic limbic encephalitis (NPLE)

Of the non-paraneoplastic causes, a syndrome of limbic encephalitis associated with voltage-gated potassium channel (VGKC) antibodies in serum (and sometimes CSF) has been reported in recent times (Buckley *et al.*, 2001; Pozo-Rosich *et al.*, 2003; Schott *et al.*, 2003; Vincent *et al.*, 2004). The antibodies are likely to be pathogenic, since target antigens are found within the molecular layer of the hippocampus. Clinically this is a subacute amnesic syndrome with associated behavioural features, epileptic seizures, and sometimes hyponatraemia due to the syndrome of inappropriate ADH secretion. The neuropsychological profile, when it can be tested, shows prominent episodic memory impairment with frontotemporal dysfunction but sparing of parietal lobe function. Despite treatment with immunosuppressive agents

(plasma exchange, IVIg, high-dose steroids), memory problems may persist, associated with medial temporal lobe atrophy, even if the other clinical features remit, and early treatment is therefore recommended. There may be other antibody-mediated limbic encephalitides with target antigens yet to be defined (Castillo *et al.*, 2006).

Cases resembling limbic encephalitis have occasionally been reported in association with connective tissue disorders such as SLE (Stubgen, 1998), Behçet's disease (Hasegawa *et al.*, 2005), and relapsing polychondritis (Fujiki *et al.*, 2004; Ohta *et al.*, 2004). Of the infective causes of limbic encephalitis, herpes simplex encephalitis is the commonest (see Section 9.1.1), but other pathogens include herpes simplex type 2 and human herpes viruses 6 and 7 (Section 9.1.5), particularly in immunocompromised patients, and neurosyphilis (Section 9.4.1; Schied *et al.*, 2005).

REFERENCES

Buckley C, Oger J, Clover L, *et al.* Potassium channel antibodies in two patients with reversible limbic encephalitis. *Ann Neurol* 2001; **50**: 73–8.

Castillo P, Woodruff B, Caselli R, *et al.* Steroid-responsive encephalopathy associated with autoimmune thyroiditis. *Arch Neurol* 2006; **63**: 197–202.

Fujiki F, Tsuboi Y, Hashimoto K, *et al.* Non-herpetic limbic encephalitis associated with relapsing polychondritis. *J Neurol Neurosurg Psychiatry* 2004; **75**: 1646–7.

Hasegawa T, Kanno S, Kato M, *et al.* Neuro-Behçet's disease presenting initially as mesiotemporal lesions mimicking herpes simplex encephalitis. *Eur J Neurol* 2005; **12**: 661–2.

Ohta Y, Nagano I, Niiya D, *et al.* Nonparaneoplastic limbic encephalitis with relapsing polychondritis. *J Neurol Sci* 2004; **220**: 85–8.

Pozo-Rosich P, Clover L, Saiz A, *et al.* Voltage-gated potassium channel antibodies in limbic encephalitis. *Ann Neurol* 2003; **54**: 530–3.

Schied R, Voltz R, Vetter T, *et al.* Neurosyphilis and paraneoplastic limbic encephalitis: important differential diagnoses. *J Neurol* 2005; **252**: 1129–32.

Schott JM, Harkness K, Barnes J, *et al.* Amnesia, cerebral atrophy, and autoimmunity. *Lancet* 2003; **361**: 1266.

Stubgen JP. Nervous system lupus mimics limbic encephalitis. *Lupus* 1998; **7**: 557–60.

Vincent A, Buckley C, Schott JM, *et al.* Potassium channel antibody-associated encephalopathy: a potentially immunotherapy-responsive form of limbic encephalitis. *Brain* 2004; **127**: 701–12.

6.13   Hashimoto's encephalopathy (HE)

This entity, first reported in the 1960s (Brain *et al.*, 1966), consists of a clinical syndrome of encephalopathy associated with stroke-like episodes, seizures, and psychosis in association with high serum titres of antithyroid autoantibodies (microsomal, thyroglobulin). Thyroid function may vary from overt hypothyroidism to overt hyperthyroidism, but most commonly there is subclinical hypothyroidism. Females are more commonly affected (4 : 1). The course may be relapsing–remitting in half of patients, for which reason some authors envisage Hashimoto's encephalopathy as a form of recurrent acute disseminated encephalomyelitis (ADEM: Chaudhuri & Behan, 2003). CSF protein is often elevated, and EEG abnormalities (diffuse slowing) are almost ubiquitous. The condition is usually (96%) responsive to steroids (Chong *et al.*, 2003). The antithyroid autoantibodies are probably epiphenomenal, unrelated to disease pathogenesis; α-enolase antibodies may be a better marker. It has been suggested by some authors that the name Hashimoto's encephalopathy be abandoned because of uncertainty about nosology, 'steroid-responsive encephalopathy' being one proposed name. Differential diagnosis encompasses mitochondrial disease, vasculitides, non-paraneoplastic limbic encephalitis due to voltage-gated potassium channel antibodies, and even Creutzfeldt–Jakob disease (Schott *et al.*, 2003).

Cases presenting with a progressive dementia have been reported on occasion (Forchetti *et al.*, 1997; Wilhelm-Gössling *et al.*, 1998; Seipelt *et al.*, 1999; Spiegel *et al.*, 2004; Creutzfeldt & Haberl,

2005), the clinical phenotype often closely resembling sporadic Creutzfeldt–Jakob disease. Cases of pathologically confirmed CJD resembling Hashimoto's encephalopathy have also been reported (Schott *et al.*, 2003). Hence, though rare, this is an important diagnosis to consider since the dementia may be reversible with steroids.

REFERENCES

Brain L, Jellinek EH, Ball K. Hashimoto's disease and encephalopathy. *Lancet* 1966; **2**: 512–14.

Chaudhuri A, Behan PO. The clinical spectrum, diagnosis, pathogenesis and treatment of Hashimoto's encephalopathy (recurrent acute disseminated encephalomyelitis). *Curr Med Chem* 2003; **10**: 1645–53.

Chong JY, Rowland LP, Utiger RD. Hashimoto encephalopathy. Syndrome or myth? *Arch Neurol* 2003; **60**: 164–71.

Creutzfeldt CJ, Haberl RL. Hashimoto encephalopathy: a do-not-miss in the differential diagnosis of dementia. *J Neurol* 2005; **252**: 1285–7.

Forchetti CM, Katsamakis G, Garron DC. Autoimmune thyroiditis and a rapidly progressive dementia: global hypoperfusion on SPECT scanning suggests a possible mechanism. *Neurology* 1997; **49**: 623–6.

Schott JM, Warren JD, Rossor MN. The uncertain nosology of Hashimoto encephalopathy. *Arch Neurol* 2003; **60**: 1812.

Seipelt M, Zerr I, Nau R, *et al.* Hashimoto's encephalitis as a differential diagnosis of Creutzfeldt–Jakob disease. *J Neurol Neurosurg Psychiatry* 1999; **66**: 172–6.

Spiegel J, Hellwig D, Becker G, Müller M. Progressive dementia caused by Hashimoto's encephalopathy: report of two cases. *Eur J Neurol* 2004; **11**: 711–13.

Wilhelm-Gössling C, Weckbecker C, Brabant EG, Dengler R. Autoimmune encephalopathy in Hashimoto's thyroiditis. A differential diagnosis in progressive dementia syndrome [in German]. *Dtsch Med Wochenschr* 1998; **123**: 279–84.

6.14   Erdheim–Chester disease

Erdheim–Chester disease is a rare, sporadic, non-Langerhans cell histiocytosis which may affect multiple organs, including the CNS (Wright *et al.*, 1999). Proposed diagnostic criteria require typical histological findings of foamy histiocytes nested among polymorphic granuloma and fibrosis or xanthogranulomatosis with CD68-positive and CD1a-negative immunohistochemical staining, with typical skeletal findings of bilateral symmetrical cortical osteosclerosis and/or increased labelling of the distal ends of the lower limb long bones on ^{99}Tc bone scintigraphy (Veyssier-Belot *et al.*, 1996). Besides skeletal involvement, common findings are diabetes insipidus, and retroperitoneal, orbital, cutaneous, and cardiac involvement. In a review of over 200 cases, Lachenal *et al.* (2006) found neurological features in about one-third, most often cerebellar and/or pyramidal signs, but in six there was dementia, cognitive impairment, or amnesia.

REFERENCES

Lachenal F, Cotton F, Desmurs-Clavel H, *et al.* Neurological manifestations and neuroradiological presentation of Erdheim–Chester disease: report of 6 cases and systematic review of the literature. *J Neurol* 2006; **253**: 1267–77.

Veyssier-Belot C, Cacoub P, Caparros-Lefebvre D, *et al.* Erdheim–Chester disease: clinical and radiologic characteristics of 59 cases. *Medicine* 1996; **75**: 757–69.

Wright RA, Hermann RC, Parisi JE. Neurological manifestations of Erdheim–Chester disease. *J Neurol Neurosurg Psychiatry* 1999; **66**: 72–5.

6.15 Bilateral vestibulopathy

The syndrome of bilateral peripheral loss of vestibular function is characterized by oscillopsia during walking and head movements, and unsteadiness of gait in the dark and on uneven ground. Although often idiopathic, some cases are associated with autoantibodies to inner ear structures. Deficits of spatial memory and navigation associated with bilateral hippocampal atrophy have been reported in bilateral vestibulopathy associated with neurofibromatosis type 2 (Brandt *et al.*, 2005).

REFERENCES

Brandt T, Schautzer F, Hamilton D, *et al.* Vestibular loss causes hippocampal atrophy and impaired spatial memory in humans. *Brain* 2005; **128**: 1579–89.

Structural brain lesions

7.1 Brain tumours and their treatment

Cognitive decline in patients with brain tumours may have many causes, including the tumour itself, concurrent tumour-related seizures, mood disorder, steroid therapy, and as a sequel of surgery, radiotherapy, and chemotherapy for the tumour, or any combination thereof (Taphoorn & Klein, 2004). Cognitive decline related to the tumour per se may be more common with certain tumour types (CNS lymphoma, gliomatosis cerebri) and with slowly, as opposed to rapidly, growing tumours (Tucha et al., 2000). Dominant as opposed to non-dominant hemisphere lesions may be associated with greater cognitive deficit, but the profile is more global than localized. Lesions located in specific eloquent structures (hippocampus, frontal lobes, fornix) may produce specific deficits. Longitudinal neuropsychological decline may be an early marker of tumour recurrence (Armstrong et al., 2003).

REFERENCES

Armstrong CL, Goldstein B, Shera D, Ledakis GE, Tallent EM. The predictive value of longitudinal neuropsychological assessment in the early detection of brain tumor recurrence. *Cancer* 2003; **97**: 649–56.

Taphoorn MJB, Klein M. Cognitive deficits in adult patients with brain tumours. *Lancet Neurol* 2004; **3**: 159–68.

Tucha O, Smely C, Preier M, Lange KW. Cognitive deficits before treatment among patients with brain tumors. *Neurosurgery* 2000; **47**: 324–33.

7.1.1 Meningiomas

Meningiomas have a predilection for certain intracranial sites, including the olfactory groove, falx, parasagittal region, and sphenoid bone, in some of which there may be prominent cognitive as well as focal neurological signs. Meningioma is recognized to be a potentially treatable cause of dementia (Erkinjuntti *et al.*, 1987; Sahadevan *et al.*, 1997). Interhemispheric parafalcine (subfrontal) meningiomas may grow to a huge size without producing neurological signs, but impaired executive function may be found on neuropsychological testing (Hanna *et al.*, 1996). Rare intraventricular meningiomas may also be associated with cognitive change (Bertalanffy *et al.*, 2006).

REFERENCES

Bertalanffy A, Roessler K, Koperek O, *et al.* Intraventricular meningiomas: a report of 16 cases. *Neurosurg Rev* 2006; **29**: 30–5.
Erkinjuntti T, Sulkava R, Kovanen J, Palo J. Suspected dementia: evaluation of 323 consecutive referrals. *Acta Neurol Scand* 1987; **76**: 359–64.
Hanna MG, Papanastassiou V, Greenhall RCD. [Minerva]. *BMJ* 1996; **313**: 502.
Sahadevan S, Pang WS, Tan NJ, Choo GK, Tan CY. Neuroimaging guidelines in cognitive impairment: lessons from 3 cases of meningiomas presenting as isolated dementia. *Singapore Med J* 1997; **38**: 339–43.

7.1.2 Gliomas

Cognitive deficits are common in survivors of low-grade glioma, whether or not they have received radiotherapy, suggesting that the tumour per se, and/or other factors (e.g. antiepileptic drug therapy), may contribute to impairment (Klein *et al.*, 2002; Torres *et al.*, 2003). In high-grade gliomas, survivors may have moderate to severe cognitive deficits. Although these may be treatment-related, nonetheless there is evidence that the tumour itself may contribute (Archibald *et al.*, 1994).

REFERENCES

Archibald YM, Lunn D, Ruttan LA, *et al.* Cognitive functioning in long-term survivors of high-grade glioma. *J Neurosurg* 1994; **80**: 247–53.
Klein M, Heimans JJ, Aaronson MK, *et al.* Effect of radiotherapy and other treatment-related factors on mid-term to long-term cognitive sequelae in low-grade gliomas: a comparative study. *Lancet* 2002; **360**: 1361–8.
Torres IJ, Mundt AJ, Sweeney PJ, *et al.* A longitudinal neuropsychological study of partial brain radiation in adults with brain tumors. *Neurology* 2003; **60**: 1113–18.

7.1.3 Pituitary tumours

Tumours of the pituitary gland usually manifest with local effects of space occupation and compression of adjacent structures (e.g. the optic chiasm) or with endocrine effects. Memory disturbance has been reported with massive pituitary tumours (Williams & Pennybacker, 1954). A potentially reversible dementia has also been mentioned on occasion. For instance, Brisman *et al.* (1993) saw a patient with personality change, labelled as depression but unresponsive to antidepressant medication, inappropriate and uninhibited behaviour which evolved to apathy, and with memory loss (5-minute recall 0/3), who on imaging had a large pituitary tumour with suprasellar extension that proved to be a macroprolactinoma. Within a month of starting treatment with a dopamine agonist (bromocriptine) the patient was subjectively normal. No detailed neuropsychological assessment was performed. Decrements in both memory and attention in comparison to normative data were observed in patients with both treated pituitary Cushing's disease and non-functioning pituitary adenomas (Heald *et al.*, 2006), perhaps reflecting an effect of pituitary tumours per se.

REFERENCES

Brisman MH, Fetell MR, Post KD. Reversible dementia due to macroprolactinoma: case report. *J Neurosurg* 1993; **79**: 135–7.

Heald A, Parr C, Gibson C, O'Driscoll K, Fowler H. A cross-sectional study to investigate long-term cognitive function in people with treated pituitary Cushing's disease. *Exp Clin Endocrinol Diabetes* 2006; **114**: 490–7.

Williams M, Pennybacker J. Memory disturbance in third ventricle tumours. *J Neurol Neurosurg Psychiatry* 1954; **17**: 115–23.

7.1.4   Craniopharyngiomas

Memory disturbances have been reported in association with craniopharyngiomas (Williams & Pennybacker, 1954). Cases of severe anterograde amnesia associated with third ventricle craniopharyngioma causing relatively selective damage to the mammillary bodies has been reported (e.g. Tanaka *et al.*, 1997; Kupers *et al.*, 2004). In one case, amnesia improved following tumour removal, although memory was still impaired, and MR brain imaging showed small atrophic mammillary bodies (Tanaka *et al.*, 1997). In another case, in which the right hippocampus was involved as well as the mammillary bodies, albeit to a lesser extent, tumour removal was associated with complete recovery of memory function. Functional imaging (PET) showed no preoperative activity in memory-related structures, but improved perfusion of anterior thalamic nuclei postoperatively (Kupers *et al.*, 2004). Relatively selective mammillary body damage may thus result in a severe anterograde amnesia, which may be partially or completely reversible.

REFERENCES

Kupers RC, Fortin A, Astrup J, Gjedde A, Ptito M. Recovery of anterograde amnesia in a case of craniopharyngioma. *Arch Neurol* 2004; **61**: 1948–52.

Tanaka Y, Miyazawa Y, Akaoka F, Yamada T. Amnesia following damage to the mammillary bodies. *Neurology* 1997; **48**: 160–5.

Williams M, Pennybacker J. Memory disturbance in third ventricle tumours. *J Neurol Neurosurg Psychiatry* 1954; **17**: 115–23.

7.1.5   Primary CNS lymphoma

The risk of developing dementia in survivors of primary CNS lymphoma has been high, possibly related to patient age, and treatment modalities (whole-brain irradiation, systemic chemotherapy). Whether tumour-related factors render these patients more susceptible to cognitive impairment, such as the tendency to seed by CSF pathways (Larner *et al.*, 1999), or to side effects of treatment, is unknown.

REFERENCES

Larner AJ, D'Arrigo C, Scaravilli F, Howard RS. Bilateral symmetrical enhancing brainstem lesions: an unusual presentation of primary CNS lymphoma. *Eur J Neurol* 1999; **6**: 721–3.

7.1.6   Splenial tumours

Tumours involving the splenium of the corpus callosum are reported to produce amnesia, thought to be related to damage to the fornix due to its anatomical propinquity to the splenium, and visual perceptual impairment due to hemispheric disconnection, whilst intellect is relatively preserved (Rudge & Warrington, 1991).

REFERENCES

Rudge P, Warrington EK. Selective impairment of memory and visual perception in splenial tumours. *Brain* 1991; **114**: 349–60.

7.1.7   Gliomatosis cerebri

Gliomatosis cerebri is a neoplastic disorder in which malignant cells widely infiltrate the brain without forming mass lesions. Clinically, the condition presents with progressive headache, gait disorder, and seizures (partial, with or without secondary generalization), with signs of raised intracranial pressure (papilloedema, ophthalmoparesis), hemiparesis, and neurobehavioural changes (Chamberlain, 2004). Neuropsychological deficits reflecting affected brain region may occur: for example, executive dysfunction and verbal memory impairment were reported in a patient with bifrontal and left temporal white matter involvement on neuroimaging (Filley *et al.*, 2003). A case with progressive cognitive decline and parkinsonism clinically resembling sporadic Creutzfeldt–Jakob disease has also been reported (Slee *et al.*, 2006). Progression to a dementia of white matter type occurs with bihemispheric white matter infiltration (Filley *et al.*, 2003).

REFERENCES

Chamberlain MC. Gliomatosis cerebri: better definition, better treatment. *Neurology* 2004; **63**: 204–5.

Filley CM, Kleinschmidt-DeMasters BK, Lillehei KO, Damek DM, Harris JG. Gliomatosis cerebri: neurobehavioral and neuropathological observations. *Cogn Behav Neurol* 2003; **16**: 149–59.

Slee M, Pretorius P, Ansorge O, Stacey R, Butterworth R. Parkinsonism and dementia due to gliomatosis cerebri mimicking sporadic Creutzfeldt–Jakob disease (CJD). *J Neurol Neurosurg Psychiatry* 2006; **77**: 283–4.

7.1.8 Radiotherapy and chemotherapy

The risk of cognitive deficits related to radiotherapy is a vexed question. The risk is known to increase with high radiation dose, large fraction and field size (whole brain versus focal), but is also related to patient age and concurrent chemotherapy. Moreover, there are potential confounders, including the malignancy per se (e.g. disease progression), comorbid medical, neurological (e.g. epilepsy), or psychiatric conditions (e.g. depression), and surgical treatment (Armstrong *et al.*, 2004; Laack & Brown, 2004; Taphoorn & Klein, 2004; Sarkissian, 2005). Recent reviews of the literature have concluded that focal radiotherapy in patients with glioma is not the main reason for cognitive deficits (Taphoorn & Klein, 2004) and that radiation effects on cognition are severe in only a minority of patients (Armstrong *et al.*, 2004).

Late delayed post-radiation cognitive decline, occurring more than 3 years post-treatment, is a rare but feared complication of treatment, and of increasing importance as an outcome measure, given improved survival from the underlying malignancy. It is associated with diffuse white matter change (leukoencephalopathy) and cortical/subcortical atrophy on brain imaging, a subcortical pattern of cognitive deficits, with psychomotor slowing, executive and memory dysfunction, sometimes sufficiently severe to constitute dementia, and pathological changes of gliosis, demyelination, and thickening of small vessels (Crossen *et al.*, 1994; Armstrong *et al.*, 2004; Omuro *et al.*, 2005). In a series of patients with primary CNS lymphoma, 5-year cumulative incidence of delayed neurotoxicity was nearly 25% (Omuro *et al.*, 2005). An annual incidence of 11% was noted in an older, retrospective, series in which relatively high doses of radiation were used (DeAngelis *et al.*, 1989).

Neurotoxicity from chemotherapeutic agents is more likely if they are given concomitantly with radiotherapy, or via intrathecal or intra-arterial routes as compared to systemically, all these factors increasing drug concentration in normal brain tissue by compromising or bypassing the blood–brain barrier.

REFERENCES

Armstrong CL, Gyato K, Awadalla AW, Lustig R, Tochner ZA. A critical review of the clinical effects of therapeutic irradiation damage to the brain: the roots of the controversy. *Neuropsychol Rev* 2004; **14**: 65–86.

Crossen JR, Garwood D, Glatstein E, Neuwelt EA. Neurobehavioral sequelae of cranial irradiation in adults: a review of radiation-induced encephalopathy. *J Clin Oncol* 1994; **12**: 627–42.

DeAngelis LM, Delattre JY, Posner JB. Radiation-induced dementia in patients cured of brain metastases. *Neurology* 1989; **39**: 789–96.

Laack NN, Brown PD. Cognitive sequelae of brain radiation in adults. *Semin Oncol* 2004; **31**: 702–13.

Omuro AMP, Ben Porat LS, Panageas KS, *et al.* Delayed neurotoxicity in primary central nervous system lymphoma. *Arch Neurol* 2005; **62**: 1595–600.

Sarkissian V. The sequelae of cranial irradiation on human cognition. *Neurosci Lett* 2005; **382**: 118–23.

Taphoorn MJB, Klein M. Cognitive deficits in adult patients with brain tumours. *Lancet Neurol* 2004; **3**: 159–68.

7.2   Hydrocephalic dementias

The association of dementia with hydrocephalus may arise in a number of situations (Benson, 1990; Esiri & Rosenberg, 2004). Hydrocephalus may be classified according to whether there is obstruction to the flow of CSF, and whether the ventricles are communicating or not. Obstructive non-communicating hydrocephalus in the context of neoplasms, inflammation (ependymitis, arachnoiditis, pachymeningitis), and acquired aqueduct stenosis may present as a subacute dementia. Non-obstructive communicating hydrocephalus may result from ex vacuo brain atrophy, perhaps in the context of parenchymal brain disease or previous brain trauma, or, extremely rarely, from CSF hypersecretion, as for example from a choroid plexus tumour. Perhaps the most challenging clinical situation, in terms of both diagnosis and management, relates to cases of communicating hydrocephalus. These may be obstructive, secondary to subarachnoid haemorrhage, trauma, meningitis or diffusely infiltrating tumour, or some other process (for example Paget's disease of the skull: Section 7.2.4); or primary or idiopathic, the condition which has come to be known as idiopathic normal pressure hydrocephalus (iNPH). Whether these latter cases represent some form of occult obstruction remains unclear. Because of the uncertainties about aetiopathogenesis, retention of the term 'occult hydrocephalus' as originally suggested by Adams *et al.* (1965), or use of the term 'chronic hydrocephalus' (Bret *et al.*, 2002), may be preferable.

REFERENCES

Adams RD, Fisher CM, Hakim S, *et al.* Symptomatic occult hydrocephalus with 'normal' cerebrospinal fluid pressure. *N Engl J Med* 1965; **273**: 117–26.

Benson DF. Hydrocephalic dementias. In: Frederiks JAM (ed.), *Handbook of Clinical Neurology. Vol. 2 (46): Neurobehavioural Disorders.* Amsterdam: Elsevier, 1990: 323–33.

Bret P, Guyotat J, Chazal J. Is normal pressure hydrocephalus a valid concept in 2002? A reappraisal in five questions and proposal for a new designation of the syndrome as 'chronic hydrocephalus'. *J Neurol Neurosurg Psychiatry* 2002; **73**: 9–12.

Esiri MM, Rosenberg GA. Hydrocephalus and dementia. In: Esiri MM, Lee VMY, Trojanowski JQ (eds.), *The Neuropathology of Dementia* (2nd edition). Cambridge: Cambridge University Press, 2004: 442–56.

7.2.1   Normal pressure hydrocephalus (NPH)

That normal pressure hydrocephalus (NPH) comprises the clinical triad of gait difficulties of parkinsonian type, urinary problems, and cognitive decline is a fact known to virtually every medical student, and a huge literature on the subject has developed since the condition was first described (Adams *et al.*, 1965; Hakim & Adams, 1965), much of it related to predicting which patients will respond to surgical shunting procedures (Vanneste, 2000; Bret *et al.*, 2002; Malm & Eklund, 2006). The advent of widespread structural neuroimaging with CT has increased the frequency with which this disorder is considered: relative preservation of cortical gyri despite ventricular expansion is suggested to point to this diagnosis, and various radiological parameters (e.g. Evans ratio) have been suggested to be helpful in predicting shunt-responsiveness. Yet, despite this 'evidence base', the condition remains in many ways obscure and perplexing, perhaps particularly for neurologists with an interest in cognitive disorders. Is it certain, for example, that at least some of these patients do not in fact have an ex vacuo non-obstructive communicating hydrocephalus due to occult primary intraparenchymal pathology causing subcortical atrophy, a well-recognized correlate of Alzheimer's disease (AD)? Very few NPH patients come to pathological analysis, either biopsy or autopsy, and when they do alternative pathologies may be found, such as AD (Golomb *et al.*, 2000; Silverberg *et al.*, 2002; Bech-Azeddine *et al.*, 2007), Parkinson's disease (Krauss *et al.*, 1997), cerebrovascular disease (Bech-Azeddine *et al.*, 2007), or progressive supranuclear palsy (Schott *et al.*, 2007), even when patients have proven to be temporarily 'shunt-responsive'. Other secondary causes of NPH have been reported, such as neuroborreliosis (see Section 9.4.3). The CSF tap test, the withdrawal of 25–30 ml of CSF with pre- and post-test assessment of gait and cognitive function, has been advocated as a predictor of shunt responsiveness, but both false negatives and false positives may occur, the latter possibly due to the presence of alternative, primary neurodegenerative, pathology (Larner & Larner, 2006).

With these diagnostic uncertainties, it is apparent that delineating the neuropsychological profile of idiopathic NPH will be difficult, yet there have been attempts (Merten, 1999; Devito *et al.*, 2005). In a very selected cohort ($n = 11$), Iddon *et al.* (1999) identified two groups: those with MMSE < 24 preoperatively, performing in the demented range, who showed significant postoperative recovery; and those showing no signs of dementia either pre- or post-shunt but who did show a specific pattern of neuropsychological impairments in comparison with healthy volunteers on tests sensitive to frontostriatal dysfunction, changes distinct from AD.

Ogino *et al.* (2006) found disproportionate impairment of frontal lobe functions (attention/concentration subtest of WMS-R; digit span, arithmetic, block design, and digit symbol substitution subtests of WAIS-R) in iNPH patients compared to AD, but disproportionately mild memory impairment (general memory and delayed recall in WAIS-R). Impaired frontal lobe function as assessed by the Frontal Assessment Battery and verbal fluency tests was also reported by the same group (Miyoshi *et al.*, 2005). Perhaps unsurprisingly, in the cohort of Golomb *et al.* (2000) more cognitive impairment was seen in those cases with greater degrees of AD pathology. Low verbal memory baseline scores were found to be predictors of poor response in a cohort of iNPH patients undergoing shunting, the more so if there was concurrent visuoconstructional deficit or executive dysfunction (Thomas *et al.*, 2005): one wonders whether these more impaired patients may have been harbouring primary neurodegenerative disease. Cognitive impairment in iNPH was reported to be more severe than in Binswanger's disease (Gallassi *et al.*, 1991). A case of NPH with transient prosopagnosia, topographical disorientation and visual object agnosia which improved after shunting has also been reported (Otani *et al.*, 2004), but without prolonged follow-up or pathological examination. Again one may wonder whether this is an example of a shunt-responsive primary neurodegenerative disorder.

Hence, there are significant methodological difficulties in defining the cognitive profile of iNPH. Nonetheless, disruption of frontal-subcortical pathways would seem the most likely pathological substrate (for example, to account for the parkinsonian gait), with a corresponding subcortical type of neuropsychological profile.

REFERENCES

Adams RD, Fisher CM, Hakim S, *et al.* Symptomatic occult hydrocephalus with 'normal' cerebrospinal fluid pressure. *N Engl J Med* 1965; **273**: 117–26.

Bech-Azeddine R, Høgh P, Juhler M, Gjerris F, Waldemar G. Idiopathic normal-pressure hydrocephalus: clinical comorbidity correlated with cerebral biopsy findings and outcome of cerebrospinal fluid shunting. *J Neurol Neurosurg Psychiatry* 2007; **78**: 157–61.

Bret P, Guyotat J, Chazal J. Is normal pressure hydrocephalus a valid concept in 2002? A reappraisal in five questions and proposal for a new designation of the syndrome as 'chronic hydrocephalus'. *J Neurol Neurosurg Psychiatry* 2002; **73**: 9–12.

Devito EE, Pickard JD, Salmond CH, *et al.* The neuropsychology of normal pressure hydrocephalus. *Br J Neurosurg* 2005; **19**: 217–24.

Gallassi R, Morreale A, Montagna P, *et al.* Binswanger's disease and normal pressure hydrocephalus: clinical and neuropsychological comparison. *Arch Neurol* 1991; **48**: 1156–9.

Golomb J, Wisoff J, Miller DC, *et al.* Alzheimer's disease comorbidity in normal pressure hydrocephalus: prevalence and shunt response. *J Neurol Neurosurg Psychiatry* 2000; **68**: 778–81.

Hakim S, Adams RD. The special clinical problem of symptomatic hydrocephalus with normal cerebrospinal fluid pressure: observations on cerebrospinal fluid hydrodynamics. *J Neurol Sci* 1965; **2**: 307–27.

Iddon JL, Pickard JD, Cross JJ, *et al.* Specific patterns of cognitive impairment in patients with idiopathic normal pressure hydrocephalus and Alzheimer's disease: a pilot study. *J Neurol Neurosurg Psychiatry* 1999; **67**: 723–32.

Krauss JK, Regel JP, Droste DW, *et al.* Movement disorders in adult hydrocephalus. *Mov Disord* 1997; **12**: 53–60.

Larner MJ, Larner AJ. Normal pressure hydrocephalus: false positives. *Pract Neurol* 2006; **6**: 264.

Malm J, Eklund A. Idiopathic normal pressure hydrocephalus. *Pract Neurol* 2006; **6**: 14–27.

Merten T. Neuropsychology of normal pressure hydrocephalus [in German]. *Nervenarzt* 1999; **70**: 496–503.

Miyoshi N, Kazui H, Ogino A, *et al.* Association between cognitive impairment and gait disturbance in patients with idiopathic normal pressure hydrocephalus. *Dement Geriatr Cogn Disord* 2005; **20**: 71–6.

Ogino A, Kazui H, Miyoshi N, *et al.* Cognitive impairment in patients with idiopathic normal pressure hydrocephalus. *Dement Geriatr Cogn Disord* 2006; **21**: 113–19.

Otani N, Nawashiro H, Ishihara S, *et al.* Normal pressure hydrocephalus manifesting as topographical disorientation and visual objective [*sic*] agnosia. *J Clin Neurosci* 2004; **11**: 313–17.

Schott JM, Williams DR, Butterworth R, *et al.* Shunt responsive progressive supranuclear palsy? *Mov Disord* 2007; **22**: 902–3.

Silverberg GD, Levinthal E, Sullivan EV, *et al.* Assessment of low-flow CSF drainage as a treatment for AD: results of a randomized pilot study. *Neurology* 2002; **59**: 1139–45.

Thomas G, McGirt MJ, Woodworth G, *et al.* Baseline neuropsychological profile and cognitive response to cerebrospinal fluid shunting for idiopathic normal pressure hydrocephalus. *Dement Geriatr Cogn Disord* 2005; **20**: 163–8.

Vanneste JA. Diagnosis and management of normal pressure hydrocephalus. *J Neurol* 2000; **247**: 5–14.

7.2.2 Aqueduct stenosis

Cases have been reported in which aqueduct stenosis is associated with schizophrenic psychosis (Roberts *et al.*, 1983; O'Flaithbheartaigh *et al.*, 1994) and delusional depression with possible diencephalic dysfunction (Motohashi *et al.*, 1990), but whether these are chance concurrences or causal associations remains unclear. No convincing report of dementia associated with congenital aqueduct stenosis has been identified.

REFERENCES

Motohashi N, Ishizuka Y, Asada T, *et al.* A case of aqueduct stenosis in adults with various neurological and psychiatric symptoms. *Eur Arch Psychiatry Clin Neurosci* 1990; **240**: 13–15.

O'Flaithbheartaigh S, Williams PA, Jones GH. Schizophrenic psychosis and associated aqueduct stenosis. *Br J Psychiatry* 1994; **164**: 684–6.

Roberts JK, Trimble MR, Robertson M. Schizophrenic psychosis associated with aqueduct stenosis in adults. *J Neurol Neurosurg Psychiatry* 1983; **46**: 892–8.

7.2.3 Colloid cyst, fornix lesions

Colloid cysts are thought to arise from ependymal cells in the vestigial paraphysis in the anterior portion of the third ventricle, where they may block the third ventricle and cause obstructive hydrocephalus. Clinical presentation is either with intermittent obstruction causing severe bifrontal-bioccipital headache, unsteady gait, incontinence, visual impairment, and drop attacks without loss of consciousness, or with a picture resembling 'normal pressure hydrocephalus'. Some cases are now found incidentally when patients undergo brain imaging for other reasons. Surgical resection of the cyst may be undertaken, although symptoms may sometimes be more easily controlled with shunting or stereotactic decompression.

Damage to the fornix as a consequence of surgery for colloid cyst may result in a persistent anterograde amnesia (Hodges & Carpenter, 1991;

Gaffan *et al.*, 1991; McMackin *et al.*, 1995; Aggleton *et al.*, 2000; Spiers *et al.*, 2001; Poreh *et al.*, 2006). Bilateral fornix interruption was a predictor of poor memory performance in one study (Aggleton *et al.*, 2000); severity of damage to the left fornix was suggested to be the most important determinant of severity of impairment in verbal memory in another (McMackin *et al.*, 1995). Recall may be less impaired than recognition (Aggleton *et al.*, 2000). Relative absence of retrograde amnesia was noted in some reports (Hodges & Carpenter, 1991; Spiers *et al.*, 2001), but in others retrograde amnesia for autobiographical episodes and for semantic memory was noted (Poreh *et al.*, 2006).

Fornix damage with subsequent neuropsychological deficits may also be a consequence of surgery for other tumours (Calabrese *et al.*, 1995; Yasuno *et al.*, 1999; Ibrahim *et al.*, 2007), focal stroke (Moudgil *et al.*, 2000; see Section 3.3.2), or carbon monoxide poisoning (Kesler *et al.*, 2001; Section 8.2.3).

REFERENCES

Aggleton JP, McMackin D, Carpenter K, *et al.* Differential cognitive effects of colloid cysts in the third ventricle that spare or compromise the fornix. *Brain* 2000; **123**: 800–15.

Calabrese P, Markowitsch HJ, Harders AG, Scholz M, Gehlen W. Fornix damage and memory: a case report. *Cortex* 1995; **31**: 555–64.

Gaffan EA, Gaffan D, Hodges JR. Amnesia following damage to the left fornix and to other sites: a comparative study. *Brain* 1991; **114**: 1297–313.

Hodges JR, Carpenter K. Anterograde amnesia with fornix damage following removal of a third ventricle colloid cyst. *J Neurol Neurosurg Psychiatry* 1991; **54**: 633–8.

Ibrahim I, Young CA, Larner AJ. Cognitive impairments associated with fornix damage caused by subependymal giant-cell astrocytoma (SEGA). *Eur J Neurol* 2007; **14** (Suppl 1): 104 (abstract P1285).

Kesler SR, Hopkins RO, Blatter DD, Edge Booth H, Bigler ED. Verbal memory deficits associated with fornix atrophy in carbon monoxide poisoning. *J Int Neuropsychol Soc* 2001; **7**: 640–6.

McMackin D, Cockburn J, Anslow P, Gaffan D. Correlation of fornix damage with memory impairment in six cases of colloid cyst removal. *Acta Neurochir Wien* 1995; **135**: 12–18.

Moudgil SS, Azzouz M, Al-Azzaz A, Haut M, Gutmann L. Amnesia due to fornix infarction. *Stroke* 2000; **31**: 1418–19.

Poreh A, Winocour G, Moscovitch M, *et al.* Anterograde and retrograde amnesia in a person with bilateral fornix lesions following removal of a colloid cyst. *Neuropsychologia* 2006; **44**: 2241–8.

Spiers HJ, Maguire EA, Burgess N. Hippocampal amnesia. *Neurocase* 2001; **7**: 357–82.

Yasuno F, Hirata M, Takimoto H, *et al.* Retrograde temporal order amnesia resulting from damage to the fornix. *J Neurol Neurosurg Psychiatry* 1999; **67**: 102–5.

7.2.4 Paget's disease of bone (osteitis deformans)

This disorder of increased bone turnover with excessive osteoclastic resorption and disorganized new bone formation has a predilection for involvement of the skull and vertebral column. Neurological complications are well recognized, particularly cranial nerve palsies due to foraminal entrapment and extradural myelopathy due to disease in vertebral bodies. Dementia as a consequence of basilar invagination is reported, producing a syndrome sometimes likened to normal pressure hydrocephalus, although there may be debate as to whether the hydrocephalus is in some sense obstructive or non-communicating, and which may be treated with ventricular shunting (Gottschalk, 1973; Culebras *et al.*, 1974; Dohrmann & Elrick, 1982; Chan *et al.*, 2000; Fereydoon *et al.*, 2005).

Paget's disease may rarely occur in association with an autosomal dominant frontotemporal dementia with or without inclusion body myopathy (IBMPFD) caused by mutations in the valosin-containing protein gene on chromosome 9 (Watts *et al.*, 2004; see Section 5.1.8).

REFERENCES

Chan YP, Shui KK, Lewis RR, Kinirons MT. Reversible dementia in Paget's disease. *J R Soc Med* 2000; **93**: 595–6.

Culebras A, Feldman RG, Fager CA. Hydrocephalus and dementia in Paget's disease of the skull. *J Neurol Sci* 1974; **23**: 307–21.

Dohrmann PJ, Elrick WL. Dementia and hydrocephalus in Paget's disease: a case report. *J Neurol Neurosurg Psychiatry* 1982; **45**: 835–7.

Fereydoon R, Mann D, Kula RW. Surgical management of hydrocephalic dementia in Paget's disease of bone: the 6-year outcome of ventriculo-peritoneal shunting. *Clin Neurol Neurosurg* 2005; **107**: 325–8.

Gottschalk PG. Normal pressure hydrocephalus with basilar impression due to Paget's disease of the skull. *Wisconsin Med J* 1973; **72**: 192.

Watts GDJ, Wymer J, Kovach MJ, *et al.* Inclusion body myopathy associated with Paget disease of bone and frontotemporal dementia is caused by mutant valosin-containing protein. *Nat Genet* 2004; **36**: 377–81.

7.3   Other structural lesions

Subdural haematoma and arachnoid cyst are considered here. Other potentially relevant structural brain lesions, such as arteriovenous malformations and fistulas, are considered elsewhere (see Section 3.5).

7.3.1   Subdural haematoma (SDH)

Cognitive sequelae associated with acute subdural haematoma (SDH) may be related to traumatic brain injury in the context of head injury, the most common cause of acute SDH; alcohol misuse may be a precipitating factor. Chronic SDH without a history of head trauma most commonly occurs in the elderly, where concurrent neurodegenerative disease (AD, dementia with Lewy bodies), with associated risk of repeated falls, may be present. Despite these possible confounding factors, SDH per se may be associated with cognitive deficits (Machulda & Haut, 2000).

Chronic SDH may present with altered mental state with features of delirium or dementia, and with or without focal neurological deficits such as hemiparesis, aphasia (Moster *et al.*, 1983), hemisensory loss, seizures, headache, and akinetic-rigid

syndrome, features which may be fixed or transient. Gerstmann syndrome has been reported (Maeshima *et al.*, 1998). Recognized risk factors for the accumulation of blood and its liquefaction in the subdural space include increasing age, history of direct head trauma (although not invariably present), use of antiplatelet or anticoagulant drugs, and alcohol misuse. A history of falls may be a particular 'red flag' (Adhiyaman *et al.*, 2002). The diagnosis may be overlooked, symptoms being attributed to other causes, such as a dementia syndrome, and brain imaging with CT may not be diagnostic if the collection is isodense, rather than hyperdense (acute) or hypodense (> 4 weeks), or if bilateral collections cause no mass effect or midline shift (Davenport *et al.*, 1994). Surgical evacuation is often the treatment of choice.

Variable mental changes have been reported in chronic SDH: lethargy and poor concentration; withdrawal; confusion with aggressive outbursts; and failing memory and intelligence reminiscent of a dementia syndrome (Luxon & Harrison, 1979). Slowed mental abilities, but with normal abbreviated mental test score, have been reported with akinetic-rigid syndrome (Abdulla & Pearce, 1999). However, there have been no prospective systematic studies. Chronic subdural haematoma is often listed in textbooks as a cause of reversible dementia, but the published evidence base for this is slim. Ishikawa *et al.* (2002) reported that nearly 70% of a series of 26 patients operated on for chronic SDH (i.e. a highly selected cohort) were demented preoperatively on the basis of their performance on MMSE, with 50% (i.e. nine patients) making a good recovery. Younger patients with a higher preoperative MMSE showed better recovery, as did patients diagnosed and evacuated early.

REFERENCES

Abdulla AJJ, Pearce VR. Reversible akinetic-rigid syndrome due to bilateral subdural haematomas. *Age Ageing* 1999; **28**: 582–3.

Adhiyaman V, Asghar M, Ganeshram KN, Bhowmick BK. Chronic subdural haematoma in the elderly. *Postgrad Med J* 2002; **78**: 71–5.

Davenport RJ, Statham PFX, Warlow CP. Detection of bilateral isodense subdural haematomas. *BMJ* 1994; **309**: 792–4.

Ishikawa E, Yanaka K, Sugimoto K, Ayuzawa S, Nose T. Reversible dementia in patients with chronic subdural haematomas. *J Neurosurg* 2002; **96**: 680–3.

Luxon LM, Harrison MJG. Chronic subdural haematoma. *Q J Med* 1979; **48** (189): 43–53.

Machulda MM, Haut MW. Clinical features of chronic subdural hematoma: neuropsychiatric and neuropsychologic changes in patients with chronic subdural hematoma. *Neurosurg Clin North Am* 2000; **11**: 473–7.

Maeshima S, Okumura Y, Nakai K, Itakura T, Komai N. Gerstmann's syndrome associated with chronic subdural haematoma: a case report. *Brain Inj* 1998; **12**: 697–701.

Moster ML, Johnston DE, Reinmuth OM. Chronic subdural hematoma with transient neurological deficits: a review of 15 cases. *Ann Neurol* 1983; **14**: 539–42.

7.3.2 Arachnoid cyst

Arachnoid cysts are not infrequent incidental findings on brain imaging, most commonly in the middle cranial fossa. Whether they sometimes have symptomatic effects related to space occupation (pressure, brain displacement, both, or other mechanisms) is debated. Some studies have found impaired learning and memory specific to the hemisphere affected (Lang *et al.*, 1985), while others have failed to show such impairments (Gallassi *et al.*, 1985). Wester and Hugdahl (1995) identified cognitive deficits affecting memory and the ability to direct attention in an auditory perceptual task (dichotic listening technique), which disappeared within hours of decompressive cyst surgery performed for symptoms such as headache, epilepsy, or hemiparesis. This was a highly selected (convenience?) sample ($n = 13$), since one of the inclusion criteria was symptomatic improvement after surgery! The symptoms listed are probably rarely encountered with arachnoid cysts, most of which are asymptomatic, incidental, findings. A case of presenile dementia associated with a left temporofrontal cyst without mass effect was reported by Richards & Lusznat (2001), but this may be simply chance concurrence: the neurological diagnosis was AD and the patient showed initial improvement with cholinesterase inhibitor treatment.

REFERENCES

Gallassi R, Ciardulli C, Ferrara R, *et al.* Asymptomatic large arachnoid cyst of the middle cranial fossa: a clinical and neuropsychological study. *Eur Neurol* 1985; **24**: 140–4.

Lang W, Lang M, Kornhuber A, Gallwitz A, Kriebel J. Neuropsychological and neuroendocrinological disturbance associated with extracerebral cysts of the anterior and middle cranial fossa. *Eur Arch Psychiatr Neurol Sci* 1985; **235**: 38–41.

Richards G, Lusznat RM. An arachnoid cyst in a patient with pre-senile dementia. *Prog Neurol Psychiatry* 2001; **5**(3): 21–2.

Wester K, Hugdahl K. Arachnoid cysts of the left temporal fossa: impaired preoperative cognition and postoperative improvement. *J Neurol Neurosurg Psychiatry* 1995; **59**: 293–8.

Endocrine, metabolic, and toxin-related disorders

8.1 Endocrine disorders

8.1.1 Diabetes mellitus

A link between diabetes mellitus per se and cognitive decline may be obscured by comorbid cerebrovascular disease (both microvascular and macrovascular), hypertension, or depression (Messier, 2005), since these conditions may confound any assessment of cognitive performance. Nonetheless, a meta-analysis of studies of cognitive performance in type 1 diabetes found evidence for slowing of mental speed and diminished mental flexibility with sparing of learning and memory (Brands *et al.*, 2005). Systematic reviews have shown a greater risk and rate of cognitive functional decline (Cukierman *et al.*, 2005) and of dementia (Biessels *et al.*, 2006) in diabetes, with processing speed and verbal memory the domains most affected (Messier, 2005). Diabetes does not appear to be a risk factor for the development of Alzheimer's disease overall, but might increase relative risk in certain subgroups (Akomolafe *et al.*, 2006).

Epidemiological studies provide some evidence that cognition may be impaired in the early stages of type 2 diabetes. In the Whitehall II study, a prospective study of the incidence of diabetes, an association was noted between diabetes and poor performance on a test of inductive reasoning (Alice Heim 4) in stroke-free patients, but verbal memory, verbal meaning, and verbal fluency tests were not affected. The study suggested that effects of diabetes on cognitive performance may be evident within 5 years of diagnosis (Kumari & Marmot, 2005). Hence, cognitive dysfunction is one of the chronic complications of diabetes, but the pathophysiology is uncertain. Possible mediating and modulating factors may include the aforementioned comorbidities and effects of glycaemic control: hyperglycaemia, insulin resistance (hyperinsulinaemia), and treatment-induced hypoglycaemia.

It might be anticipated that, as for neuropathic and nephropathic complications of diabetes, stricter glycaemic control might reduce the risk of cognitive impairment. Observational studies suggest that acute hyperglycaemia is associated with a slowing of cognitive performance in some subjects with either type 1 or type 2 diabetes, with a possible threshold around 15 mmol/l (Cox *et al.*, 2005). Whether this is a consequence of hyperglycaemia per se or of underlying insulin resistance is not certain: hyperinsulinaemia is reported in epidemiological studies to be a risk factor for the development of dementia and memory decline (Luchsinger *et al.*, 2004).

A management strategy of strict glycaemic control may exacerbate the risk of episodes of treatment-induced hypoglycaemia, which might also contribute to cognitive impairment. Hypoglycaemia is recognized to cause acute neuropsychiatric features as a consequence of neuroglycopaenia, with or without concurrent features of autonomic activation. Severe hypoglycaemia is also a recognized cause of acute amnesia (Fisher, 2002). An amnesic syndrome has on occasion been reported in patients with diabetes experiencing profound hypoglycaemia as a consequence of intensive insulin treatment, for example using a subcutaneous pump, in the absence of confounding epileptic seizures. Bilateral high-signal-intensity hippocampal lesions on MR brain imaging have been noted in some patients (Holemans *et al.*, 2001) but are not invariably found (Larner *et al.*, 2003). Prognosis is variable: the amnesia may be completely reversible (Holemans *et al.*, 2001) or partially reversible (Larner *et al.*, 2003). Amnesia for hypoglycaemia is reported to be a common feature in patients with insulinomas (Dizon *et al.*, 1999). Presumably this amnesia induced by profound hypoglycaemia reflects hippocampal vulnerability to the effects of neuroglycopaenia. Whether repeated episodes of hypoglycaemia cause persistent cognitive deficits in diabetes remains an open question. Small studies have suggested that adults with a history of severe hypoglycaemia (i.e. episodes requiring assistance from another person to be reversed) scored lower on some neuropsychological tests than those who had never experienced severe hypoglycaemia (Wredling *et al.*, 1990; Sachon *et al.*, 1992). Cohort studies have also suggested a modest association between reported frequency of severe hypoglycaemia, lower IQ, and slowed and more variable reaction times (Langan *et al.*, 1991; Lincoln *et al.*, 1996). In contrast, however, longitudinal studies have failed to find any deleterious cognitive effects of repeated severe hypoglycaemia (Reichard & Pihl, 1994; Diabetes Control and Complications Trial Research Group, 1996). This is a vexed question, with currently no clear-cut answer (Deary & Frier, 1996).

REFERENCES

Akomolafe A, Beiser A, Meigs JB, *et al.* Diabetes mellitus and risk of developing Alzheimer disease: results from the Framingham Study. *Arch Neurol* 2006; **63**: 1551–5

Biessels GJ, Staekenborg S, Brunner E, Brayne C, Scheltens P. Risk of dementia in diabetes mellitus: a systematic review. *Lancet Neurol* 2006; **5**: 64–74.

Brands AMA, Biessels GJ, De Haan EHF, Kappelle LJ, Kessels RPC. The effects of type 1 diabetes on cognitive performance. *Diabetes Care* 2005; **28**: 726–35.

Cox DJ, Kovatchev B, Gonder-Frederick LA, *et al.* Relationships between hyperglycemia and cognitive performance among adults with type 1 and type 2 diabetes. *Diabetes Care* 2005; **28**: 71–7.

Cukierman T, Gerstein HC, Williamson JD. Cognitive decline and dementia in diabetes: systematic overview of progressive observational studies. *Diabetologia* 2005; **48**: 2460–9.

Deary IJ, Frier BM. Severe hypoglycaemia and cognitive impairment in diabetes. *BMJ* 1996; **313**: 767–8.

Diabetes Control and Complications Trial Research Group. Effects of intensive diabetes therapy on neuropsychological function in adults in the diabetes control and complications trial. *Ann Intern Med* 1996; **124**: 379–88.

Dizon AM, Kowalyk S, Hoogwerf BJ. Neuroglycopenic and other symptoms in patients with insulinomas. *Am J Med* 1999; **106**: 307–10.

Fisher CM. Unexplained sudden amnesia. *Arch Neurol* 2002; **59**: 1310–13.

Holemans X, Dupuis M, Missan N, Vanderijst JF. Reversible amnesia in a type 1 diabetic patient and bilateral hippocampal lesions on magnetic resonance imaging (MRI). *Diabet Med* 2001; **18**: 761–3.

Kumari M, Marmot M. Diabetes and cognitive function in a middle-aged cohort: findings from the Whitehall II study. *Neurology* 2005; **65**: 1597–603.

Langan SJ, Deary IJ, Hepburn DA, Frier BM. Cumulative cognitive impairment following severe hypoglycaemia in adult patients with insulin-treated diabetes mellitus. *Diabetologia* 1991; **34**: 337–44.

Larner AJ, Moffat MA, Ghadiali E, *et al.* Amnesia following profound hypoglycaemia in a type 1 diabetic patient. *Eur J Neurol* 2003; **10** (Suppl 1): 92 (abstract P1170).

Lincoln NB, Faleiro RM, Kelly C, Kirk BA, Jeffcoate WJ. Effect of long-term glycemic control on cognitive function. *Diabetes Care* 1996; **19**: 656–8.

Luchsinger JA, Tang-Ming X, Shea S, Mayeux R. Hyperinsulinemia and risk of Alzheimer disease. *Neurology* 2004; **63**: 1187–92.

Messier C. Impact of impaired glucose tolerance and type 2 diabetes on cognitive aging. *Neurobiol Aging* 2005; **26** (Suppl 1): 26–30.

Reichard P, Pihl M. Mortality and treatment side effects during long-term intensified conventional insulin treatment in Stockholm Diabetes Intervention Study. *Diabetes* 1994; **43**: 313–17.

Sachon C, Grimaldi A, Digy JP, *et al.* Cognitive function, insulin-dependent diabetes and hypoglycaemia. *J Intern Med* 1992; **231**: 471–5.

Wredling R, Levander S, Adamson U, Lins P. Permanent neuropsychological impairment after recurrent episodes of severe hypoglycaemia in man. *Diabetologia* 1990; **33**: 152–7.

8.1.2 Thyroid disorders

Hypothyroidism

Hypothyroidism is well recognized to have neuropsychiatric features, popularized by Richard Asher in his 1949 paper as 'myxoedematous madness'; interestingly, a number of his cases were stated to have dementia (cases 4, 6, 13), one was initially referred with a suspected diagnosis of Alzheimer's disease, and others were mentally slow, becoming more alert with treatment (Asher, 1986). Hypothyroidism now features ubiquitously in the textbook rubric of 'reversible dementia', and few patients complaining of memory problems escape

having their thyroid function tests checked. An examination of the evidence base, however, tells a rather different story. In a literature search of studies on the aetiology of dementia, Clarnette and Patterson (1994) found only a single case due to hypothyroidism in 2781 cases of reversible dementia. Nonreversible cases have also been reported (Mennemeier *et al.*, 1993). Dugbartey (1998) noted that hypothyroidism has been associated with deficits in general intelligence, complex attention and concentration, memory, perceptual and visuoperceptual function, expressive and receptive language, and executive/frontal functions. A study of thyroid cancer patients on and off thyroxine suggested that the memory defect in delayed recall of verbal information could not be solely attributed to reduced attentional resources (Burmeister *et al.*, 2001).

Subclinical hypothyroidism (SCH) is characterized by low levels of thyroid-stimulating hormone (TSH) but normal levels of T4, T3, free T4, and free T3, and may reflect incipient hypothyroidism. Some studies have suggested cognitive impairments in SCH, including logical memory (Baldini *et al.*, 1997) and working memory (Zhu *et al.*, 2006), whereas others have found cognitive performance to be within the normal range (Bono *et al.*, 2004). Verbal fluency (and mood) may improve after thyroxine treatment in asymptomatic individuals with mild biochemical hypothyroidism (Bono *et al.*, 2004), as may memory and working memory performance. A positive correlation between plasma thyroid hormone (T4) level and cognitive function as assessed with MMSE has been noted in euthyroid older women (Volpato *et al.*, 2002).

Since the risk of hypothyroidism, like dementia, increases with age, the possibility that cognitive impairment is a comorbid rather than a causal factor in some cases cannot be ruled out. Mood may also need to be taken into account (Mennemeier *et al.*, 1993; Bono *et al.*, 2004). Currently there seems little justification in submitting all cognitively impaired patients to thyroid function tests unless there are other somatic and/or neurological symptoms and signs pointing to the possibility of thyroid dysfunction, although TSH remains a mandatory test in the revised guidelines for dementia investigation promulgated by the European Federation of Neurological Societies (Waldemar *et al.*, 2006).

Thyroid dysfunction may also be seen in association with cognitive disorder in Hashimoto's encephalopathy (see Section 6.13).

Hyperthyroidism

Occasional reports of dementia associated with hyperthyroidism with reversal upon correction of thyroid status have appeared (Bulens, 1981). An epidemiological study suggesting that subclinical hyperthyroidism is a risk factor for dementia and Alzheimer's disease has appeared (Kalmijn *et al.*, 2000). A case–control study of patients with newly diagnosed thyrotoxicosis of Graves' type (a condition originally described by Parry: Larner, 2005) found subjective reports of cognitive deficits in the toxic phase, but no impairment was found on comprehensive neuropsychological testing (Vogel *et al.*, 2007), contrasting with a case report of impairments of attention, memory, and constructive skills in a man with Graves' disease, whose symptoms and temporoparietal hypoperfusion on SPECT scanning improved with a return to euthyroidism (Fukui *et al.*, 2001).

REFERENCES

Asher R. Myxoedematous madness. In: Avery Jones F (ed.), *Richard Asher Talking Sense.* Edinburgh: Churchill Livingstone, 1986: 77–95.

Baldini IM, Vita A, Mauri MC, *et al.* Psychopathological and cognitive features in subclinical hypothyroidism. *Prog Neuropsychopharmacol Biol Psychiatry* 1997; **21**: 925–35.

Bono G, Fancellu R, Blandini F, Santoro G, Mauri M. Cognitive and affective status in mild hypothyroidism and interactions with L-thyroxine treatment. *Acta Neurol Scand* 2004; **110**: 59–66.

Bulens C. Neurological complications of hyperthyroidism: remission of spastic paraplegia, dementia, and optic neuropathy. *Arch Neurol* 1981; **38**: 669–70.

Burmeister LA, Ganguli M, Dodge HH, *et al.* Hypothyroidism and cognition: preliminary evidence for a specific defect in memory. *Thyroid* 2001; **11**: 1177–85.

Clarnette RM, Patterson CJ. Hypothyroidism: does treatment cure dementia? *J Geriatr Psychiatry Neurol* 1994; **7**: 23–7.

Dugbartey AT. Neurocognitive aspects of hypothyroidism. *Arch Intern Med* 1998; **158**: 1413–18.

Fukui T, Hasegawa Y, Takenaka H. Hyperthyroid dementia: clinicoradiological findings and response to treatment. *J Neurol Sci* 2001; **184**: 81–8.

Kalmijn S, Mehta KM, Pols HA, *et al.* Subclinical hyperthyroidism and the risk of dementia: the Rotterdam study. *Clin Endocrinol (Oxf)* 2000; **53**: 733–7.

Larner AJ. Caleb Hillier Parry (1755–1822): clinician, scientist, friend of Edward Jenner (1749–1823). *J Med Biogr* 2005; **13**: 189–94.

Mennemeier M, Garner RD, Heilman KM. Memory, mood and measurement in hypothyroidism. *J Clin Exp Neuropsychol* 1993; **15**: 822–31.

Vogel A, Elberling TV, Hørding M, *et al.* Affective symptoms and cognitive functions in the acute phase of Graves' thyrotoxicosis. *Psychoneuroendocrinology* 2007; **32**: 36–43.

Volpato S, Guralnik JM, Fried LP, *et al.* Serum thyroxine level and cognitive decline in euthyroid older women. *Neurology* 2002; **58**: 1055–61.

Waldemar G, Dubois B, Emre M, *et al.* Alzheimer's disease and other disorders associated with dementia. In: Hughes R, Brainin M, Gilhus NE (eds.), *European Handbook of Neurological Management.* Oxford: Blackwell, 2006: 266–98.

Zhu DF, Wang ZX, Zhang DR, *et al.* fMRI revealed neural substrate for reversible working memory dysfunction in subclinical hypothyroidism. *Brain* 2006; **129**: 2923–30.

8.1.3 Parathyroid disorders

Idiopathic hypoparathyroidism, probably an immune diathesis of the parathyroid glands, may result in a variety of systemic and neurological disorders, the latter including seizures, extrapyramidal signs, altered mental state, and signs of raised intracranial pressure including papilloedema, neuromuscular hyperactivity (carpopedal spasm, muscle cramps, Chvostek's and Trousseau's signs), as well as dementia. Many of these features may be explained by the accompanying hypocalcaemia, and reverse with its correction. Dementia has on occasion been reported as the presenting sign of hypoparathyroidism (Robinson *et al.*, 1954; Eraut, 1974;

Slyter, 1979), which may respond to treatment with 1,25-dihydroxycholecalciferol (Mateo & Gimenez-Roldan, 1982). A case of dementia associated with hypoparathyroidism but normocalcaemia which proved reversible with treatment with 1,25-dihydroxycholecalciferol has also been presented (Stuerenburg *et al.*, 1996).

Occasional cases of cognitive impairment associated with hypercalcaemia due to primary hyperparathyroidism have been reported, with reversal after parathyroidectomy (Logullo *et al.*, 1998).

REFERENCES

Eraut D. Idiopathic hypoparathyroidism presenting as dementia. *BMJ* 1974; **1**: 429–30.

Logullo F, Babbini MT, Di Bella P, Provinciali L. Reversible combined cognitive impairment and severe polyneuropathy resulting from primary hyperparathyroidism. *Ital J Neurol Sci* 1998; **19**: 86–9.

Mateo D, Gimenez-Roldan S. Dementia in idiopathic hypoparathyroidism: rapid efficacy of alfacalcidol. *Arch Neurol* 1982; **39**: 424–5.

Robinson KC, Kallberg MH, Crowley MF. Idiopathic hypoparathyroidism presenting as dementia. *BMJ* 1954; **2**: 1203–6.

Slyter H. Idiopathic hypoparathyroidism presenting as dementia. *Neurology* 1979; **29**: 393–4.

Stuerenburg HJ, Hansen HC, Thie A, Kunze K. Reversible dementia in idiopathic hypoparathyroidism associated with normocalcemia. *Neurology* 1996; **47**: 474–6.

8.1.4   Cushing's syndrome (hypercortisolism)

Most cases of Cushing's syndrome, due to hypercortisolaemia, result from pituitary adenomas secreting adrenocorticotrophic hormone (ACTH), others from ectopic ACTH-producing tumours (most often in the lung), and adrenal cortex tumours. Exogenous steroid, most often given therapeutically for a wide variety of diseases, neurological and otherwise, can also result in cushingoid features. Complications include hypertension, impaired glucose tolerance or diabetes, osteoporosis, cushingoid habitus, cutaneous striae, myopathy, and neu-ropsychiatric features such as depression. Cognitive dysfunction may also occur: experimental animal studies have shown the hippocampus to be vulnerable to glucocorticoid excess.

The cognitive impairments identified in Cushing's syndrome patients have varied between studies: selective memory impairments were documented in one case–control study (Mauri *et al.*, 1993), whereas selective attention and visual spatial processing seemed most affected in another report (Forget *et al.*, 2000). Hence, cognitive dysfunction may be variable from case to case (Whelan *et al.*, 1980). Another study showed no differences in cognitive function between patients with pituitary Cushing's disease and a control group composed of patients with non-functioning pituitary adenomas, although the scores of both groups for memory and attention showed significant decrements compared to normative data (Heald *et al.*, 2006), perhaps reflecting an effect of pituitary tumours per se (see Section 7.1.3). Some studies report cognitive improvement after pituitary surgery (Mauri *et al.*, 1993), while others document little or no change in performance, suggesting long-lasting deleterious effects of hypercortisolism (Forget *et al.*, 2002). Reduced hippocampal volume on structural brain imaging has been reported in Cushing's syndrome, and this correlated with memory dysfunction as measured by verbal recall (Starkman *et al.*, 1992). Similar findings have also been reported in elderly individuals with elevated cortisol as compared to those with normal cortisol (Lupien *et al.*, 1998).

REFERENCES

Forget H, Lacroix A, Cohen H. Persistent cognitive impairment following surgical treatment of Cushing's syndrome. *Psychoneuroendocrinology* 2002; **27**: 367–83.

Forget H, Lacroix A, Somma M, Cohen H. Cognitive decline in patients with Cushing's syndrome. *J Int Neuropsychol Soc* 2000; **6**: 20–9.

Heald A, Parr C, Gibson C, O'Driscoll K, Fowler H. A cross-sectional study to investigate long-term cognitive function in people with treated pituitary Cushing's disease. *Exp Clin Endocrinol Diabetes* 2006; **114**: 490–7.

Lupien SJ, de Leon M, de Santi S, *et al.* Cortisol levels during human aging predict hippocampal atrophy and memory deficits. *Nat Neurosci* 1998; **1**: 69–73.

Mauri M, Sinforiani E, Bono G, *et al.* Memory impairment in Cushing's disease. *Acta Neurol Scand* 1993; **87**: 52–5.

Starkman MN, Gebarski SS, Berent S, Schteingart DE. Hippocampal formation volume, memory dysfunction, and cortisol levels in patients with Cushing's syndrome. *Biol Psychiatry* 1992; **32**: 756–65.

Whelan TB, Schteingart DE, Starkman MN, Smith A. Neuropsychological deficits in Cushing's syndrome. *J Nerv Ment Dis* 1980; **168**: 753–7.

8.1.5 Conn's syndrome (primary hyperaldosteronism)

Gudin *et al.* (2000) reported a 64-year-old woman with a confusional state, disorientation, and apathy, with investigation findings of hypokalaemia, metabolic alkalosis, and raised aldosterone levels and radiological evidence of a suprarenal adenoma. A 7-year history of decline in cognitive function had been noted 2 years earlier, ascribed to vascular dementia because of hypertension and CT evidence of cerebrovascular change. The patient's confusional state improved with ion replacement and spironolactone, and following surgical removal of the adenoma the pre-existing cognitive decline also improved. The authors suggested Conn's syndrome is a treatable cause of dementia, albeit extremely rare.

REFERENCES

Gudin M, Sanabria C, Legido B, *et al.* Cognitive dysfunction related to hormonal and ionic levels in a patient diagnosed of [*sic*] Conn syndrome. *J Neurol* 2000; **247** (Suppl 3): III/75 (abstract P275).

8.2 Metabolic disorders

Included here are cognitive disorders related to vitamin deficiencies not covered elsewhere (for thiamine deficiency, see Wernicke–Korsakoff Syndrome, Section 8.3.1), electrolyte-related problems, and impairment or failure of specific organs.

8.2.1 Central pontine (and extrapontine) myelinolysis, osmotic demyelination syndrome

Central pontine myelinolysis was first described as such by Adams *et al.* (1959) as a relatively symmetrical destruction of myelin sheaths in the basal pons, sometimes extending beyond (hence 'extrapontine myelinolysis'), often associated with hyponatraemia or its treatment, particularly but not exclusively seen in chronic alcoholics or other patients with chronic undernourishment (Kleinschmidt-DeMasters *et al.*, 2006). Since change in serum osmolality is common to many of the recognized precipitating factors, the terms osmotic demyelination or osmotic myelinolysis are preferred by some authors (Sterns *et al.*, 1986).

Although a range of neuropsychiatric disorders complicating this syndrome are well recognized, neuropsychological studies have been rare (Ruchinskas, 1998; Vermetten *et al.*, 1999; Lee *et al.*, 2003). Findings include mildly reduced IQ and impaired attention, information processing speed, memory (especially retrieval), and executive function, with relatively spared language, features more suggestive of a 'white matter' than a cortical dementia. Deficits do not necessarily reverse with clinical recovery. In one case such changes, accompanied by pathological crying and laughter, occurred with lesions confined to the pons (Lee *et al.*, 2003), in which context it may be noted that cognitive dysfunction with exclusively pontine pathology has also been reported with cerebrovascular disease (van Zandvoort *et al.*, 2003; see Section 3.3.8).

'Callosal dementia' (see Section 1.12), a disconnection syndrome, has been described in association with central and extrapontine myelinolysis (Ghika Schmid *et al.*, 1999).

REFERENCES

Adams RD, Victor M, Mancall EL. Central pontine myelinolysis: a hitherto undescribed disease occurring in alcoholic and malnourished patients. *Arch Neurol Psychiatr Chicago* 1959; **81**: 154–72.

Ghika Schmid F, Ghika J, Assal G, Bogousslavsky J. Callosal dementia: behavioral disorders related to central and extrapontine myelinolysis [in French]. *Rev Neurol Paris* 1999; **155**: 367–73.

Kleinschmidt-DeMasters BK, Rojiani AM, Filley CM. Central and extrapontine myelinolysis: then ... and now. *J Neuropathol Exp Neurol* 2006; **65**: 1–11.

Lee TMC, Cheung CCY, Lau EYY, Mak A, Li LSW. Cognitive and emotional dysfunction after central pontine myelinolysis. *Behav Neurol* 2003; **14**: 103–7.

Ruchinskas R. Cognitive dysfunction after central pontine myelinolysis. *Neurocase* 1998; **4**: 173–9.

Sterns RH, Riggs JE, Schochet SS. Osmotic demyelination syndrome following correction of hyponatremia. *N Engl J Med* 1986; **314**: 1535–42.

van Zandvoort M, de Haan E, van Gijn J, Kappelle LJ. Cognitive functioning in patients with a small infarct in the brainstem. *J Int Neuropsychol Soc* 2003; **9**: 490–4.

Vermetten E, Rutten SJ, Boon PJ, Hofman PA, Leentjens AF. Neuropsychiatric and neuropsychological manifestations of central pontine myelinolysis. *Gen Hosp Psychiatry* 1999; **21**: 296–302.

8.2.2 Gastrointestinal disease

Cobalamin (vitamin B_{12}) deficiency

Addison's original description of pernicious anaemia in 1853 included the clinical observation that 'the mind occasionally wanders'. Cobalamin (vitamin B_{12}) is a cofactor in several metabolic pathways, and its deficiency may be associated with dementia; indeed this may be the sole manifestation (no anaemia). The belief that vitamin B_{12} deficiency is a reversible cause of dementia became prevalent in the 1950s. Practically every textbook of neurology lists vitamin B_{12} deficiency as a reversible cause of dementia or cognitive impairment. Recommendations that all patients attending memory clinics should have their vitamin B_{12} level checked are not hard to find. Yet the evidence base for such definitive statements and recommendations is, at best, weak. Reversible dementias in general are increasingly rare (Clarfield, 2003), and convincing documentation of cognitive impairment associated with vitamin B_{12} deficiency with reversal on repletion is simply not to be found in the literature.

A low vitamin B_{12} is not an uncommon finding in patients with dementia or cognitive decline. For example, in 170 consecutive patients diagnosed with dementia, Teunisse *et al.* (1996) found low vitamin B_{12} in 26 (15%), all but one of whom fulfilled diagnostic criteria for Alzheimer's disease (AD). At the group level, no patient improved with vitamin B_{12} repletion, nor was there any evidence for slowing of AD progression. One patient with a sudden onset of cognitive decline after a respiratory tract infection did improve, but this may have been coincidental with recovery from the infection. Likewise, Eastley *et al.* (2000) found low vitamin B_{12} in 125 of 1432 consecutive clinic attenders (8.7%). No demented patient improved with repletion. Hence, these studies would seem to suggest that in most cases a low vitamin B_{12} in a demented patient is a coexistent, rather than a causal, abnormality, perhaps related to prolonged dietary neglect. Other studies have found low vitamin B_{12} and folate and elevated levels of total homocysteine in AD patients, independent of nutritional status (Clarke *et al.*, 1998; McCaddon *et al.*, 1998), and epidemiological studies suggest that low vitamin B_{12} may increase the risk of developing AD (Wang *et al.*, 2001). The mechanism is not known, but an hypothesis has been proposed suggesting that functional vitamin B_{12} deficiency contributes to the pathogenesis of AD (McCaddon *et al.*, 2002). Current guidelines from the American Academy of Neurology advise that vitamin B_{12} levels should be assessed in cases of dementia, since this is a common comorbidity and may influence cognitive function (Knopman *et al.*, 2001), but revised guidelines from the European Federation of Neurological Societies state only that vitamin B_{12} level will often be required in individual cases (Waldemar *et al.*, 2006).

Individual cases and case series of dementia and vitamin B_{12} deficiency are few. In a 17-year study of cobalamin deficiency, Healton *et al.* (1991) recorded 18 cases of mental impairment in 143 cases, 8 with global dementia and 9 with recent memory loss; 11/18 recovered completely with repletion. Another study suggested that improvement may be related to symptom duration, as for other neurological consequences of vitamin B_{12} deficiency (Martin *et al.*, 1992). Chiu (1996) found 25 cases of dementia attributed to B_{12} deficiency reported between 1958 and 1995, 10 with marked improvement on repletion; all had some haematological abnormality (anaemia, raised MCV, hypersegmented neutrophils) or neurological signs in addition to cognitive impairment.

Reports with careful and sequential neuropsychological assessment are also lacking. The case reported by Meadows *et al.* (1994) was confounded by a history of alcohol misuse. Another patient, a health professional with marked clinical improvement after repletion therapy, declined repeat neuropsychological assessment (Larner *et al.*, 1999; Larner & Rakshi, 2001). A report claiming a subcortical dementia pattern associated with vitamin B_{12} deficiency was based on clinical observations, unsubstantiated by neuropsychological assessment (Saracaceanu *et al.*, 1997).

Eastley *et al.* (2000) found that patients with cognitive decline but without dementia did, at the group level, show improvement in verbal fluency with vitamin B_{12} repletion, leading them to suggest that vitamin B_{12} may improve frontal lobe and language function in patients with cognitive impairment. Studies of vitamin B_{12} in mild cognitive impairment might be of interest, but none has been identified, and it is not amongst recommended biomarkers for mild cognitive impairment (see Section 2.6).

Hence, in the view of this author, it would seem that if vitamin B_{12} deficiency does cause cognitive decline, this is an extremely rare occurrence, with only a handful of reversible cases of sometimes dubious authenticity recorded in the literature, much less common than non-pathogenic coexistence of dementia with vitamin B_{12} deficiency. This may simply reflect the low positive predictive value of a low vitamin B_{12} measurement (Chiu, 1996; Connick *et al.*, 2006).

Defective cobalamin transport and/or metabolism secondary to impaired biosynthesis of methylcobalamin and adenosylcobalamin produces a functional deficiency of methylmalonyl CoA mutase and methionine synthase with resulting methylmalonic aciduria and homocystinuria. Most cases present before 2 months of age, but cases in children and even young adults have been reported, presenting with a rapidly progressive dementia and myelopathy, of which the dementia is on occasion responsive to hydroxycobalamin injections (Shinnar & Singer, 1984; Al-Memar *et al.*, 1998; Augoustides Savvopoulou *et al.*, 1999).

Gluten sensitivity and coeliac disease

The neurological associations of gluten sensitivity, with or without bowel disease (coeliac disease) are protean, the most common being epilepsy, cerebellar ataxia, axonal neuropathy, myelopathy, myoclonus, intracerebral (especially occipital) calcification, migraine, and cerebral vasculitis with encephalopathy (Pengiran Tengah *et al.*, 2002), as well as neurological sequelae following dissemination of enteropathy-type T-cell lymphoma, which may complicate the disease (Doran *et al.*, 2005). Although a presenile dementia of uncertain aetiology has also been reported on occasion (Collin *et al.*, 1991), a review of the neurological complications of coeliac disease concluded that there was no firm evidence of a link between dementia and gluten sensitivity (Pengiran Tengah *et al.*, 2002). However, Hu *et al.* (2006) reported a series of 13 patients seen over a 35-year period with cognitive impairment coincident with gastrointestinal symptom onset or exacerbation. A frontal subcortical pattern of cognitive impairment was typical; many patients had concurrent ataxia or neuropathy. In three patients cognitive function was reported to improve or stabilize on gluten withdrawal.

Pellagra

This condition, a deficiency of vitamins of the B group, including but not necessarily confined to niacin (nicotinic acid, nicotinamide), is sometimes remembered as the '3 Ds': diarrhoea, dermatitis, dementia; or sometimes the 4 Ds (+ death). As far as can be ascertained, the nature of this dementia has not been fully described. A pellagra encephalopathy of alcoholic aetiology has been described (Serdaru *et al.*, 1988), but of course alcohol per se may contribute to any cognitive impairment irrespective of vitamin status.

REFERENCES

Al-Memar AY, Preece MA, Ross C, Green S, Pall HS. Combined methylmalonic aciduria and homocystinuria: a defect in cellular metabolism of cobalamin and a treatable cause of dementia. *J Neurol Neurosurg Psychiatry* 1998; **65**: 420 (abstract).

Augoustides Savvopoulou P, Mylonas I, Sewell AC, Rosenblatt DS. Reversible dementia in an adolescent with cblC disease: clinical heterogeneity within the same family. *J Inherit Metab Dis* 1999; **22**: 756–8.

Chiu HFK. Vitamin B_{12} deficiency and dementia. *Int J Geriatr Psychiatry* 1996; **11**: 851–8.

Clarfield AM. The decreasing prevalence of reversible dementia: an updated meta-analysis. *Arch Intern Med* 2003; **163**: 2219–29.

Clarke R, Smith AD, Jobst KA, *et al.* Folate, vitamin B12, and serum total homocysteine in confirmed Alzheimer disease. *Arch Neurol* 1998; **55**: 1449–55.

Collin P, Pirttilä T, Nurmikko T, *et al.* Celiac disease, brain atrophy, and dementia. *Neurology* 1991; **41**: 372–5.

Connick P, Cooper S, Grosset D. Investigating B_{12} deficiency amongst neurological patients. *J Neurol Neurosurg Psychiatry* 2006; **77**: 126 (abstract 002).

Doran M, du Plessis DG, Larner AJ. Disseminated enteropathy-type T-cell lymphoma: cauda equina syndrome complicating coeliac disease. *Clin Neurol Neurosurg* 2005; **107**: 517–20.

Eastley R, Wilcock GK, Bucks RS. Vitamin B_{12} deficiency in dementia and cognitive impairment: the effects of treatment on neuropsychological function. *Int J Geriatr Psychiatry* 2000; **15**: 226–33.

Healton EB, Savage DG, Brust JCM, *et al.* Neurologic aspects of cobalamin deficiency. *Medicine (Baltimore)* 1991; **70**: 229–45.

Hu WT, Murray JA, Greenaway MC, Parisi JE, Josephs KA. Cognitive impairment and celiac disease. *Arch Neurol* 2006; **63**: 1440–6.

Knopman DS, DeKosky ST, Cummings JL, *et al.* Practice parameter: diagnosis of dementia (an evidence-based review). Report of the Quality Standards Subcommittee of the American Academy of Neurology. *Neurology* 2001; **56**: 1143–53.

Larner AJ, Janssen JC, Cipolotti L, Rossor MN. Cognitive profile in dementia associated with vitamin B_{12} deficiency due to pernicious anaemia. *J Neurol* 1999; **246**: 317–9.

Larner AJ, Rakshi JS. Vitamin B_{12} deficiency and dementia. *Eur J Neurol* 2001; **8**: 730.

McCaddon A, Davies G, Hudson P, Tandy S, Cattell H. Total serum homocysteine in senile dementia of Alzheimer type. *Int J Geriatr Psychiatry* 1998; **13**: 235–9.

McCaddon A, Regland B, Hudson P, Davies G. Functional vitamin B_{12} deficiency and Alzheimer disease. *Neurology* 2002; **58**: 1395–9.

Martin DC, Francis J, Protetch J, Huff FJ. Time dependency of cognitive recovery with cobalamin replacement: report of a pilot study. *J Am Geriatr Soc* 1992; **40**: 168–72.

Meadows ME, Kaplan RF, Bromfield EB. Cognitive recovery with vitamin B_{12} therapy: a longitudinal neuropsychiatric assessment. *Neurology* 1994; **44**: 1764–5.

Pengiran Tengah DSNA, Wills AJ, Holmes GKT. Neurological complications of coeliac disease. *Postgrad Med J* 2002; **78**: 393–8.

Saracaceanu E, Tramoni AV, Henry JM. An association between subcortical dementia and pernicious anaemia: a psychiatric mask. *Compr Psychiatry* 1997; **38**: 349–51.

Serdaru M, Hausser-Hauw C, Laplane D, *et al.* The clinical spectrum of alcoholic pellagra encephalopathy. *Brain* 1988; **111**: 829–42.

Shinnar S, Singer HS. Cobalamin C mutation (methylmalonic aciduria and homocystinuria) in adolescence: a treatable cause of dementia and myelopathy. *N Engl J Med* 1984; **311**: 451–4.

Teunisse S, Bollen AE, van Gool WA, Walstra GJM. Dementia and subnormal levels of vitamin B_{12}: effects of replacement therapy on dementia. *J Neurol* 1996; **243**: 522–9.

Waldemar G, Dubois B, Emre M, *et al.* Alzheimer's disease and other disorders associated with dementia. In: Hughes R, Brainin M, Gilhus NE (eds.), *European Handbook of Neurological Management*. Oxford: Blackwell, 2006: 266–98.

Wang HX, Wahlin A, Basun H, *et al.* Vitamin B_{12} and folate in relation to the development of Alzheimer's disease. *Neurology* 2001; **56**: 1188–94.

8.2.3 Respiratory disorders

Chronic obstructive pulmonary disease (COPD)

A study by Grant et al. (1982) found that patients with chronic obstructive pulmonary disease (COPD) were worse than control patients on all neuropsychological tests prior to treatment, especially 'higher' functions such as abstracting ability and complex perceptual–motor integration. There was some evidence that performance was worse the greater the degree of hypoxaemia, and this was confirmed in a later study (Grant et al., 1987). Chronic oxygen therapy was associated with a small improvement in neuropsychological functioning, with a suggestion that continuous therapy was better than solely nocturnal treatment (Heaton et al., 1983).

A study of 36 patients with COPD reported that just under half had a specific pattern of cognitive deterioration characterized by impairments of verbal and visual memory tasks despite preserved visual attention, and with diffuse worsening of other functions. These changes were distinct from those seen in AD patients, and were correlated with age and duration of respiratory failure (Incalzi et al., 1993). In a further study from this group, decline of verbal memory was found to parallel that of overall cognitive function, due to impairment of both active recall and passive recognition of learned material. Poor adherence to medication was associated with abnormal delayed recall scores (Incalzi et al., 1997). In a follow-up study, onset of depression was a risk factor for cognitive decline (Incalzi et al., 1998). Roehrs et al. (1995) found deficits in complex reasoning and memory in COPD patients as well as motor skills, the latter sensitive to hypoxaemia. Another group reported MMSE abnormalities in 62% of COPD patients, affecting recent memory, construction, attention, language, and orientation, the cognitive abnormalities correlating with functional abnormalities (Özge et al., 2004). However, a study by Kozora et al. (1999) found that most COPD patients studied were similar to controls on most tests, and easily distinguishable from

mild AD, the exception being a reduced letter fluency. The fact that three-quarters of the patients were receiving supplementary oxygen therapy may account for the preservation of cognitive function in this study.

In a community-based longitudinal study of cognitive impairment and dementia, COPD was noted to be more likely in patients with non-progressive cognitive decline, i.e. in those patients in whom an original diagnosis of dementia was not confirmed at follow-up (Schofield et al., 1995).

Obstructive sleep apnoea–hypopnoea syndrome (OSAHS)

Obstructive sleep apnoea–hypopnoea syndrome (OSAHS) is caused by critical narrowing of the upper airway during sleep when reduced muscle tone leads to increased resistance to the flow of air, and partial obstruction often results in loud snoring. Sleep is restless due to successive episodes of apnoea, often witnessed by the bed partner, which are relieved by brief arousal from sleep. A narrow anteroposterior pharyngeal diameter, obesity, high alcohol intake, and male sex seem to be risk factors. As a consequence of sleep fragmentation, the commonest daytime symptom is excessive somnolence, manifest as a tendency to fall asleep in monotonous or inappropriate situations. OSAHS is diagnosed using nocturnal polysomnography or, more practically in routine clinical work, pulse oximetry. The severity of OSAHS may be measured using the apnoea/hypopnoea index (AHI), or respiratory disturbance index (RDI), which is calculated from polysomnographic recordings as the number of apnoeas/hypopnoeas per hour of sleep. AHI or RDI of 10–20 indicates mild, 20–50 moderate, and > 50 severe disease. With pulse oximetry, a desaturation index (DI) may be calculated as the number of desaturations (decrease in oxygen saturation by $\geq 4\%$) per hour of sleep or, if the recording is unattended, per time of recording. $DI \geq 5$ may be used to define sleep-disordered breathing (Redline et al., 2000).

OSAHS may present with various neurological symptoms besides excessive daytime sleepiness, including blackouts and headache, sometimes with features suggestive of raised intracranial pressure, and may be mistaken for narcolepsy, epilepsy, and idiopathic intracranial hypertension, respectively. Apparent intellectual decline, which may be mistaken for dementia, is also reported to be a recognized feature of OSAHS, which may improve after appropriate treatment of the underlying condition (Douglas, 2003; Larner, 2003).

Findley *et al.* (1986) found impairments in measures of attention, concentration, complex problem solving, and short-term recall of verbal and spatial information in OSAHS patients with hypoxaemia as compared with OSAHS patients without hypoxaemia; cognitive impairment did not correlate with measures of sleep fragmentation, suggesting that it was hypoxia rather than sleep disturbance (a recognized cause of cognitive dysfunction: Durmer & Dinges, 2005) that accounted for the cognitive deficits. A patient reported by Scheltens *et al.* (1991), in whom cognitive impairment was the presenting feature of a sleep apnoea syndrome, had impaired learning and retention, impaired sustained attention, impaired visuospatial reasoning, vulnerability to interference, impaired verbal fluency, but no aphasia, apraxia, or agnosia. Polysomnography showed a mixed picture of central and obstructive apnoeas in this patient. The authors suggested that both cerebral hypoxia and sleep fragmentation contributed to cognitive impairment, which reversed with appropriate treatment (nocturnal continuous positive airway pressure). Mild cognitive impairment with slight reductions in verbal reasoning and verbal comprehension performance, poor performance on tests of short-term memory and learning, reduced verbal fluency, and mild attentional problems, but with intact non-verbal reasoning, language, visuospatial, and constructional functions were noted in another patient (Larner & Ghadiali, unpublished observations), deficits more typical of subcortical pathology due to interruption of frontal-subcortical circuits. This neuropsychological profile may correlate with white matter cerebral metabolic impairments seen with magnetic resonance spectroscopy in OSAHS patients (Kamba *et al.*, 2001).

An overview of case–control studies of neuropsychological function in patients with sleep-disordered breathing found that impairment was generally greater with increasing severity of disease (Engelman *et al.*, 2000), recognizing that some tasks are more sensitive to hypoxaemia, and others more sensitive to sleepiness. Comparing groups of patients with OSAHS and COPD, Roehrs *et al.* (1995) found that deficits in complex reasoning and memory were not specific to diagnosis, whereas sustained attention was worse in the OSAHS group, reflecting its sensitivity to sleepiness, and motor skills were worse in the COPD group, reflecting their sensitivity to hypoxaemia. A study comparing OSAHS patients with AD, multi-infarct dementia, and COPD found a distinctive cognitive profile suggestive of subcortical damage (Antonelli Incalzi *et al.*, 2004).

Central sleep apnoea is characterized by periodic apnoea due to loss of ventilatory motor output, due to an unstable ventilatory control system, resulting in lack of inspiratory muscle effort (Abad & Guilleminault, 2004; Badr, 2005). There are diverse causes, including neurological diseases such as multiple system atrophy, but some cases remain idiopathic. We have encountered a patient with central sleep apnoea presenting with cognitive complaints, whose neuropsychological profile showed marked impairments in non-verbal reasoning and processing speed, indicative of a subcortical type dementia, but the interpretation was confounded by prior radiotherapy for a malignant brain tumour (Larner & Ghadiali, unpublished observations).

Carbon monoxide poisoning

A delayed encephalopathy may develop a few days to weeks after carbon monoxide (CO) poisoning, with or without a history of acute poisoning, sometimes with extrapyramidal or pyramidal signs and psychosis (Ernst & Zibrak, 1998). MR imaging abnormalities occur in about 12% of patients, most typically widespread periventricular white matter changes, although basal ganglia involvement is also reported.

A prospective study of episodes of CO poisoning found cognitive deficits in 30% of patients (Parkinson *et al.*, 2002). Occasionally these deficits may be very focal, as for example in a renowned case of visual-form agnosia (Goodale & Milner, 2004), and a case of apparent visual motion blindness (akinetopsia) has been reported (Larner, 2005). Delayed onset of cognitive, including memory, problems by up to 30 days after acute poisoning may occur, associated with extensive diffuse white matter change (Balla *et al.*, 2005). Delayed atrophy of the fornix, correlating with decline on tests of verbal memory, has also been reported in patients poisoned with CO (Kesler *et al.*, 2001).

The complications of CO poisoning typically improve with time, but patients may sometimes be left with permanent neurological and/or neuropsychological sequelae (e.g. Goodale & Milner, 2004).

REFERENCES

Abad VC, Guilleminault C. Neurological perspective on obstructive and nonobstructive sleep apnea. *Semin Neurol* 2004; **24**: 261–9.

Antonelli Incalzi R, Marra C, Salvigni BL, *et al.* Does cognitive dysfunction conform to a distinctive pattern in obstructive sleep apnea syndrome? *J Sleep Res* 2004; **13**: 79–86.

Badr MS. Central sleep apnea. *Prim Care* 2005; **32**: 361–74.

Balla C, Kanta O, Paschalidou M, Artemis N, Milonas I. Delayed encephalopathy of carbon monoxide (CO) poisoning. *Eur J Neurol* 2005; **12** (Suppl 2): 290 (abstract P2484).

Douglas NJ. The obstructive sleep apnoea/hypopnoea syndrome. *Pract Neurol* 2003; **3**: 22–8.

Durmer JS, Dinges DF. Neurocognitive consequences of sleep deprivation. *Semin Neurol* 2005; **25**: 117–29.

Engelman HM, Kingshott RN, Martin SE, Douglas NJ. Cognitive function in the sleep apnea/hypopnea syndrome (SAHS). *Sleep* 2000; **23** (Suppl 4): S102–8.

Ernst A, Zibrak JD. Carbon monoxide poisoning. *N Engl J Med* 1998; **339**: 1603–8.

Findley LJ, Barth JT, Powers DC, *et al.* Cognitive impairment in patients with obstructive sleep apnea and associated hypoxemia. *Chest* 1986; **90**: 686–90.

Goodale MA, Milner AD. *Sight Unseen: an Exploration of Conscious and Unconscious Vision.* Oxford: Oxford University Press, 2004.

Grant I, Heaton RK, McSweeny AJ, Adams KM, Timms RM. Neuropsychologic findings in hypoxemic chronic obstructive pulmonary disease. *Arch Intern Med* 1982; **142**: 1470–6.

Grant I, Prigatano GP, Heaton RK, *et al.* Progressive neuropsychologic impairment and hypoxemia: relationship in chronic obstructive pulmonary disease. *Arch Gen Psychiatry* 1987; **44**: 999–1006.

Heaton RK, Grant I, McSweeny AJ, Adams KM, Petty TL. Psychologic effects of continuous and nocturnal oxygen therapy in hypoxemic chronic obstructive pulmonary disease. *Arch Intern Med* 1983; **143**: 1941–7.

Incalzi RA, Chiappini F, Fuso L, *et al.* Predicting cognitive decline in patients with hypoxaemic COPD. *Respir Med* 1998; **92**: 527–33.

Incalzi RA, Gemma A, Marra C, *et al.* Chronic obstructive pulmonary disease: an original model of cognitive decline. *Am Rev Respir Dis* 1993; **148**: 418–24.

Incalzi RA, Gemma A, Marra C, *et al.* Verbal memory impairment in COPD: its mechanisms and clinical relevance. *Chest* 1997; **112**: 1506–13.

Kamba M, Inoue Y, Higami S, *et al.* Cerebral metabolic impairments in patients with obstructive sleep apnoea: an independent association of obstructive sleep apnoea with white matter change. *J Neurol Neurosurg Psychiatry* 2001; **71**: 334–9.

Kesler SR, Hopkins RO, Blatter DD, Edge Booth H, Bigler ED. Verbal memory deficits associated with fornix atrophy in carbon monoxide poisoning. *J Int Neuropsychol Soc* 2001; **7**: 640–6.

Kozora E, Filley CM, Julian LJ, Cullum CM. Cognitive functioning in patients with chronic obstructive pulmonary disease and mild hypoxemia compared with patients with mild Alzheimer disease and normal controls. *Neuropsychiatry Neuropsychol Behav Neurol* 1999; **12**: 178–83.

Larner AJ. Obstructive sleep apnoea syndrome presenting in a neurology outpatient clinic. *Int J Clin Pract* 2003; **57**: 150–2.

Larner AJ. Delayed motor and visual complications after attempted suicide. *Lancet* 2005; **366**: 1826.

Özge C, Ünal O, Özge A, Saraçoglu M. Cognitive and functional deterioration in patients with severe COPD. *Eur J Neurol* 2004; **11** (Suppl 2): 24–5 (abstract SC221).

Parkinson RB, Hopkins RO, Cleavinger HB, *et al.* White matter hyperintensities and neuropsychological outcome following carbon monoxide poisoning. *Neurology* 2002; **58**: 1525–32.

Redline S, Kapur VK, Sanders MH, *et al.* Effects of varying approaches for identifying respiratory disturbances on sleep apnea assessment. *Am J Respir Crit Care Med* 2000; **161**: 369–74.

Roehrs T, Merrion M, Pedrosi B, *et al.* Neuropsychological function in obstructive sleep apnea syndrome (OSAS) compared to chronic obstructive pulmonary disease (COPD). *Sleep* 1995; **18**: 382–8.

Scheltens P, Visscher F, Van Keimpema ARJ, *et al.* Sleep apnea syndrome presenting with cognitive impairment. *Neurology* 1991; **41**: 155–6.

Schofield PW, Tang M, Marder K, *et al.* Consistency of clinical diagnosis in a community-based longitudinal study of dementia and Alzheimer's disease. *Neurology* 1995; **45**: 2159–64.

8.3   Toxin-related disorders

8.3.1   Alcohol-related disorders

Alcohol is probably the most widely available and socially tolerated neuroactive substance. Although epidemiological studies suggest it to be protective against dementia in modest dosage (Ruitenberg *et al.*, 2002), escalating dosage unequivocally increases the risk of late-life dementia (Saunders *et al.*, 1991). Wernicke–Korsakoff syndrome is the best known of the syndromes of cognitive impairment related to alcohol, although it can on occasion occur in the absence of a history of alcohol overuse. Other syndromes of cognitive impairment which might also be encompassed under the rubric of 'alcohol-related', since alcohol overuse is a risk factor for their development, include subdural haematoma (see Section 7.3.1), pellagra (Section 8.2.2), and obstructive sleep apnoea–hypopnoea syndrome (Section 8.2.3).

Wernicke–Korsakoff syndrome (WKS)

The neurological and neuropsychological consequences of the Wernicke–Korsakoff syndrome (WKS), due to thiamine (vitamin B_1) deficiency, have been extensively studied (Victor *et al.*, 1989). Although most cases relate to alcohol misuse with consequent undernutrition, WKS may also occur in the context of malnutrition from other causes, such as prolonged vomiting in pregnancy or parenteral nutrition with inadequate supplementation (Monaghan *et al.*, 2006), or with other diencephalic lesions such as tumours or trauma.

Initially WKS was characterized as a neurological disorder with nystagmus, ophthalmoplegia, and ataxia, and a neuropsychological syndrome of selective anterograde amnesia with relative preservation of intelligence, sometimes complicated by confabulations (Butters & Cermak, 1980). For this reason, Korsakoff patients have often been used in group studies to compare their cognitive profile with that seen in other cognitive disorders such as Alzheimer's disease and Huntington's disease (Butters, 1984). However, with the development of new diagnostic criteria (Caine *et al.*, 1997) the spectrum of WKS has broadened to include patients without the classical neurological signs. In this broader group there is evidence for generalized cognitive impairment or dementia ('thiamine dementia') rather than selective ('diencephalic') amnesia (Bowden & Ritter, 2005). Because of the potential reversibility of cognitive deficits with thiamine repletion, and the fact that many cases were previously overlooked on clinical grounds, there is a strong case for making a presumptive diagnosis of WKS in any patient with a history suggestive of alcohol dependence.

Neuropathologically there is shrinkage of the mammillary bodies, structures around the third and fourth ventricles (i.e. the diencephalon), and the medial thalamus. Which of these is the substrate of the cognitive impairments has been argued, but generally the mammillary bodies are not thought to be relevant (Victor, 1987), with better correlations for the medial thalamus, although the exact nuclei involved (mediodorsal, centromedial, anterior) may vary (Mayes *et al.*, 1988; Halliday *et al.*, 1994; Harding *et al.*, 2000). There may be loss of hippocampal volume but without neuronal loss (Harper

& Scolyer, 2004), but this does not necessarily imply normal hippocampal function: functional imaging studies have suggested loss of hippocampal memory encoding in WKS patients, possibly as a consequence of hippocampal–thalamic involvement (Caulo *et al.*, 2005). Neuronal loss in the nucleus basalis of Meynert might also be relevant (Butters, 1985).

Alcohol-related dementia, primary alcoholic dementia

Whether alcohol (i.e. ethanol) per se is neurotoxic, and may cause cognitive decline independent of thiamine deficiency, remains a subject of debate (Moriyama *et al.*, 2006). Although provisional diagnostic criteria for alcohol-related dementia have been proposed (Oslin *et al.*, 1998), others suggest that this syndrome may be better conceptualized as a multifactorial 'alcohol-induced dementia', related to comorbidities such as nutritional deficiency (perhaps causing prior episodes of WKS); damage to other organs, particularly liver, with repeated episodes of hepatic encephalopathy; head injury, subdural haematoma, epileptic seizures, hydrocephalus, Marchiafava–Bignami disease, obstructive sleep apnoea; and pre-existing cognitive status. Concurrent morbidity such as cerebrovascular disease and/or Alzheimer's disease may also contribute to cognitive decline. Many patients conforming to the proposed criteria might also conform to the criteria for WKS (Caine *et al.*, 1997). An important differential diagnosis is frontal variant frontotemporal dementia (see Section 2.2.1), in which hyperorality may include alcohol overconsumption.

Neuropathological studies have shown cerebral atrophy due to white matter loss, and neuronal and synaptic losses in some areas such as frontal association cortex (Harper, 1998); these frontal changes are likened by some authors to those seen in frontotemporal dementia (Brun & Andersson, 2001). There is relative sparing of other areas including the hippocampus (Harper & Scolyer, 2004). However, a specific neuropathological substrate for alcohol-related dementia has not yet been defined (Bowden & Ritter, 2005).

It is therefore not surprising that no specific neuropsychological profile for alcohol-related dementia has been defined. Working memory and executive deficits may occur, perhaps reflecting frontal neuropathological changes, as may declines in memory and aspects of crystallized intelligence (Bates *et al.*, 2002).

Marchiafava–Bignami disease

Marchiafava–Bignami disease is a rare alcohol-associated disorder characterized by demyelination and necrosis of the corpus callosum; lesions may also occur in the putamen. Clinically a distinction may be drawn between those cases in which impaired consciousness occurs, with a poorer prognosis, and those in which consciousness is preserved. Cognitive impairment may occur in both the prodrome and recovery phase of the former, as may interhemispheric disconnection syndromes (Kohler *et al.*, 2000; Heinrich *et al.*, 2004). The latter may include combinations of apraxia, agraphia, and Balint syndrome, along with neurobehavioural features (Kalckreuth *et al.*, 1994), the syndrome which has been labelled 'callosal dementia' (Ghika Schmid *et al.*, 1999).

Acquired non-Wilsonian hepatocerebral degeneration

This condition has been characterized as a syndrome of fixed or progressive neurological deficits, including dementia, dysarthria, gait ataxia, intention tremor, parkinsonism, spastic paraparesis, and choreoathetosis, as a consequence of cerebral degeneration in the context of repeated episodes of hepatic encephalopathy, the liver damage usually following alcohol misuse. It is argued that individually such episodes of hepatic encephalopathy may be reversible, but that cumulatively there is a degenerative effect on neural tissue, with microcavitary changes in layers V and VI of the cortex, underlying white matter, basal ganglia, and cerebellum (Victor *et al.*, 1965). Others have doubted whether this condition exists as a separate entity. Cases with features overlapping those of extrapontine myelinolysis (see Section 8.2.1) have been reported (Kleinschmidt-DeMasters *et al.*, 2006). Functional imaging may show reduced parieto-occipital perfusion, and structural imaging typically shows abnormal signal in the pallidum and midbrain, although cerebellar involvement has also been reported (Park & Heo, 2004). Clinical and radiological changes have been improved with branched chain amino acids (Ueki *et al.*, 2002), but there is no report of cognitive improvement.

REFERENCES

Bates ME, Bowden SC, Barry D. Neurocognitive impairment associated with alcohol use disorders: implications for treatment. *Exp Clin Psychopharmacol* 2002; **10**: 193–212.

Bowden SC, Ritter AJ. Alcohol-related dementia and the clinical spectrum of Wernicke–Korsakoff syndrome. In: Burns A, O'Brien J, Ames D (eds.), *Dementia* (3rd edition). London: Hodder Arnold, 2005: 738–44.

Brun A, Andersson J. Frontal dysfunction and frontal cortical synapse loss in alcoholism: the main cause of alcohol dementia? *Dement Geriatr Cogn Disord* 2001; **12**: 289–94.

Butters N. The clinical aspects of memory disorders: contributions from experimental studies of amnesia and dementia. *J Clin Neuropsychol* 1984; **6**: 17–36.

Butters N. Alcoholic Korsakoff's syndrome: some unresolved issues concerning etiology, neuropathology, and cognitive deficits. *J Clin Exp Neuropsychol* 1985; **7**: 181–210.

Butters N, Cermak LS. *Alcoholic Korsakoff's Syndrome: an Information-Processing Approach to Amnesia*. London: Academic Press, 1980.

Caine D, Halliday GM, Kril JJ, Harper CG. Operational criteria for the classification of chronic alcoholics: identification of Wernicke's encephalopathy. *J Neurol Neurosurg Psychiatry* 1997; **62**: 51–60.

Caulo M, Van Hecke J, Toma L, *et al.* Functional MRI study of diencephalic amnesia in Wernicke–Korsakoff syndrome. *Brain* 2005; **128**: 1584–94.

Ghika Schmid F, Ghika J, Assal G, Bogousslavsky J. Callosal dementia: behavioral disorders related to central and extrapontine myelinolysis [in French]. *Rev Neurol Paris* 1999; **155**: 367–73.

Halliday G, Cullen K, Harding A. Neuropathological correlates of memory dysfunction in the Wernicke–Korsakoff syndrome. *Alcohol Alcohol Suppl* 1994; **2**: 245–51.

Harding A, Halliday G, Caine D, Kril J. Degeneration of anterior thalamic nuclei differentiates alcoholics with amnesia. *Brain* 2000; **123**: 141–54.

Harper C. The neuropathology of alcohol-specific brain damage, or does alcohol damage the brain? *J Neuropathol Exp Neurol* 1998; **57**: 101–10.

Harper C, Scolyer RA. Alcoholism and dementia. In: Esiri MM, Lee VMY, Trojanowski JQ (eds.), *The Neuropathology of Dementia* (2nd edition). Cambridge: Cambridge University Press, 2004: 427–41.

Heinrich A, Runge U, Khaw AV. Clinicoradiologic subtypes of Marchiafava-Bignami disease. *J Neurol* 2004; **251**: 1050–9.

Kalckreuth W, Zimmermann P, Preilowski B, Wallesch CW. Incomplete split-brain syndrome in a patient with chronic Marchiafava–Bignami disease. *Behav Brain Res* 1994; **64**: 219–28.

Kleinschmidt-DeMasters BK, Filley CM, Rojiani AM. Overlapping features of extrapontine myelinolysis and acquired chronic (non-Wilsonian) hepatocerebral degeneration. *Acta Neuropathol (Berl)* 2006; **112**: 605–16.

Kohler CG, Ances BM, Coleman AR, *et al.* Marchiafava–Bignami disease: literature review and case report. *Neuropsychiatry Neuropsychol Behav Neurol* 2000; **13**: 67–76.

Mayes AR, Mendell PR, Mann D, Pickering A. Location of lesions in Korsakoff's syndrome: neuropsychological and neuropathological data on two patients. *Cortex* 1988; **24**: 367–88.

Monaghan TS, Murphy DT, Tubridy N, Hutchinson M. The woman who mistook the past for the present. *Adv Clin Neurosci Rehabil* 2006; **6** (3); 27–8.

Moriyama Y, Mimura M, Kato M, Kashima H. Primary alcoholic dementia and alcohol-related dementia. *Psychogeriatrics* 2006; **6**: 114–8.

Oslin D, Atkinson RM, Smith DM, *et al.* Alcohol related dementia: proposed clinical criteria. *Int J Geriatr Psychiatry* 1998; **13**: 203–12.

Park SA, Heo K. Prominent cerebellar symptoms with unusual magnetic resonance imaging findings in acquired hepatocerebral degeneration. *Arch Neurol* 2004; **61**: 1458–60.

Ruitenberg A, van Swieten JC, Witteman JCM, *et al.* Alcohol consumption and risk of dementia: the Rotterdam Study. *Lancet* 2002; **359**: 281–6.

Saunders PA, Copeland JR, Dewey ME, *et al.* Heavy drinking as a risk factor for depression and dementia in elderly men. Findings from the Liverpool longitudinal community study. *Br J Psych* 1991; **159**: 213–16.

Ueki Y, Isozaki E, Miyazaki Y, *et al.* Clinical and neuroradiological improvement in chronic acquired hepatocerebral degeneration after branched-chain amino acid therapy. *Acta Neurol Scand* 2002; **106**: 113–16.

Victor M. The irrelevance of the mammillary body lesions in the causation of the Korsakoff amnesic state. *Int J Neurol* 1987; **21–22**: 51–7.

Victor M, Adams RD, Cole M. The acquired (non-Wilsonian) type of chronic hepatocerebral degeneration. *Medicine (Baltimore)* 1965; **44**: 345–95.

Victor M, Adams RD, Collins GH. *The Wernicke–Korsakoff Syndrome and Related Neurologic Disorders Due to Alcoholism and Malnutrition* (2nd edition). Philadelphia: Davis, 1989.

8.3.2 Solvent exposure

Long and intense occupational exposure to certain organic solvents may cause chronic organic-solvent neurotoxicity (e.g. painter's encephalopathy), manifested as neuropsychiatric symptoms and cognitive decline, particularly slowed information processing and reaction time, easy fatigue, and impairments on tests of frontal lobe function and memory for new material (Arlien-Soberg *et al.*, 1979; Ogden, 1993; Dryson & Ogden, 2000). Whether chronic low-level exposure can also cause cognitive decline is less certain (Ridgway *et al.*, 2003). Recreational solvent inhalation ('glue sniffing') may produce impairments in memory, attention and concentration, and non-verbal intelligence in the long term (Allison & Jerrom, 1984), as well as neuropsychiatric symptoms.

REFERENCES

Allison WM, Jerrom DW. Glue sniffing: a pilot study of the cognitive effects of long-term use. *Int J Addict* 1984; **19**: 453–8.

Arlien-Soberg P, Bruhn P, Gyldensted C, Melgaard B. Chronic painters' syndrome: toxic encephalopathy in house painters. *Acta Neurol Scand* 1979; **60**: 149–56.

Dryson E, Ogden JA. Organic solvent induced chronic toxic encephalopathy: extent of recovery and associated factors, following cessation of exposure. *Neurotoxicology* 2000; **21**: 659–66.

Ogden JA. The psychological and neuropsychological assessment of chronic occupational solvent neurotoxicity: a case series. *NZ J Psychol* 1993; **23**: 83–94.

Ridgway P, Nixon TE, Leach JP. Occupational exposure to organic solvents and long-term nervous system damage detectable by brain imaging, neurophysiology or histopathology. *Food Chem Toxicol* 2003; **41**: 153–87.

8.3.3 Domoic acid poisoning (amnesic shellfish poisoning)

In Prince Edward Island, Canada, in 1987, an outbreak of food poisoning following ingestion of mussels occurred (Perl *et al.*, 1990. Patients presented within hours of eating mussels with diarrhoea, vomiting, abdominal cramps, with or without headaches. Other features included delirium, seizures, myoclonus, ataxia, alternating hemiparesis, and complete external ophthalmoplegia. In the acute stages EEG showed slowing and PET scanning showed hypometabolism of the amygdala and hippocampus. Gradual and spontaneous recovery occurred over 3 months, but some patients were left with residual anterograde amnesia, temporal lobe epilepsy, and motor neuronopathy or sensorimotor axonal neuropathy. Autopsy studies of non-survivors showed cell loss and astrocytosis in the amygdala and hippocampus. The syndrome of amnesic shellfish poisoning was shown to be due to production of domoic acid, an excitotoxin which binds to kainate-type glutamate receptors, produced in mussels infested with the phytoplankton *Nitzschia pungens*. The diagnosis can be made using a mouse bioassay for the toxin, although the condition is no longer seen in Canada as shellfish are now screened for the toxin.

REFERENCES

Perl TM, Bédard L, Kosatsky T, *et al.* An outbreak of toxic encephalopathy caused by eating mussels contaminated with domoic acid. *N Engl J Med* 1990; **322**: 1775–80.

Infective disorders

The spectrum of infectious diseases causing cognitive impairment and dementia has changed over the past century. Whereas neurosyphilis was once common, now infection with human immunodeficiency virus and herpes viruses, and diseases caused by prions (see Section 2.5), are perhaps the most notable infectious causes of cognitive decline and dementia (Almeida & Lautenschlager, 2005).

REFERENCES

Almeida OP, Lautenschlager NT. Dementia associated with infectious diseases. *Int Psychogeriatr* 2005; **17** (Suppl 1): S65–77.

9.1 Encephalitides and meningoencephalitides

Infection of the brain parenchyma with or without involvement of the surrounding meninges may be caused by a wide variety of organisms, most usually viral, but sometimes protozoan, rickettsial, or fungal (Anderson, 2001). Despite intensive investigation, a causative organism is not always found and treatment may of necessity be empirical, covering the most likely candidate organisms.

Encephalitis is often a medical emergency, requiring intensive supportive care and control of epileptic seizures. With the advent of antiviral agents such as aciclovir, mortality has declined considerably, leaving increased numbers of survivors who may have neuropsychological sequelae.

Encephalitides and meningoencephalitides covered elsewhere include Rasmussen's syndrome of chronic encephalitis and epilepsy (see Section 4.2.2), in which an infective aetiology remains a possibility, and chronic inflammatory meningoencephalitis, a term sometimes used for Sjögren's syndrome (Section 6.5).

REFERENCES

Anderson M. Encephalitis and other brain infections. In: Donaghy M (ed.), *Brain's Diseases of the Nervous System* (11th edition). Oxford: Oxford University Press, 2001: 1117–80.

9.1.1 Herpes simplex encephalitis (HSE)

Herpes simplex virus type 1 (HSV) is the commonest recognized cause of encephalitis, producing an acute necrotizing encephalitis of orbitofrontal and temporal lobes, sometimes involving insular and cingulate cortices, with an overlying meningitis. Typically the presentation is with fever and headache, sometimes with behavioural changes which may progress to clouding of consciousness and coma, sometimes complicated by focal or secondary generalized seizures (Kennedy & Chaudhuri, 2002). However, presentation with isolated memory impairment has been described (Young *et al.*, 1992). MR brain imaging may show focal oedema in the medial temporal lobes, orbital surface of the frontal lobes, insular and cingulate cortex, sometimes asymmetrically, with gadolinium enhancement. CSF is typically under raised pressure with a lymphocytic pleocytosis (10–200 cells/mm³), with a raised protein (0.6–6.0 g/l) but a normal glucose level. CSF PCR for HSV is a highly sensitive and specific test for confirmation of the diagnosis, although false negatives may be encountered early (< 48 hours) or late (> 10 days) in the disease process. EEG is invariably abnormal, showing non-specific disorganized and slow background rhythm in the early stages, with epileptiform abnormalities such as high-voltage periodic lateralizing epileptiform discharges (PLEDs) appearing later. Since early and appropriate treatment of HSE (e.g. aciclovir) has been shown to reduce mortality and morbidity significantly, brain biopsy may be considered to establish the diagnosis in atypical cases, or when a tumour in the temporal lobe is considered part of the differential diagnosis.

Cognitive sequelae of HSE have been recognized for some time (Gordon *et al.*, 1990; Kapur *et al.*, 1994; Caparros-Lefebvre *et al.*, 1996; Utley *et al.*, 1997). The typical pattern of impairment is of new learning in both verbal and visual domains. The severity of the amnesic syndrome is related to the severity of damage, judged neuroradiologically, to medial limbic structures (hippocampus and amygdala). Amnesia may occur despite appropriate treatment of HSE with aciclovir, but shorter delay between symptom onset and treatment may be associated with better outcome. In addition to amnesia, deficits may less frequently be found in retrograde memory, executive functions, and language (with mild anomia). Impaired autobiographical memory may occur in patients with bilateral damage (Eslinger, 1998). Intractable epilepsy and affective disorder may contribute to neuropsychological outcome. It should be pointed out that cognitive recovery occurs in many patients (Hokkanen & Launes, 1997a).

Although persistent anterograde and retrograde (global) amnesia after HSE is well described in patients selected for symptoms of memory impairment, it seems to be an unusual complication, although the risk is greater (by 2–4 times) than in non-herpetic encephalitis. Greater deficits in verbal memory, verbal semantic functions, and visuoperceptual functions have been noted in herpetic as compared to non-herpetic encephalitis (Hokkanen *et al.*, 1996a,b). Executive deficits may also been seen following recovery from HSE, presumably reflecting orbitofrontal injury (Utley *et al.*, 1997). Duration of transient encephalitic amnesia correlates with neuropsychological outcome (Hokkanen & Launes, 1997b).

REFERENCES

Caparros-Lefebvre D, Girard-Buttoz I, Reboul S, *et al.* Cognitive and psychiatric impairment in herpes simplex virus encephalitis suggest involvement of the amygdalo-frontal pathways. *J Neurol* 1996; **243**: 248–56.

Eslinger PJ. Autobiographical memory after temporal and frontal lobe lesions. *Neurocase* 1998; **4**: 481–95.

Gordon B, Selnes OA, Hart J, Hanley DF, Whitley RJ. Long-term cognitive sequelae of acyclovir-treated herpes simplex encephalitis. *Arch Neurol* 1990; **47**: 646–7.

Hokkanen L, Launes J. Cognitive recovery instead of decline after acute encephalitis: a prospective follow up study. *J Neurol Neurosurg Psychiatry* 1997a; **63**: 222–7.

Hokkanen L, Launes J. Duration of transient amnesia correlates with cognitive outcome in acute encephalitis. *Neuroreport* 1997b; **8**: 2721–5.

Hokkanen L, Poutiainen E, Valanne L, *et al.* Cognitive impairment after acute encephalitis: comparison of herpes simplex and other aetiologies. *J Neurol Neurosurg Psychiatry* 1996a; **61**: 478–84.

Hokkanen L, Salonen O, Launes J. Amnesia in acute herpetic and nonherpetic encephalitis. *Arch Neurol* 1996b; **53**: 972–8.

Kapur N, Barker S, Burrows EH, *et al.* Herpes simplex encephalitis: long term magnetic resonance imaging and neuropsychological profile. *J Neurol Neurosurg Psychiatry* 1994; **57**: 1334–42.

Kennedy PGE, Chaudhuri A. Herpes simplex encephalitis. *J Neurol Neurosurg Psychiatry* 2002; **73**: 237–8.

Utley TFM, Ogden JA, Gibb A, McGrath N, Anderson NE. The long-term neuropsychological outcome of herpes simplex encephalitis in a series of unselected survivors. *Neuropsychiatry Neuropsychol Behav Neurol* 1997; **10**: 180–9.

Young CA, Humphrey PR, Ghadiali EJ, Klapper PE, Cleator GM. Short-term memory impairment in an alert patient as a presentation of herpes simplex encephalitis. *Neurology* 1992; **42**: 260–1.

9.1.2 Herpes zoster encephalitis

Varicella zoster virus (VZV), a herpes virus, may lie dormant for many years after a primary infection, to be reactivated as herpes zoster or shingles, and this may sometimes be complicated by encephalitis (herpes zoster encephalitis, HZE).

Neuropsychological sequelae of HZE were reported by Hokkanen *et al.* (1997) in nine immunocompetent patients. These included forgetfulness, slowing of thought processes, emotional and personality changes, and impaired cognitive ability, suggesting a subcortical type of impairment. In contrast, a report of eight patients undergoing neuropsychological assessment 4–52 months after onset of HZE found no significant differences between patients and controls (Wetzel *et al.*, 2002). The discrepancy in these studies may relate to the timing of assessment, which was carried out in most of the patients in the Hokkanen *et al.* (1997) study directly after they were able to cooperate adequately after the acute stage of infection.

REFERENCES

Hokkanen L, Launes J, Poutiainen E, *et al.* Subcortical type cognitive impairment in herpes zoster encephalitis. *J Neurol* 1997; **244**: 239–45.

Wetzel K, Asholt I, Herrmann E, *et al.* Good cognitive outcome of patients with herpes zoster encephalitis: a follow-up study. *J Neurol* 2002; **249**: 1612–14.

9.1.3 Adenovirus encephalitis

Cases with severe amnesia, resembling herpes simplex encephalitis, have been reported (Hokkanen *et al.*, 1996).

REFERENCES

Hokkanen L, Poutiainen E, Valanne L, *et al.* Cognitive impairment after acute encephalitis: comparison of herpes simplex and other aetiologies. *J Neurol Neurosurg Psychiatry* 1996; **61**: 478–84.

9.1.4 Coxsackie virus encephalitis

A possible case of subcortical type cognitive impairment has been described following encephalitis due to this RNA virus (Peatfield, 1987).

REFERENCES

Peatfield RC. Basal ganglia damage and subcortical dementia after possible insidious Coxsackie virus encephalitis. *Acta Neurol Scand* 1987; **76**: 340–5.

9.1.5 Human herpes virus 6 infection

Infection with human herpes virus 6 (HHV-6) causes fever and a rash (exanthema subitum) in children, a benign, self-limiting condition. Seropositivity occurs in most children by age 3 years, with decline after the age of 40 years. Symptomatic infection in adults is very rare, mostly occurring in the context of immunosuppression. Cases of persistent amnesia (anterograde and retrograde) have been reported as a consequence of HHV-6 infection (Kapur & Brooks, 1999; Bollen *et al.*, 2001; Wainwright *et al.*, 2001), for example in the context of immunosuppression associated with lung transplantation (Bollen *et al.*, 2001) or stem cell transplantation (Wainwright *et al.*,

2001). High-intensity signal change has been seen on MR brain imaging in the medial temporal lobe including the hippocampus, and hence this may be considered a form of non-paraneoplastic limbic encephalitis (see Section 6.12.2). Similar cases have been seen rarely with human herpes virus 7 infection (Dewhurst, 2004).

REFERENCES

Bollen AE, Wartan AN, Krikke AP, Haaxma-Reiche H. Amnestic syndrome after lung transplantation by human herpes virus-6 encephalitis. *J Neurol* 2001; **248**: 619–20.

Dewhurst S. Human herpesvirus type 6 and human herpesvirus type 7 infections of the central nervous system. *Herpes* 2004; **11**: 105A–11A.

Kapur N, Brooks DJ. Temporally-specific retrograde amnesia in two cases of discrete bilateral hippocampal pathology. *Hippocampus* 1999; **9**: 247–54.

Wainwright MS, Martin PL, Morse RP, *et al.* Human herpesvirus 6 limbic encephalitis after stem cell transplantation. *Ann Neurol* 2001; **50**: 612–19.

9.1.6 Rotavirus encephalitis

A case with cognitive impairment has been reported (Hokkanen *et al.*, 1996), although this is likely to be the exception rather than the rule.

REFERENCES

Hokkanen L, Poutiainen E, Valanne L, *et al.* Cognitive impairment after acute encephalitis: comparison of herpes simplex and other aetiologies. *J Neurol Neurosurg Psychiatry* 1996; **61**: 478–84.

9.1.7 Subacute sclerosing panencephalitis (SSPE)

Subacute sclerosing panencephalitis (SSPE) is usually a disorder of late childhood or early adolescence, due to reactivation of measles virus infection causing progressive inflammation and gliosis of the brain. The clinical phenotype is characterized by behavioural change, myoclonic jerks, seizures, and progressive dementia, followed by pyramidal signs, stupor, decorticate postures, and death. Characteristic investigation findings include antibodies against measles virus and oligoclonal bands in CSF, a pathognomonic EEG signature with periodic bursts of high-voltage waves at a rate of 2–3 per second, and periventricular and subcortical white matter change on MR imaging. Only occasional adult-onset cases have been reported (Singer *et al.*, 1997), usually with the characteristic clinical picture, but one atypical case presenting with a 'pure cortical dementia' without movement disorder has been described (Frings *et al.*, 2002). The clinical description was of initial apathy, disorientation in time, psychomotor slowing, and depression, followed 3 years later by verbal perseverations, anomia, phonemic paraphasia, dysgraphia, dyslexia, ideomotor and ideational apraxia, with MMSE score of 9.5/30. No more detailed neuropsychological assessment was presented. Serial MR brain imaging showed progressive generalized cerebral atrophy.

REFERENCES

Frings M, Blaeser I, Kastrup O. Adult-onset subacute sclerosing panencephalitis presenting as a degenerative dementia syndrome. *J Neurol* 2002; **249**: 942–3.

Singer C, Lang AE, Suchowersky O. Adult-onset subacute sclerosing panencephalitis: case reports and review of the literature. *Mov Disord* 1997; **12**: 342–53.

9.1.8 Tick-borne encephalitis

Cognitive impairment has been described as a long-term complication of tick-borne encephalitis, specifically deficits in memory, concentration, verbal fluency, and verbal learning (Günther *et al.*, 1997).

REFERENCES

Günther G, Haglund M, Lindquist L, Forsgren M, Skoldenberg B. Tick-borne encephalitis in Sweden in relation to aseptic meningo-encephalitis of other etiology: a prospective study of clinical course and outcome. *J Neurol* 1997; **244**: 230–8.

9.1.9 Japanese encephalitis

According to one review, 20% of survivors of Japanese encephalitis have severe cognitive and language, as well as motor, impairment (Solomon *et al.*, 2000).

REFERENCES

Solomon T, Dung NM, Kneen R, *et al.* Japanese encephalitis. *J Neurol Neurosurg Psychiatry* 2000; **68**: 405–15.

9.1.10 Post-encephalitic parkinsonism, encephalitis lethargica, von Economo disease

The exact relationship of this condition, which occurred in epidemic proportions following the First World War, to brain infection remains uncertain: a suspected relationship to influenza infection has not been corroborated by examination of archival tissues. Basal ganglia autoimmunity may play a role in pathogenesis (as in Sydenham's chorea: Section 6.11). Occasional cases of encephalitis lethargica still occur, generally dominated clinically by movement disorders (parkinsonism, dystonia, oculogyric crises, myoclonus) and neuropsychiatric features. Neuropsychological features have been little studied, but in one case a general cognitive decline was seen initially, particularly affecting memory and executive functions, which improved over time concurrent with cognitive rehabilitation strategies (Dewar & Wilson, 2005).

REFERENCES

Dewar BK, Wilson BA. Cognitive recovery from encephalitis lethargica. *Brain Inj* 2005; **19**: 1285–91.

9.2 Meningitides

9.2.1 Bacterial meningitis

Although neurological recovery is now the norm when bacterial meningitis is promptly diagnosed and appropriately treated in adults, nonetheless functional impairments precluding return to employment may persist, particularly in the cognitive domain. Cohort studies have indicated impairments in psychomotor performance, concentration, visuoconstructive capacity, and memory functions compared to healthy controls, a pattern resembling the subcortical type of cognitive impairment (Merkelbach *et al.*, 2000). Deficits were found in 73% of patients in this study, whereas only 27% were impaired in another study (van de Beek *et al.*, 2002), although both suggested that pneumococcal meningitis had a worse cognitive outcome than meningococcal meningitis. This differential outcome according to infecting organism was not found in the study of Schmidt *et al.* (2006), in which a history of alcoholism, a recognized predisposing cause for pneumococcal meningitis, was an exclusion criterion. This study found impairments in short-term and working memory and in executive tasks, with additional difficulties in language and visuoconstructive function. Reduced brain volume and increased ventricular volume was noted in neuroradiological studies, and white matter lesions correlated negatively with short-term and working memory performance.

REFERENCES

Merkelbach S, Sittinger H, Schweizer I, Müller M. Cognitive outcome after bacterial meningitis. *Acta Neurol Scand* 2000; **102**: 118–23.

Schmidt H, Heimann B, Djukic M, *et al.* Neuropsychological sequelae of bacterial and viral meningitis. *Brain* 2006; **129**: 333–45.

van de Beek D, Schmand B, de Gans J, *et al.* Cognitive impairment in adults with good recovery after bacterial meningitis. *J Infect Dis* 2002; **186**: 1047–52.

9.2.2 Viral meningitis

Viral meningitis is generally considered a benign, self-limiting condition without cognitive sequelae. A postal questionnaire controlled study reported that survivors of viral meningitis showed a slight, non-significant, increase in prevalence of chronic fatigue syndrome compared to controls who had had non-enteroviral, non-CNS viral infections, but this disappeared on correction for age, sex, and duration of follow-up (Hotopf *et al.*, 1996). Mild cognitive impairment has been reported following viral meningitis due to enterovirus, myxovirus, and herpes virus infection (Sittinger *et al.*, 2002). Follow-up studies to see whether such deficits progress, reverse, or remain static are awaited. Schmidt *et al.* (2006) found impairments in cognitive performance in viral meningitis patients in similar domains to bacterial meningitis patients, but these were less severe and without the neuroradiological correlates found in bacterial meningitis.

REFERENCES

Hotopf M, Noah N, Wessely S. Chronic fatigue and minor psychiatric morbidity after viral meningitis: a controlled study. *J Neurol Neurosurg Psychiatry* 1996; **60**: 504–9.

Schmidt H, Heimann B, Djukic M, *et al.* Neuropsychological sequelae of bacterial and viral meningitis. *Brain* 2006; **129**: 333–45.

Sittinger H, Müller M, Schweizer I, Merkelbach S. Mild cognitive impairment after viral meningitis in adults. *J Neurol* 2002; **249**: 554–60.

9.2.3 Fungal meningitis

Meningitis due to the fungus *Cryptococcus neoformans*, in which the clinical picture was thought to mimic vascular dementia, has been reported (Aharon-Peretz *et al.*, 2004).

REFERENCES

Aharon-Peretz J, Kilot D, Finkelstein R, *et al.* Cryptococcal meningitis mimicking vascular dementia. *Neurology* 2004; **62**: 2135.

9.3   Human immunodeficiency virus (HIV) and related conditions

Human immunodeficiency virus (HIV, originally named human T-lymphotropic virus type III, HTLV-III) is the best known of the retroviruses, responsible for the AIDS pandemic. In the body, the virus is spread haematogenously and is thought to enter the brain within blood-derived macrophages. Neurological complications are prominent in HIV infection (Harrison & McArthur, 1995; Gendelman *et al.*, 2005), and their pathogenesis is thought to be multifactorial, related to primary HIV infection, opportunistic CNS infection (toxoplasmosis, cryptococcal meningitis, CMV encephalitis, tuberculous meningitis, neurosyphilis, progressive multifocal leukoencephalopathy related to JC virus activation), or tumour formation (CNS lymphoma), sometimes resulting in dementia. Concurrent substance misuse and mood disorder may contribute to cognitive impairment in some cases.

REFERENCES

Gendelman HE, Grant I, Everall IP, Lipton SA, Swindells S (eds.). *The Neurology of AIDS* (2nd edition). Oxford: Oxford University Press, 2005.

Harrison MJG, McArthur JC. *AIDS and Neurology*. Edinburgh: Churchill Livingstone, 1995.

9.3.1   HIV dementia, AIDS dementia

Cognitive impairment associated with HIV infection in the absence of mood disorder or opportunistic infection was recognized soon after the epidemic was first defined, ranging from psychomotor slowing and mental dullness through to frank dementia (Grant *et al.*, 2005). Dementia may sometimes be the initial manifestation of HIV infection (Navia *et al.*, 1986), but seems to progress more rapidly when there is concurrent advanced immunosuppression (CD4 count < 200) and hence in parallel with progressive systemic disease (Price *et al.*, 1988; McArthur *et al.*, 1993). Criteria for the

diagnosis of HIV dementia and of lesser degrees of HIV-associated cognitive impairment have been proposed (American Academy of Neurology AIDS Task Force, 1991; Grant & Atkinson, 1995). The frequency of neurocognitive impairments in seropositive asymptomatic individuals remains uncertain (Grant *et al.*, 2005). Other factors which might contribute to neuropsychological impairment in HIV positive individuals include drug and alcohol misuse, educational attainment, and head injury.

The neuropsychological profile of HIV dementia is characterized by psychomotor slowing, memory impairment (typically impaired free recall with relatively preserved recognition recall), and executive dysfunction, all suggestive of a subcortical pattern of dementia. There may be concurrent motor problems with gait and postural reflexes, and impaired reaction times. Neuropsychological deficits correlate with neuroradiological and neuropathological studies indicating frontostriatal involvement, although cortical areas may also be affected with disease evolution (Oechsner *et al.*, 1993; Power & Johnson, 1995).

Treatment with antiretrovirals, and particularly combination highly active antiretroviral treatment (HAART), has resulted in a dramatic decline in the incidence of HIV dementia (Catalan & Thornton, 1993; Sacktor *et al.*, 2002). However, with increased survival, aging may emerge as a risk factor for HIV-associated cognitive disorder. HAART has been reported to reverse partially clinical and spectroscopic features in AIDS patients with subcorticofrontal cognitive impairment (Stankoff *et al.*, 2001).

REFERENCES

American Academy of Neurology AIDS Task Force. Nomenclature and research case definitions for neurologic manifestations of human immunodeficiency virus-type 1 (HIV-1) infection: report of a Working Group of the American Academy of Neurology AIDS Task Force. *Neurology* 1991; **41**: 778–85.

Catalan J, Thornton S. Whatever happened to HIV dementia? *Int J STD AIDS* 1993; **4**: 1–4.

Grant I, Atkinson J. Psychiatric aspects of acquired immune deficiency syndrome. In: Sadock B (ed.), *Comprehensive Textbook of Psychiatry*. Baltimore: Williams & Wilkins, 1995: 1644–69.

Grant I, Sacktor N, McArthur J. HIV and neurocognitive disorders. In: Gendelman HE, Grant I, Everall IP, Lipton SA, Swindells S (eds.), *The Neurology of AIDS* (2nd edition). Oxford: Oxford University Press, 2005: 357–73.

McArthur JC, Hoover DR, Bacellar H, *et al.* Dementia in AIDS patients: incidence and risk factors. *Neurology* 1993; **43**: 2245–52.

Navia BA, Jordan BD, Price RW. The AIDS dementia complex: I. Clinical features. *Ann Neurol* 1986; **19**: 517–24.

Oechsner M, Möller AA, Zaudig M. Cognitive impairment, dementia and psychological functioning in human immunodeficiency virus infection: a prospective study based on DSM-III-R and ICD-10. *Acta Psychiatr Scand* 1993; **87**: 13–17.

Power C, Johnson RT. HIV-1 associated dementia: clinical features and pathogenesis. *Can J Neurol Sci* 1995; **22**: 92–100.

Price RW, Brew B, Sidtis J, *et al.* The brain in AIDS: central nervous system HIV-1 infection and AIDS dementia complex. *Science* 1988; **239**: 586–92.

Sacktor N, McDermott MP, Marder K, *et al.* HIV-associated cognitive impairment before and after the advent of combination therapy. *J Neurovirol* 2002; **8**: 136–42.

Stankoff B, Tourbah A, Suarez S, *et al.* Clinical and spectroscopic improvement in HIV-associated cognitive impairment. *Neurology* 2001; **56**: 112–15.

9.3.2 Progressive multifocal leukoencephalopathy (PML)

Progressive multifocal leukoencephalopathy (PML) is a white matter disorder related to JC virus activation, rarely seen outside the context of HIV-induced immunosuppression. Hemiparesis, hemianopia, and dementia are common clinical features. One series examining the initial symptoms of PML in AIDS patients found cognitive disorders in 36% and speech disturbance in 40% (Berger *et al.*, 1998).

REFERENCES

Berger JR, Pall L, Lanska D, Whiteman M. Progressive multifocal leukoencephalopathy in patients with HIV infection. *J Neurovirol* 1998; **4**: 59–68.

9.3.3 HTLV-1

The retrovirus HTLV-1 classically causes a myelopathy (HTLV-1-associated myelopathy, HAM, or tropical spastic paraparesis, TSP), but other features have been described including cognitive decline and even subcortical dementia. Silva *et al.* (2003) reported psychomotor slowing, verbal and visual memory deficits, impaired attention, and visuomotor problems in both asymptomatic HTLV-1 carriers and patients with HAM/TSP, but there was no association with degree of motor disability.

REFERENCES

Silva MTT, Mattos P, Alfano A, Araújo AQC. Neuropsychological assessment in HTLV-1 infection: a comparative study among TSP/HAM, asymptomatic carriers and healthy controls. *J Neurol Neurosurg Psychiatry* 2003; **74**: 1085–9.

9.4 Other disorders of infective aetiology

9.4.1 Neurosyphilis

Neurosyphilis of the parenchymatous, rather than meningovascular, type has long been recognized to cause dementia: as 'general paresis [or paralysis] of the insane' (GPI), it was once a common cause of cognitive and behavioural decline (Dewhurst, 1969; Nieman, 1991). The advent of the antibiotic era saw a dramatic decline in cases, but now the disease is once again being seen more frequently, in part associated with HIV infection and AIDS (Carr, 2003). In a recent series of cases of neurosyphilis, defined by a positive CSF fluorescent treponemal antibody absorption test, very few with concurrent HIV positivity, the most common presentation (50%) was with 'neuropsychiatric' disease (= psychosis, delirium, dementia). Stroke, spinal cord disease (myelopathy), and seizures were the other typical presentations. No neuropsychological data were presented and hence the pattern, if any, of cognitive deficits was not disclosed. Residual cognitive loss was reported in nearly 50% of patients for whom outcome was known. The authors suggested that the term 'syphilitic encephalitis' was preferable to GPI (Timmermans & Carr, 2004). Syphilis has always been described as the great mimic of other conditions, and one important differential diagnosis is with limbic encephalitis (Schied *et al.*, 2005). Dementia related to meningovascular neurosyphilis in the context of HIV infection (see Section 9.3) has been reported (Fox *et al.*, 2000).

REFERENCES

Carr J. Neurosyphilis. *Pract Neurol* 2003; **3**: 328–41.

Dewhurst K. The neurosyphilis psychoses today: a survey of 91 cases. *Br J Psychiatry* 1969; **115**: 31–8.

Fox PA, Hawkins DA, Dawson S. Dementia following an acute presentation of meningovascular neurosyphilis in an HIV-1 positive patient. *AIDS* 2000; **14**: 2062–3.

Nieman EA. Neurosyphilis yesterday and today. *J R Coll Physicians Lond* 1991; **25**: 321–4.

Schied R, Voltz R, Vetter T, *et al.* Neurosyphilis and paraneoplastic limbic encephalitis: important differential diagnoses. *J Neurol* 2005; **252**: 1129–32.

Timmermans M, Carr J. Neurosyphilis in the modern era. *J Neurol Neurosurg Psychiatry* 2004; **75**: 1727–30.

9.4.2   Tuberculosis

Recent years have seen a resurgence in cases of tuberculosis as an opportunistic infection in the context of HIV infection, and this association needs to be considered when assessing cognitive sequelae of tuberculosis. Studies from the Indian subcontinent list tuberculosis as a cause of dementia (Jha & Patel, 2004). Dementia has also been associated with a dorsal midbrain tuberculous granuloma (Meador *et al.*, 1996). Disseminated brain tuberculomas may cause cognitive features (Akritidis *et al.*, 2005), and a pure amnesic syndrome has been reported following recovery from probable tuberculous meningitis with evidence of medial temporal lobe and mammillary body involvement (Ceccaldi *et al.*, 1995).

REFERENCES

Akritidis N, Galiatsou E, Kakadellis J, Dimas K, Paparounas K. Brain tuberculomas due to miliary tuberculosis. *South Med J* 2005; **98**: 111–13.

Ceccaldi M, Belleville S, Royere ML, Poncet M. A pure reversible amnesic syndrome following tuberculous meningoencephalitis. *Eur Neurol* 1995; **35**: 363–7.

Jha S, Patel R. Some observations on the spectrum of dementia. *Neurol India* 2004; **52**: 213–14.

Meador KJ, Loring DW, Sethi KD, *et al.* Dementia associated with dorsal midbrain lesion. *J Int Neuropsychol Soc* 1996; **2**: 359–67.

9.4.3   Neuroborreliosis (Lyme disease)

Infection with the spirochaete *Borrelia burgdorferi*, transmitted by the bite of infected *Ixodes* ticks, causes the zoonosis borreliosis, which may produce multi-system disease with dermatological, cardiological, and neurological sequelae. Neuroborreliosis may include aseptic meningitis, with or without multiple radicular or peripheral nerve lesions; myelitis; cranial neuropathy, especially involving the facial nerve; and meningoradiculitis of the cauda equina (Steere, 1989; Halperin *et al.*, 1991). Cognitive complications may also occur, in late (stage III) Lyme disease. Guidelines for the diagnosis of neuroborreliosis have been published (American Academy of Neurology Quality Standards Subcommittee, 1996).

Lyme encephalopathy occurring years after the acute illness was reported in one series to produce defects in verbal memory, mental flexibility, verbal associative functions, and articulation, but with preserved intellectual and problem-solving skills, sustained attention, visuoconstructive abilities, and mental speed (Benke *et al.*, 1995). Mental activation speed, as measured by response times, was found to be slower in Lyme patients, but perceptual and motor speed was preserved (Pollina *et al.*, 1999). Involvement primarily of frontal systems was the conclusion of one review of neuropsychological function in Lyme disease (Westervelt & McCaffrey, 2002), and a case of rapidly progressive frontal-type dementia has been reported (Waniek *et al.*, 1995). Although depression may complicate the presentation, memory impairment does seem to be associated with evidence of CNS involvement (CSF intrathecal antibodies to *B. burgdorferi*, elevated protein, or positive PCR for *B. burgdorferi* DNA: Kaplan *et al.*, 1999). Children when appropriately treated seem to have an excellent cognitive prognosis (Adams *et al.*, 1999). Few cases have come to autopsy: one showed evidence of spongiform change, neuronal loss, and microglial activation, along with silver-impregnated organisms strongly suggesting *B. burgdorferi* in both cortex and thalamus to account for the cognitive changes (Kobayashi *et al.*, 1997).

Occasional cases of borreliosis have been reported presenting as 'normal pressure hydrocephalus' (see Section 7.2.1), cognitive impairments reversing after appropriate antibiotic treatment (Danek *et al.*, 1996; Etienne *et al.*, 2003).

REFERENCES

Adams WV, Rose CD, Eppes SC, Klein JD. Long-term cognitive effects of Lyme disease in children. *Appl Neuropsychol* 1999; **6**: 39–45.

American Academy of Neurology Quality Standards Subcommittee. Practice parameter: diagnosis of patients with nervous system Lyme borreliosis (Lyme disease). Summary statement. *Neurology* 1996; **46**: 881–2.

Benke T, Gasse T, Hittmair Delazer M, Schmutzhard E. Lyme encephalopathy: long-term neuropsychological deficits years after acute neuroborreliosis. *Acta Neurol Scand* 1995; **91**: 353–7.

Danek A, Uttner I, Yousry T, Pfister HW. Lyme neuroborreliosis disguised as normal pressure hydrocephalus. *Neurology* 1996; **46**: 1743–5.

Etienne M, Carvalho P, Fauchais AL, *et al.* Lyme neuroborreliosis revealed as a normal pressure hydrocephalus: a cause of reversible dementia. *J Am Geriatr Soc* 2003; **51**: 579–80.

Halperin JJ, Volkman DJ, Wu P. Central nervous system abnormalities in Lyme neuroborreliosis. *Neurology* 1991; **41**: 1571–82.

Kaplan RF, Jones Woodward L, Workman K, *et al.* Neuropsychological deficits in Lyme disease patients with and without other evidence of central nervous system pathology. *Appl Neuropsychol* 1999; **6**: 3–11.

Kobayashi K, Mizukoshi C, Aoki T, *et al. Borrelia burgdorferi*-seropositive chronic encephalomyelopathy: Lyme neuroborreliosis? An autopsied report. *Dement Geriatr Cogn Disord* 1997; **8**: 384–90.

Pollina DA, Sliwinski M, Squires NK, Krupp LB. Cognitive processing speed in Lyme disease. *Neuropsychiatry Neuropsychol Behav Neurol* 1999; **12**: 72–8.

Steere AC. Lyme disease. *N Engl J Med* 1989; **321**: 586–96.

Waniek C, Prohovnik I, Kaufman MA, Dwork AJ. Rapidly progressive frontal-type dementia associated with Lyme disease. *J Neuropsychiatry Clin Neurosci* 1995; **7**: 345–7.

Westervelt HJ, McCaffrey RJ. Neuropsychological functioning in chronic Lyme disease. *Neuropsychol Rev* 2002; **12**: 153–77.

9.4.4 Neurocysticercosis

Infection with the larval stage (cysticercus) of the helminth cestode *Taenia solium*, the pork tapeworm, usually results from eating undercooked pork. Various neurological syndromes may occur when cysticerci reach the CNS: intraparenchymal disease typically induces focal or generalized epilepsy, extraparenchymal disease causes mass effect and intracranial hypertension (Garcia & Del Brutto, 2005; Garcia *et al.*, 2006).

Cognitive decline is occasionally reported, sometimes sufficient to cause dementia. A study from Mexico City found 15% of patients with untreated neurocysticercosis fulfilled DSM-IV criteria for dementia, more than three-quarters of whom no longer fulfilled criteria after treatment with albendazole and steroids, suggesting that this is a reversible cause of dementia. Dementia was associated with the number of parasitic lesions seen in frontal, temporal, and parietal lobes (Ramirez Bermudez *et al.*, 2005). In a study from Brazil, patients with mesial temporal lobe epilepsy due to hippocampal sclerosis with incidental calcified neurocysticercosis had no greater cognitive deficits than those without, suggesting that these chronic lesions do not contribute to cognitive performance (Terra Bustamente *et al.*, 2005).

REFERENCES

Garcia HH, Del Brutto OH. Neurocysticercosis: updated concepts about an old disease. *Lancet Neurol* 2005; **4**: 653–61.

Garcia HH, Gonzalez AE, Tsang VCW, Gilman RH, for the Cysticercosis Working Group in Peru. Neurocysticercosis: some of the essentials. *Pract Neurol* 2006; **6**: 288–97.

Ramirez Bermudez J, Higuera J, Sosa AL, *et al.* Is dementia reversible in patients with neurocysticercosis? *J Neurol Neurosurg Psychiatry* 2005; **76**: 1164–6.

Terra Bustamente VC, Coimbra ER, Rezek KO, *et al.* Cognitive performance of patients with mesial temporal lobe epilepsy and incidental calcified neurocysticercosis. *J Neurol Neurosurg Psychiatry* 2005; **76**: 1080–3.

9.4.5   Whipple's disease

Although extremely rare, Whipple's disease is a diagnosis which is often considered by neurologists, because of the possibility of reversing the movement and cognitive disorder which results from infection with the causative organism, *Tropheryma whippelii*. It is a multisystem granulomatous disorder, the clinical phenotype of which is pleomorphic, but neurological signs may occur in isolation from the more familiar gastrointestinal and systemic symptoms (Anderson, 2000). Diagnostic guidelines for neurological Whipple's have been published and it has been estimated that 11% of CNS Whipple's disease cases present with cognitive decline in the absence of other neurological symptoms and signs (Louis *et al.*, 1996). Cognitive features may be prominent in primary Whipple's disease of the brain along with other symptoms such as seizures and ataxia (Panegyres *et al.*, 2006).

Detailed reports of the cognitive impairments in Whipple's disease are few. Manzel *et al.* (2000) reported a biopsy-confirmed case with impairments in sustained attention, memory, executive function, and constructional praxis, with behavioural disinhibition and confabulation, features which correlated with MR imaging changes in the mesial temporal lobe and basal forebrain. The cognitive picture was thought to resemble that seen after herpes simplex encephalitis or subarachnoid haemorrhage from a ruptured anterior communicating artery aneurysm.

REFERENCES

Anderson M. Neurology of Whipple's disease. *J Neurol Neurosurg Psychiatry* 2000; **68**: 2–5.

Louis ED, Lynch T, Kaufmann P, Fahn S, Odel J. Diagnostic guidelines in central nervous system Whipple's disease. *Ann Neurol* 1996; **40**: 561–8.

Manzel K, Tranel D, Cooper G. Cognitive and behavioral abnormalities in a case of central nervous system Whipple disease. *Arch Neurol* 2000; **57**: 399–403.

Panegyres PK, Edis R, Beaman M, Fallon M. Primary Whipple's disease of the brain: characterization of the syndrome and molecular diagnosis. *Q J Med* 2006; **99**: 609–23.

Neuromuscular disorders

It may seem odd that disease of muscle or neuromuscular junction, these most distal outposts of the neurological system, might be associated with dysfunction of higher cortical function. However, diseases manifesting with neuropathy or myopathy may in fact be multisystem disorders with a broad phenotype that also encompasses cognitive processes, sometimes related to expression of abnormal or dysfunctional proteins (D'Angelo & Bresolin, 2006). Myotonic dystrophy is the classic example, but other neuropathic and myopathic disorders with concurrent cognitive features covered elsewhere include mitochondrial disorders (see Section 5.5.1), acid maltase deficiency and Anderson–Fabry disease (Section 5.5.3), neurofibromatosis (Section 5.6.1), and adult polyglucosan body disease (Section 5.5.7).

REFERENCES

D'Angelo MG, Bresolin N. Cognitive impairment in neuromuscular disorders. *Muscle Nerve* 2006; **34**: 16–33.

10.1 Myotonic dystrophy (Steinert disease)

Advances in the understanding of the genetic basis of myotonic dystrophy have led to a new classification. Classical dystrophia myotonica, Steinert's disease, associated with expansions of the CTG trinucleotide in the myotonic dystrophy protein kinase gene (*DMPK*) on chromosome 19, is now known as myotonic dystrophy type 1 (DM1); the entity previously known as proximal myotonic myopathy (PROMM, Ricker's disease), now known to be associated with expansions of the CCTG tetranucleotide in the *ZIP9* gene on chromosome 3q, is now known as myotonic dystrophy type 2 (DM2) (International Myotonic Dystrophy Consortium, 2000; Udd *et al.*, 2003). Adult-onset DM1 is a pleiotropic disorder, one feature of which may be cognitive impairment. Features such as cognitive dysfunction, visuospatial deficits, behavioural abnormalities, and hypersomnia, are reported to be more prominent in DM1 than DM2 (Harper *et al.*, 2004).

The most commonly observed cognitive impairments in DM1 relate to executive (frontal lobe) dysfunction, with lack of initiative and apathy despite preserved general intelligence. Features may be static, or progressive, with temporal lobe (memory) impairments. Some studies have found no correlation between cognitive impairment and CTG repeat number or severity of muscle involvement (Rubinsztein *et al.*, 1997; Modoni *et al.*, 2004), whilst others have found a correlation with CTG expansion size (Perini *et al.*, 1999). Atypical presentation of DM1 as apparent primary dementia may occur. There is noted to be a high risk of cognitive impairments in childhood-onset disease, particularly associated with maternal inheritance, whereas adult-onset disease is at lower risk. Wilson *et al.* (1999) reported an adult patient with paternal inheritance and an 11-year decline in cognitive function, for which no cause other than DM1 was identified.

DM1 may be accompanied by white matter changes on MR brain imaging (Di Costanzo *et al.*, 2002), which may (Censori *et al.*, 1994) or may not (Sinforiani *et al.*, 1991) correlate with neuropsychological impairment. Sophisticated neuroimaging techniques indicate neocortical damage in DM1 brains even in the absence of white matter change (Giorgio *et al.*, 2006), which might conceivably be related to cognitive deficits. Concurrent hypersomnia might also be relevant. Neurofibrillary tangles comparable to those seen in Alzheimer's disease have been observed in DM1 brain (Kiuchi *et al.*, 1991), perhaps related to the altered splicing patterns of the gene encoding tau in DM1 brain (Sergeant *et al.*, 2001).

In DM2 impaired visuospatial recall and construction has been noted, more prevalent than in DM1 (Meola *et al.*, 1999).

REFERENCES

Censori B, Provinciali L, Danni M, *et al.* Brain involvement in myotonic dystrophy: MRI features and their relationship to clinical and cognitive conditions. *Acta Neurol Scand* 1994; **90**: 211–17.

Di Costanzo A, Di Salle F, Santoro L, *et al.* Pattern and significance of white matter abnormalities in myotonic dystrophy type 1: an MRI study. *J Neurol* 2002; **249**: 1175–82.

Giorgio A, Dotti MT, Battaglini M, *et al.* Cortical damage in brains of patients with adult-form of myotonic dystrophy type 1 and no or minimal MRI abnormalities. *J Neurol* 2006; **253**: 1471–7.

Harper PS, van Engelen B, Eymard B, Wilcox DE (eds.). *Myotonic Dystrophy: Present Management, Future Therapy.* Oxford: Oxford University Press, 2004.

International Myotonic Dystrophy Consortium (IDMC). New nomenclature and DNA testing guidelines for myotonic dystrophy type 1 (DM1). *Neurology* 2000; **54**: 1218–21.

Kiuchi A, Otsuka N, Namba Y, Nakano I, Tomonaga M. Presenile appearance of abundant Alzheimer's neurofibrillary tangles without senile plaques in the brain in myotonic dystrophy. *Acta Neuropathol (Berl)* 1991; **82**: 1–5.

Meola G, Sansone V, Perani D, *et al.* Reduced cerebral blood flow and impaired visual–spatial function in proximal myotonic myopathy. *Neurology* 1999; **53**: 1042–50.

Modoni A, Silvestri G, Pomponi MG, *et al.* Characterization of the pattern of cognitive impairment in myotonic dystrophy type 1. *Arch Neurol* 2004; **61**: 1943–7.

Perini GI, Menegazzo E, Ermani M, *et al.* Cognitive impairment and (CTG)n expansion in myotonic dystrophy patients. *Biol Psychiatry* 1999; **46**: 425–31.

Rubinsztein JS, Rubinsztein DC, McKenna PJ, Goodburn S, Holland AJ. Mild myotonic dystrophy is associated with memory impairment in the context of normal general intelligence. *J Med Genet* 1997; **34**: 229–33.

Sergeant N, Sablonniere B, Schraen-Maschke S, *et al.* Dysregulation of human brain microtubule-associated tau mRNA maturation in myotonic dystrophy type 1. *Hum Mol Genet* 2001; **10**: 2143–55.

Sinforiani E, Sandrini G, Martelli A, *et al.* Cognitive and neuroradiological findings in myotonic dystrophy. *Funct Neurol* 1991; **6**: 377–84.

Udd B, Meola G, Krahe R, *et al.* Report of the 115th ENMC workshop: DM2/PROMM and other myotonic dystrophies. 3rd workshop, 14–16 February 2003, Naarden, The Netherlands. *Neuromuscul Disord* 2003; **13**: 589–96.

Wilson BA, Balleny H, Patterson K, Hodges JR. Myotonic dystrophy and progressive cognitive decline: a common condition or two separate problems? *Cortex* 1999; **35**: 113–21.

10.2   Myasthenia gravis (MG)

A central cholinergic deficit resulting in impaired memory has been suggested in myasthenia gravis (Tucker *et al.*, 1988; Davidov-Lusting *et al.*, 1992), mirroring the peripheral (neuromuscular junction) cholinergic transmission deficit responsible for the characteristic fatiguable weakness, particularly of extraocular, bulbar, and proximal limb muscles. Central cholinergic dysfunction is, after all, thought to be central to the pathophysiology of cognitive deficits in Alzheimer's disease and, possibly, dementia with Lewy bodies (see Sections 2.1 and 2.4). Tucker *et al.* (1988) found MG subjects to be impaired relative to both healthy controls and subjects with chronic non-neurological disease on the Boston Naming Test, WMS Logical Memory, and WMS Design Reproduction. Moreover, one patient with MG showed improvement in memory after treatment with plasmapheresis. However, others have found no evidence for memory impairments in MG patients in comparison with normal controls, and hence no support for the idea of impaired central cholinergic mechanisms (Glennerster *et al.*, 1996).

REFERENCES

Davidov-Lusting M, Klinghoffer V, Kaplan DA, Steiner I. Memory abnormalities in myasthenia gravis: possible fatigue of central nervous system cholinergic circuits. *Autoimmunity* 1992; **14**: 85–6.

Glennerster A, Palace J, Warburton D, Oxbury S, Newsom-Davis J. Memory in myasthenia gravis: neuropsychological tests of cerebral cholinergic function before and after effective immunologic treatment. *Neurology* 1996; **46**: 1138–42.

Tucker DM, Roeltgen DP, Wann PD, Wertheimer RI. Memory dysfunction in myasthenia gravis: evidence for central cholinergic effects. *Neurology* 1988; **38**: 1173–7.

Index